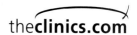

CLINICS IN
SPORTS MEDICINE

Spor y

GUEST EDITOR
Teodor T. Postolache, MD

CONSULTING EDITOR
Mark D. Miller, MD

April 2005 • Volume 24 • Number 2

SAUNDERS

An Imprint of Elsevier, Inc.
PHILADELPHIA   LONDON   TORONTO   MONTREAL   SYDNEY   TOKYO

W.B. SAUNDERS COMPANY
A Division of Elsevier Inc.

1600 John F. Kennedy Blvd. • Suite 1800 • Philadelphia, Pennsylvania 19103

http://www.theclinics.com

CLINICS IN SPORTS MEDICINE
April 2005
Editor: Debora Dellapena

volume 24, Number 2
ISSN 0278-5919
ISBN 1-4160-2769-6

Reprints: For copies of 100 or more, of articles in this publication, please contact the Commercial Reprints Department, Elsevier Inc., 360 Park Avenue South, New York, New York 10010-1710. Tel. (212) 633-3813; Fax: (212) 462-1935 e-mail: reprints@elsevier.com.

The ideas and opinions expressed in *Clinics in Sports Medicine* do not necessarily reflect those of the Publisher. The Publisher does not assume any responsibility for any injury and/or damage to persons or property arising out of or related to any use of the material contained in this periodical. The reader is advised to check the appropriate medical literature and the product information currently provided by the manufacturer of each drug to be administered to verify the dosage, the method and duration of administration, or contraindications. It is the responsibility of the treating physician or other health care professional, relying on independent experience and knowledge of the patient, to determine drug dosages and the best treatment for the patient. Mention of any product in this issue should not be construed as endorsement by the contributors, editors, or the Publisher of the product or manufacturers' claims.

Clinics in Sports Medicine (ISSN 0278-5919) is published quarterly by W.B. Saunders Company. Corporate and Editorial Offices: 1600 John F. Kennedy Blvd., Suite 1800, Philadelphia, PA 19103-2899. Accounting and Circulation Offices: 6277 Sea Harbor Drive, Orlando, FL 32887-4800. Periodicals postage paid at Orlando, FL 32862, and additional mailing offices. Subscription prices are $180.00 per year (US individuals), $277.00 per year (US institutions), $90.00 per year (US students), $203.00 per year (Canadian individuals), $333.00 per year (Canadian institutions), $118.00 (Canadian students), $235.00 per year (foreign individuals), $333.00 per year (foreign institutions), and $118.00 per year (foreign students). Foreign air speed delivery is included in all *Clinics* subscription prices. All prices are subject to change without notice. POSTMASTER: Send address changes to *Clinics in Sports Medicine*, W.B. Saunders Company, Periodicals Fulfillment, Orlando, FL 32887-4800. **Customer Service: 1-800-654-2452 (US). From outside of the US, call 1-407-345-4000.** E-mail: hhspcs@harcourt.com.

Clinics in Sports Medicine is covered in *Index Medicus, Current Contents/Clinical Medicine, Excerpta Medica, and ISI/Biomed.*

Printed in the United States of America.

CONSULTING EDITOR

MARK D. MILLER, MD, Associate Professor, Department of Orthopaedics, Co-Director, Department of Sports Medicine, University of Virginia Health System, Charlottesville, Virginia

GUEST EDITOR

TEODOR T. POSTOLACHE, MD, Associate Professor; Director, Mood and Anxiety Program, Department of Psychiatry, University of Maryland School of Medicine, Baltimore, Maryland; Director, Institute for Sports Chronobiology, Washington, DC

CONTRIBUTORS

GREG ATKINSON, PhD, Professor, Research Institute for Sport and Exercise Sciences, Liverpool John Moores University, Liverpool, United Kingdom

CHRISTIAN CAJOCHEN, PhD, Professor, Psychiatric University Clinic, Centre for Chronobiology, Basel, Switzerland

MARY A. CARSKADON, PhD, Professor, Psychiatry and Human Behavior, Division of Child and Adolescent Psychiatry, Brown Medical School, Providence; Director, Sleep and Chronobiology Research Laboratory, E.P. Bradley Hospital, East Providence, Rhode Island

DOMINIQUE CHOUDAT, MD, Professor of Occupational Medicine, Head of Department of Occupational Medicine, Hopital Cochin, Université Paris V, School of Medicine, Paris, France

ROGER J. COLE, PhD, Psychobiologist, Synchrony Applied Health Sciences, Del Mar, California

NAAMA W. CONSTANTINI, MD, DFM, Dip Sport Med, FACSM, Chairman, Medical Commission, The Olympic Committee of Israel, Department of Physiology, Tel-Aviv Medical School, Tel-Aviv University-Sackler Faculty of Medicine, Tel Aviv, Israel

WILLIAM C. DEMENT, MD, PhD, Lowell W. and Josephine Q. Berry Professor of Psychiatry and Sleep Medicine, Department of Psychiatry and Behavioral Sciences; Director, The Stanford Sleep Disorders Clinic and Research Center, Stanford University, Stanford, California

DAVID F. DINGES, PhD, Professor of Psychology, Division of Sleep and Chronobiology, Department of Psychiatry; Director, Unit for Experimental Psychiatry, Department of Psychiatry, University of Pennsylvania School of Medicine, Philadelphia, Pennsylvania

BARRY DRUST, PhD, Senior Lecturer, Research Institute for Sport and Exercise Sciences, Liverpool John Moores University, Liverpool, United Kingdom

GAL DUBNOV, MD, Msc, Department of Human Nutrition and Metabolism Hebrew University–Hadassah Medical School, Jerusalem, Israel

BEN EDWARDS, BSc, MSc, PhD, Research Institute for Sport and Exercise Sciences, Liverpool John Moores University, Liverpool, England

HELENE A. EMSELLEM, MD, Medical Director, The Center for Sleep and Wake Disorders, Chevy Chase, Maryland; Associate Clinical Professor of Neurology, The George Washington School of Medicine, Washington, DC

TSUNG-MIN HUNG, PhD, Professor, Graduate Institute of Exercise and Sport Science, Taipei Physical Education College, Taipei, Taiwan, Republic of China

HIRSH D. KOMAROW, MD, Staff Clinician, Laboratory of Allergic Disease, National Institute of Allergy and Infectious Disease, National Institutes of Health, Bethesda; Assistant Professor, Mood and Anxiety Program, Department of Psychiatry, University of Maryland School of Medicine, Baltimore, Maryland

KURT KRÄUCHI, Psychiatric University Clinic, Centre for Chronobiology, Basel, Switzerland

CONSTANCE M. LEBRUN, MDCM, MPE, CCFP, Dip Sport Med, FACSM, Director, Primary Care Sport Medicine and Research, Fowler Kennedy Sport Medicine Clinic, University of Western Ontario, London, Ontario, Canada

DAMIEN LEGER, MD, Biol D, Department of Occupational Medicine, Hopital Cochin, Université Paris V, School of Medicine; Head of Sleep Center, Sleep Disorders Center, Hotel Dieu de Paris, Assistance Publique Hopitaux de Paris, Université Paris V, and Paris Sleep Group (PSG), Paris, France

ARNAUD METLAINE, MD, Practician, Sleep Disorders Center, Hotel Dieu de Paris, Assistance Publique Hopitaux de Paris, Université Paris V, and Paris Sleep Group (PSG), Paris, France

TIMOTHY H. MONK, PhD, DSc, Professor of Psychiatry; Director, Human Chronobiology Research Program, Western Psychiatric Institute and Clinic, University of Pittsburgh Medical Center, Pittsburgh, Pennsylvania

FERNANDO MONTES, Director of Strength and Conditioning, Texas Rangers Baseball Club, Arlington, Texas

KAREN E. MURTAGH, CRNP, Nurse Practitioner, The Center for Sleep and Wake Disorders, Chevy Chase, Maryland

DAN A. OREN, Associate Professor, Department of Psychiatry, Yale University School of Medicine, New Haven, Connecticut

TEODOR T. POSTOLACHE, MD, Associate Professor; Director, Mood and Anxiety Program, Department of Psychiatry, University of Maryland School of Medicine, Baltimore, Maryland; Director, Institute for Sports Chronobiology, Washington, DC

THOMAS REILLY, BA, MSc, PhD, DSc, FErgS, FIBiol, DHC, Professor and Director, Research Institute for Sport and Exercise Sciences, Liverpool John Moores University, Liverpool, England

NAOMI L. ROGERS, PhD, Senior Research Fellow, Sleep and Circadian Research Group, Woolcock Institute of Medical Research, University of Sydney, Sydney, NSW, Australia

RICHARD N. ROSENTHAL, MD, Professor, Columbia University College of Physicians and Surgeons; Chairman, Department of Psychiatry, St. Luke's Roosevelt Hospital Center, New York, New York

JOSEPH J. SORIANO, Senior Programmer/Research Analyst, Mood and Anxiety Program, Department of Psychiatry, University of Maryland School of Medicine, Baltimore, Maryland

ROBERT STICKGOLD, PhD, Center for Sleep and Cognition, Department of Psychiatry, Harvard Medical School, Beth Israel Deaconess Medical Center, Boston, Massachusetts

JOHN W. STILLER, MD, Co-Director of Neurology, St. Elizabeth's Hospital, Washington, DC; Clinical Faculty, Mood and Anxiety Program, Department of Psychiatry, University of Maryland School of Medicine, Baltimore, Maryland; Consultant, Institute for Sports Chronobiology, Washington, DC; Consultant, Maryland State Athletic Commission, Baltimore, Maryland

SHAWN D. YOUNGSTEDT, PhD, Assistant Professor, Department of Exercise Science, Norman J. Arnold School of Public Health, University of South Carolina, Columbia, South Carolina

HANS P.A. VAN DONGEN, PhD, Research Associate Professor of Sleep and Chronobiology, Department of Psychiatry, University of Pennsylvania School of Medicine, Philadelphia, Pennsylvania

MATTHEW P. WALKER, PhD, Sleep and Neuroimaging Laboratory, Center for Sleep and Cognition, Department of Psychiatry, Harvard Medical School, Beth Israel Deaconess Medical Center, Boston, Massachusetts

JIM WATERHOUSE, DPhil, Professor, Research Institute for Sport and Exercise Sciences, Liverpool John Moores University, Liverpool, England

ANNA WIRZ-JUSTICE, PhD, Professor, Psychiatric University Clinic, Centre for Chronobiology, Basel, Switzerland

CONTENTS

two processes cause performance to deteriorate progressively over days, modulated within days by further performance reductions at night and relative improvements during the daytime. As the homeostatic pressure for sleep builds up higher across prolonged wakefulness, the rate of dissipation of that pressure during subsequent sleep is enhanced exponentially, so that even brief periods of sleep provide significant performance recuperation. Nevertheless, sleep restriction practiced on a chronic basis induces cumulative performance deficits of the same order of magnitude as observed during total sleep deprivation. There are also considerable individual differences in the degree of vulnerability to performance impairment from sleep loss, and these differences represent a trait.

Sleep Extension: Getting as Much Extra Sleep as Possible 251
William C. Dement

Nearly all people, whether they consider themselves sleep deprived or not, can initially obtain extra sleep. However, as accumulating extra sleep reduces carryover sleep debt, a point is reached where it is no longer possible to obtain extra sleep. If there were a practical method to make a precise measurement of a person's daily sleep requirement, it may be possible to show that most individuals are carrying a very large sleep debt. Several observations and studies demonstrate that almost everyone is sleep deprived and carries some amount of sleep debt. How long such an indebtedness will persist without change if no extra sleep is obtained is not known.

Insomnia and Sleep Disruption: Relevance for Athletic Performance 269
Damien Leger, Arnaud Metlaine, and Dominique Choudat

Insomnia is a common sleep complaint even in young adults and has important daytime consequences. Several subjective and objective tools are recommended to assess the magnitude of the problem and to try to find a cause. Chronic insomnia is often caused by precipitating factors, such as acute stress, work conditions, illness, and travel, and perpetuating factors, such as poor sleep hygiene, anxiety, and medications. Insomnia may have implications in athletic performance resulting from physical and cognitive effects. Several pharmacologic and nonpharmacologic approaches are employed in the management of insomnia that have proven effective for short-term treatment. The pharmacologic approaches include the use of zolpidem and specific GABA agonists, benzodiazepines for specific indications, antidepressants, and melatonin. The nonpharmacologic approaches include stimulus control, sleep restriction, relaxation strategies, and cognitive behavioral therapy.

Thermophysiologic Aspects of the Three-Process-Model of Sleepiness Regulation

Kurt Kräuchi, Christian Cajochen, and Anna Wirz-Justice

The following overview reconsiders the three-process model of sleepiness regulation (homeostatic, circadian, and sleep inertia) from a thermophysiologic point of view. Our results gathered over the last decade indicate that the homeostatic aspect of sleepiness regulation (ie, buildup of sleepiness during wakefulness and its decay during sleep) is not related to the thermoregulatory system, whereas the two other processes of sleepiness regulation (ie, circadian and sleep inertia process) are clearly related to thermoregulation in humans. Distal skin temperature of hands and feet seems to be the crucial variable for the association between thermophysiology, sleepiness, and sleep. Increased distal skin temperature before a nocturnal sleep episode is a good predictor for short sleep-onset latency. The disappearance of sleep inertia after sleep or a nap episode shows very similar kinetics as distal vasoconstriction. Furthermore, relaxation-induced sleepiness (eg, after lying down, at lights-off, with thermal biofeedback training) also evokes an increase in distal skin temperatures. The reverse effect occurs at lights-on or a posture change from supine to standing, Therefore, in terms of thermophysiology, sleep inertia can be explained as the reverse of a relaxation process (ie, decrease in distal skin temperatures). Our results reinterpret the so-called "sleep-evoked" reduction of core body temperature as a consequence of relaxation-induced vasodilatation after lights-off. Sleep per se has no further thermoregulatory effect. Taken together, a thermophysiologic approach may provide a successful strategy to treat sleep-onset insomnia and alleviate sleep inertia.

It's Practice, with Sleep, that Makes Perfect: Implications of Sleep-Dependent Learning and Plasticity for Skill Performance

Matthew P. Walker and Robert Stickgold

Although there is no consensus regarding the functions of sleep, one exciting hypothesis is that sleep contributes importantly to learning and memory. Over the last decade, several studies have provided substantive evidence supporting the role of sleep in memory processing. This article focuses on sleep-dependent learning and brain plasticity in humans, specifically in the development of skill performance that is the foundation of many sports actions. The different forms and stages of human memory are discussed, then evidence of sleep-dependent skill learning and associated sleep-dependent brain plasticity is described. In conclusion, a consideration of the fundamental importance of sleep in real-life skill learning is provided.

paper outlines the known sites of caffeine activity in the body, and discusses these with respect to the effects of caffeine observed during performance assessments.

Nonpharmacologic Techniques for Promoting Sleep

Roger J. Cole

Athletes could benefit from simple, self-administered, nonpharmacologic techniques for promoting sleep onset. A wealth of physiologic evidence and limited clinical data support several potential methods that might be conveniently applied at or near bedtime. These include inverted posture, skin warming/core cooling, motor relaxation, sensory withdrawal/masking, breathing techniques, and cognitive relaxation. Each holds promise as a possible element of a comprehensive sleep management program, but all need further investigation to confirm their efficacy or to determine optimal methods of application.

Effects of Exercise on Sleep

Shawn D. Youngstedt

Historically, perhaps no daytime behavior has been more closely associated with better sleep than exercise. The assumption that exercise promotes sleep has also been central to various hypotheses about the functions of sleep. Hypotheses that sleep serves an energy conservation function, a body tissue restitution function, or a temperature down-regulation function have all predicted a uniquely potent effect of exercise on sleep because no other stimulus elicits greater depletion of energy stores, tissue breakdown, or elevation of body temperature, respectively. Exercise offers a potentially attractive alternative or adjuvant treatment for insomnia. Sleeping pills have a number of adverse effects and are not recommended for long-term use, partly on the basis of a significant epidemiologic association of chronic hypnotic use with mortality. Other behavioral/cognitive treatments are more effective for chronic insomnia treatment, but difficult and costly to deliver. By contrast, exercise could be a healthy, safe, inexpensive, and simple means of improving sleep.

The Post-Lunch Dip in Performance @ doi:10.1016/j.csm.2004.12.002

Timothy H. Monk

For some performance variables, and some individuals, there is a dip in performance during the midafternoon hours (referred to as the *post-lunch dip*) that is linked to an increase in sleep propensity at that time of day. The post-lunch dip is a real phenomenon that can occur even when the individual has had no lunch and is unaware of the time of day. This dip has its roots in human biology, and may be linked to the size of the 12-hour harmonic in the circadian system. It is certainly exacerbated by a high-carbohydrate lunch, and may be more likely to occur in extreme morning-type individuals.

This review focuses on travel stress in athletes. An outline of the circadian system is presented, followed by an explanation of how disturbances to its regulation are related to jet lag. There are consequences of jet lag that affect exercise performance and health. Measures to ameliorate adverse effects of jet lag include behavioral or pharmacologic strategies. Coaches and mentors and the athletes they support should be considered when preparing for long-haul flights across multiple meridians.

Bright light treatment is the most potent melatonin suppressor and circadian phase shifter and is a safe nonpharmacologic antidepressant for seasonal depression. In addition, bright light treatment may restore performance in conditions of sleep debt and misalignment between peak performance and the athletic event. This article discusses the therapeutic use of bright light treatment, its side effects, and mechanisms of action.

Levels of leisure-time physical activity and physical fitness are generally higher in the summer than in the winter months for most people living away from the equator. The notion that an abrupt increase in physical activity in the spring, after a period of relative inactivity, can trigger sudden cardiac events has not been confirmed. There are seasonal variations in the physiological responses to exercise and the occurrence of injuries during participation in sports, but it is not known whether these changes are explained by fluctuations in activity levels and environmental conditions, or by any endogenous circannual rhythms in the human. There are indications of endogenous control for some physiological processes (eg, the metabolic responses to a given intensity of exercise) that seem to mediate more favorable effects of exercise on body composition in the winter. Well-trained athletes show obvious seasonality in their competitive performances, generally in line with adopted annual periodization strategies, although these strategies can be disrupted by external seasonal factors, such as heat stress or the susceptibility to upper respiratory tract infections. Maximal oxygen consumption and other physiological indicators of exercise performance might not mirror seasonal variation in real performances, which suggests that top-class athletes maintain a good level of general physical conditioning throughout the year.

Seasonal Allergy and Seasonal Decrements in Athletic Performance @ doi:10.1016/j.csm.2004.12.006

Hirsh D. Komarow and Teodor T. Postolache

Allergic diseases are common in all age groups and locations around the world. In the United States, allergic diseases affect 20 to 40 million people annually, including 10% to 30% of adults and close to 40% of children. An estimated 15 million people in the United States have been diagnosed as having asthma, with this number on the rise. Concomitant asthma affects 67% of patients who have allergic rhinitis. As a result of the increase in ventilation during exercise, athletes in particular experience significant symptoms of allergy triggered by exposure to aeroallergens. The allergic response causes nasal and conjunctival congestion, tearing, breathing difficulties, pruritus, fatigue, and mood changes, which affect athletic performance. Systemic symptoms of anaphylaxis from allergy, although rare, can be life threatening. Several decades ago it was inconceivable that an athlete who had asthma could perform competitively, let alone win Olympic gold medals. Today, with proper diagnosis, education, and optimal therapeutic management, the allergic athlete can achieve great strides in all sports endeavors. To avoid seasonal allergic flares and maximize performance, the physician providing care for an athlete who has seasonal allergies must be aware of the climatic patterns of aeroallergen expression, and adjust exercise and pharmacologic regimens accordingly. This article summarizes the effects of allergic disease on exercise and highlights the challenges that seasonal allergy place on athletic performance. Doping considerations grant additional complexity to this issue and underscore the need for a competent, skillful, informed, and ethical approach to treating seasonal allergy in the competitive athlete.

The Menstrual Cycle and Sport Performance @ doi:10.1016/ j.csm.2005.01.003

Naama W. Constantini, Gal Dubnov, and Constance M. Lebrun

The female sex steroid hormones estrogen and progesterone have potential effects on exercise capacity and performance through numerous mechanisms, such as substrate metabolism, cardiorespiratory function, thermoregulation, psychologic factors, and injuries. Consequently, hormone level changes may theoretically lead to either improved or decreased performance at various times throughout the menstrual cycle. Numerous methodological issues and a paucity of studies have precluded evidence-based conclusions in almost every area of research in this field. In addition, there appears to be a great degree of inter- and intraindividual variability in these hormonal responses. Using oral contraceptives may be advantageous for female athletes who are negatively affected by their menstrual cycle, as they may provide a stable yet controllable hormonal milieu for training and competition.

Sports Chronobiology Consultation: From the Lab to the Arena

This final article, coauthored by a chronobiology consultant, a sports psychologist who applied a chronobiology-based program to an Olympic national team, a clinical neurologist, a performance data analyst, a training–conditioning coach from a major league baseball team who applied chronobiology principles to major league pitchers, and a substance abuse expert, discusses practical aspects of a sports chronobiology consultation, including the goals and current arsenal of available interventions. Short vignettes of actual cases are presented for edification, and references are made to appropriate reviews found elsewhere in this issue.

FORTHCOMING ISSUE

RECENT ISSUES

CLINICS
IN SPORTS
MEDICINE

Clin Sports Med 24 (2005) xvii–xviii

Foreword

Sports Chronobiology

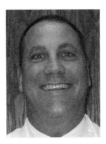

Mark D. Miller, MD
Consulting Editor

This is an issue that won't put you to sleep! I had to go to Dorland's Medical Dictionary to figure out exactly what *chronobiology* means: "The scientific study of the effect of time on living systems." Because I've been blessed with the ability to fall asleep as soon as my head hits the pillow, I really haven't thought much about this subject. I found it interesting, however, that sleep (or lack thereof) can affect athletic performance–now you've got my attention!

This issue, expertly edited by Dr. Teodor T. Postolache, provides a detailed review of the current state of the art on chronobiology. Chapters on circadian rhythms (that expression I've heard of), sleep debt, insomnia, sleep apnea, effects of various factors (including environmental factors), and substances on sleep, and seasonal variations are all thoroughly covered. The issue includes a discussion of various controversies in chronobiology, so hopefully we can put some of these issues to bed.

We are also pleased to introduce the concept of Web-based learning to this issue of *Clinics in Sports Medicine*. Five articles listed in the Table of Contents are accessible only through the Internet (sportsmed.theclinics.com). These articles include a discussion of sleep memory processing, sleep in children and adolescents (which is usually until noon in my house), post-lunch performance

doi:10.1016/j.csm.2005.01.004

drops (yes, they are real), and the affect of menstrual cycles and seasonal allergies on athletic performance.

A lot to cover, and a lot to learn–see if you can find the time!

Mark D. Miller, MD
Department of Sports Medicine
University of Virginia
McCue Center, 3rd Floor
Emmet Street & Massie Road
Charlottesville, VA 22903-0753, USA
E-mail address: mdm3p@virginia.edu

CLINICS
IN SPORTS
MEDICINE

Clin Sports Med 24 (2005) xix–xxii

Preface

Sports Chronobiology

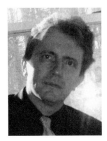

Teodor T. Postolache, MD
Guest Editor

Not uncommon scenarios: athlete A is the heavy favorite but athlete B wins; team X is an overwhelming favorite but team Y wins. "How could this happen?" many of us, often the fans of the beaten favorites, wonder. The explanation is sometimes simple. Although athlete A is most of the time better than athlete B, athlete B at his peak is better than athlete A at his trough. Similarly, although team X is usually stronger than team Y, team Y is stronger at their best than team X at their worst.

Everyone's performance level has rhythmic variation, although the amplitude of these rhythms varies from one person to another. Based on their period, rhythms are classified as circadian (with a period of approximately of 24 hours), ultradian (with a period of considerably less than 24 hours), and infradian (with a period of considerably more than 24 hours, such as menstrual and annual) rhythms. For instance, basic components of performance, such as flexibility, muscular strength, and reaction time, in almost every sport have rhythmic peaks and troughs that follow a circadian pattern.

Asking for the definition of "chronobiology" became one of the subtle signs of improvement in patients in my clinical practice. New patients referred to me for treatment of anxiety or depression often look at a poster on the wall: it features swimmers arching their back in a supreme effort to try to gain an edge of a few millimeters immediately after the start of a backstroke competition. The poster, with large letters, reads "Sports Chronobiology." Patients look at the poster, but ask no questions. Only after several weeks, after depression has lifted or anxiety improved, do patients ask, "OK, Doc, but what's Chronobiology?" Chronobiology is the science of rhythms in biological processes, a science of time and timing.

I am honored to serve as Guest Editor for the first issue of the *Clinics in Sports Medicine* dedicated to biological rhythms in sports. I have invited as contributors a distinguished group of internationally recognized researchers in sleep and chronobiology, some of whom focus on sports and exercise. I am very pleased that several "patriarchs" and "matriarchs" of the field agreed to contribute to this issue. I have also invited gifted teachers and practitioners to contribute, including some who have worked directly with Olympic or professional athletes. My deep appreciation goes to all contributors for their effort and enthusiasm. I would also like to thank Deb Dellapena from Elsevier for her continuous assistance and Mark Goldstein for his energetic help in the early stages of the project. I am grateful to my mother for pointing out during my early childhood the interdependency between us and our environment, and to my father who may have sparked my interest in biological rhythms with his interest in economical cycles. Finally, I need to thank Tatiana Tarasova, coach of many Olympic and world champions, who helped me overcome my doubts about taking chronobiology from the lab to the arena—from very controlled to very "noisy" conditions inherent to competitive sports.

A long time ago, at bedtime, my grandmother told me a story about a prince who helped an ant queen when she was in deep trouble. The grateful queen gave him a wing to rub when he was in trouble. Much later in the story, he faced the following choice: build a gold castle in one night, in which case he would marry the princess and live happily ever after, or be beheaded. After working hard for several hours, he realized he could not finish in time.

Suddenly he remembered the queen's wing. He rubbed it, and she appeared. When she understood what needed to be done, she said, "Prince, just go to sleep. And I will take care of it. You see, they (pointing toward the many ants that began appearing from all directions) cannot work while they are being watched." It was hard for the prince to fall asleep, as he was worrying about his neck. The queen saw this. "Prince, open your eyes, look at the sky, breath slowly, and count the stars," she said. He counted the stars, his eyes slowly closed, and he fell into a deep sleep. When he awoke in the morning, the gold towers of the castle shone in the light of the rising sun. And the ants, nocturnal creatures that they are, had disappeared.

This story from my childhood resonates well with the intent of this volume. First, because sleeping right, especially before the test of our lifetime, is enormously important. And second, because sleep is not a passive but an active phenomenon that is necessary for our somatic and mental functioning, including memory consolidation of learned psychomotor skills, which is of special importance for athletes.

The goals of a sports chronobiology consultation are to reduce impairments of sports performance related to circadian adversity (eg, early morning, early afternoon or late evening dips in performance, jet lag) and seasonal and menstrual rhythms, and to prevent and minimize sleep debt. Both goals can be accomplished with appropriate schedules that integrate practice, rest/activity, sleep/wake, meals, travel, and, for shifting circadian rhythms, timed light exposure and avoidance.

The readers may notice certain differences of opinions between reviewers, reflecting the richness of perspectives in the field. As in many areas of medicine, there are disagreements between the clinical (applicative) versus the fundamental research perspective. For instance, well-designed laboratory experiments in chronobiology are very time consuming, and it seems unlikely that elite athletes, given their busy schedules, will ever be subject to standardized research on the effects of sleep and biological rhythms on performance. Nevertheless, a great deal of theoretical and practical knowledge has now been gained on elite performers in challenging circumstances, such as astronauts and pilots, in addition to normal individuals in simulated adverse chronobiologic circumstances in the lab. Should we wait to recommend certain noninvasive and safe interventions until conclusive research has been completed on elite or highly trained athletes? Not in my opinion.

Applying sports chronobiology requires mindfulness of individual differences. For instance, one in ten people is a morning type, and one in ten people is an evening type. Younger athletes, especially adolescents, tend to have delayed circadian rhythms, go to bed later, and need to wake up later, and can easily become sleep deprived if awakened early in the morning for practice or school. Although the seminal work of my mentor, Thomas Wehr, has shown that the required duration of sleep in humans, after several weeks of paying accumulated sleep debt, is slightly above 8 hours, later studies led by my ex-colleague and friend, Daniel Aeschbach, show that short sleepers, who sleep less than 6 hours per night, and long sleepers, who sleep more than 9 hours daily, are quite different based on electroencephalographic and hormonal parameters. Therefore, although applying chronobiologic interventions to a team as a whole is expected to improve the performance of the team, better results are obtained if chronobiologic interventions are tailored to each team member.

My expectation is that our volume will contribute to at least three outcomes. First, I hope that through teaching certain natural, safe, legal, and ethical alternatives to sustain and increase stamina and vigilance, the present volume will contribute to successfully fighting doping, a major plague in contemporary sports. Second, as athletes are important role models for many people, the use of sleep hygiene and chronobiology in sports may contribute to making our increasingly 'round-the-clock society more receptive to the idea that sleep and timing are essential for performance and health.

Finally, and most of all, I hope that this volume will expand the awareness in the world of sports of the importance of sleep and circadian rhythms. It's not only practice, practice, practice that counts, but also adequate sleep and timing, timing, timing. In my view, the timing is right for certain chronobiologic principles and skills to be included in the arsenal of far-sighted sports physicians, conditioning coaches, trainers, and sports psychologists to help their athletes stay healthy, maintain competitive longevity, and perform at the peak of their abilities when most needed.

Teodor T. Postolache, MD
University of Maryland School of Medicine
Mood and Anxiety Program
685 West Baltimore Street
Washington, DC 21201, USA
E-mail address: tpostolache@psych.umaryland.edu

ELSEVIER
SAUNDERS

CLINICS
IN SPORTS
MEDICINE

Clin Sports Med 24 (2005) 205–235

Sleep-wake and Other Biological Rhythms: Functional Neuroanatomy

John W. Stiller, MD[a,b,c,d,*], Teodor T. Postolache, MD[a,b]

[a]Mood and Anxiety Program, Department of Psychiatry, University of Maryland School of Medicine, 685 West Baltimore Street, Baltimore, MD 21201, USA
[b]Institute for Sports Chronobiology, 2423 Pennsylvania Avenue, NW, Washington, DC 20037, USA
[c]Neurology Consultation Service, St. Elizabeth's Hospital, 2700 Martin Luther King Jr. Avenue, Washington, DC 20032, USA
[d]Maryland State Athletic Commission, 500 North Calvert Street, Room 304, Baltimore, MD 21202, USA

Biological rhythms consist of regularly recurring physiologic and certain behavioral phenomena. An endogenous biological rhythm is one that is intrinsically determined and persists in the absence of external influences. However, it is ultimately the interaction of environmental influences with these rhythms that determines the timing and level of functioning. Biological rhythms are often classified by their period, which is the interval for completion of one cycle. Circadian rhythms occur approximately every 24 hours. Ultradian rhythms have periods considerably shorter than 24 hours, whereas infradian rhythms have periods considerably longer than 24 hours. Ultradian rhythms include breathing and heart rate; seasonal and menstrual rhythms are two examples of infradian rhythms. Common circadian rhythms include rhythmic fluctuations in body temperature and the levels of certain hormones. We start with a discussion of sleep.

Functional neuroanatomy of sleep and wakefulness

Sleep, once regarded as a passive state determined by a decrease in activity of the arousal systems of the brain collectively referred to as the reticular acti-

This review was supported by the Institute for Sports Chronobiology, Washington, DC.
* Corresponding author. Mood and Anxiety Program, Department of Psychiatry, University of Maryland School of Medicine, 685 West Baltimore Street, Baltimore, MD 21201.
E-mail address: john.stiller@dc.gov (J.W. Stiller).

vating system, is now understood to also have an active neurophysiologic (ie, sleep-promoting) component. In the early 1900s, Viennese neurologist Constantin von Economo [1] observed that patients suffering from encephalitis lethargica could manifest either excessive sleepiness or wakefulness depending on what part of the brain was injured. Specifically, patients who had lesions of the posterior hypothalamus/rostral midbrain region suffered from excessive sleepiness and those who had lesions of the anterior hypothalamus/preoptic area, unremitting insomnia. Since von Economo's time there has been an abundance of research which has more precisely defined the anatomic pathways and neurochemical systems that subserve the behavioral states of wakefulness and sleep. For our purposes it is helpful to look at these anatomic regions/neurochemical systems separately. However, it is the dynamic interaction among these systems that determines the behavioral state (ie, stage of sleep or level of alertness).

Stages of sleep

In the normal adult, sleep is divided into rapid eye movement (REM) and non–rapid eye movement (NREM) types which cycle throughout the night [2]. REM sleep episodes become longer as sleep progresses, with the longest REM episodes typically occurring in early morning. In normal adults 20% to 25% of total sleep time is spent in REM. REM and NREM sleep are differentiated by brain-wave patterns, eye movements, and muscle tone (Table 1). The electroencephalogram (EEG) of wakefulness is made up of an admixture of low-voltage fast activity in the beta range (13–30 Hz) and faster, with superimposed alpha activity (8–12 Hz) that is most noticeable during relaxation with eye closure.

Table 1
Sleep stage and physiologic activity

	Wakefulness	NREM sleep	REM sleep
EEG	Fast, low voltage	Slow, high voltage	Fast, low voltage
Eye movement	Vision related	Slow, infrequent	Rapid
Muscle tone	↑↑	↑	0
LDT/PPT	↑	0	↑↑
LC/DR/TMN	↑↑	↑	0
VLPO cluster	0	↑↑	↑?
VLPO extended	0	↑?	↑↑
Orexin/hyprocretin	↑↑	0?	0?

↑↑, rapid firing rate (or increased muscle tone); ↑, slower firing rate (or less muscle tone); 0, little or no firing (or atonia); ?, hypothesized firing patterns that have not yet been unequivocally proven. *Abbreviations:* DR, dorsal raphe nucleus; EEG, electroencephalogram; LC, locus coeruleus; LDT, laterodorsal tegmental nuclei; PPT, pedunculopontine tegmental nuclei; TMN, tuberomammillary nucleus; VLPO, ventrolateral preoptic nucleus. *From* Saper CB, Chou TC, Scammell TE. The sleep switch: hypothalamic control of sleep and wakefulness. Trends Neurosci 2001;24:726–31; with permission.

REM sleep is characterized by fast low-voltage brain waves on the EEG (similar to that of wakefulness), muscle atonia, rapid eye movements, and fluctuations of autonomic function (ie, blood pressure, heart rate, respiration) [3].

NREM sleep includes four stages roughly correlated with the depth of sleep. Stage 1 is characterized by light sleep and Stage 4 by deep sleep. Stage 1 (2%–5% of total sleep time) is the transition from a waking state to sleep (Fig. 1). It is characterized initially by slow conjugate eye movements, loss of posterior alpha activity, and mild generalized slowing of mixed frequency low- to medium-amplitude background rhythms. Stage 2 (45%–55% of total sleep time) is

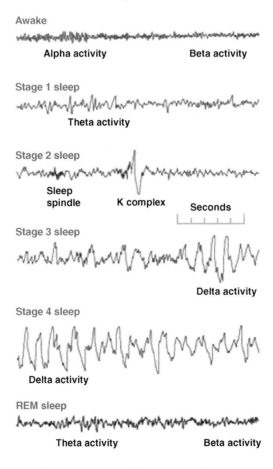

Fig. 1. EEG activity associated with stages of sleep. Awake: low voltage, random, fast activity with superimposed alpha. Stage 1: 4–7 Hz theta activity. Stage 2: 11–15 Hz sleep spindles and K complexes. Stage 3: 20%–50% high-voltage activity in the delta band (<2 Hz). Stage 4: >50% high-voltage activity in the delta band (<2 Hz). REM: low-voltage fast activity with superimposed theta (similar to the awake state). (*From* Horne JA. Why we sleep: the functions of sleep in humans and other animals. Oxford, England: Oxford University Press, 1988; with permission.)

characterized by an increase in slow waves and the presence of sleep spindles (episodic generalized symmetrical complexes usually of 12–15 Hz that last 1–2 seconds). K complexes (sharp transients characterized by an initial negative and then positive component) may or may not accompany spindle activity. Although spindles help define Stage 2 sleep, they can occur in other stages [4]. Stage 3 and 4 together are referred to as slow-wave sleep (SWS) and occupy 10% to 20% of total sleep time. As opposed to REM sleep, SWS is greatest early in the sleep period. Stage 3 is made up of 20% to 50% high-voltage slow-wave activity (2 Hz or less) and Stage 4 is characterized by more than 50% of similar slow-wave activity [3,5].

Wakefulness/arousal promoting regions

An understanding of the arousal systems of the brain can be challenging because these systems consist of multiple neuronal circuits, with significant redundancy, and involve many neurochemical systems [6]. The arousal systems include ascending activating projections to the cerebral cortex (Fig. 2) and descending projections to the spinal cord. The neuronal circuitries of the activating systems are located in the brainstem, hypothalamus, thalamus, and basal forebrain (BF).

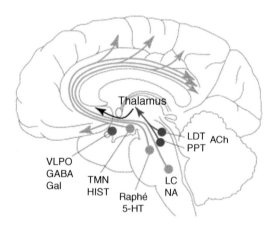

Fig. 2. The ascending arousal system sends projections from the brainstem and posterior hypothalamus diffusely to the forebrain. Neurons of the laterodorsal tegmental nuclei and pedunculopontine nuclei (LDT and PPT, *blue circles*) send cholinergic fibers (Ach) to many forebrain targets, including the thalamus, which then regulate cortical activity. Aminergic nuclei (*green circles*) project diffusely throughout the forebrain, regulating the activity of cortical and hypothalamic targets directly. Neurons of the tuberomammillary nucleus (TMN) contain histamine (HA), neurons of the raphe nuclei contain 5-HT, and neurons of the locus coeruleus (LC) contain noradrenaline (NA). Sleep-promoting neurons of the ventrolateral preoptic nucleus (VLPO, *red circle*) contain GABA and galanin (Gal). (*From* Saper CB, Chou TC, Scammell TE. The sleep switch: hypothalamic control of sleep and wakefulness. Trends Neurosci 2001;24:726–31; with permission.)

Brain stem arousal systems

Brain stem arousal systems may be divided into the following anatomic regions/neurochemical systems:

Reticular formation (RF)
Pontomesencephalic cholinergic neurons
Locus coeruleus (LC) noradrenergic neurons
Ventral mesencephalic dopaminergic neurons
Raphe serotonergic neurons

Reticular formation
The RF is made up of neuronal cell bodies and fiber tracts in the central core of the brain stem from the medulla to the midbrain. Although these neurons may receive multiple somatic and visceral sensory signals that may contribute to an awake or alert state, the RF does not require these external stimuli to maintain an awake state. The RF can maintain wakefulness of the individual by an endogenous or intrinsic self-sustaining mechanism [7]. Ascending excitatory signals project by way of a dorsal pathway to the thalamus and by way of a ventral pathway to the hypothalamus and BF [6]. Increased discharge rates of these ascending pathways are associated with cortical activation. Many of the reticular neurons contain the excitatory amino acid glutamate, which is likely necessary for wakefulness [8,9].

Pontomesencephalic cholinergic neurons
The pedunculopontine (PPT) and laterodorsal tegmental (LDT) regions contain groups of cholinergic neurons located in the dorsal midbrain and pons (see Fig. 2) and give rise to ascending pathways similar to those in the RF (ie, projections to thalamus, hypothalamus, BF) [10]. These cholinergic neuronal groups actively discharge during wakefulness and REM sleep (see Table 1) and are therefore associated with increased thalamocortical activity and cortical activation that accompany these states [11,12].

Locus coeruleus noradrenergic neurons
LC noradrenergic neurons synthesize norepinephrine (NE). This group of neurons is located in the mid/rostral pons near the floor of the fourth ventricle and gives rise to diffuse projections to cortex, hippocampus, and multiple subcortical regions including thalamus, hypothalamus, and BF (see Fig. 2) [13,14]. LC neurons fire maximally during wakefulness (particularly during stress), stop firing during REM sleep, and discharge at a rate somewhere between these two levels during SWS (see Table 1) [15–17]. Although LC clearly activates the cortex and causes increased arousal associated with other activating systems, it is

not absolutely necessary for activation/arousal, as demonstrated by the lack of a lasting effect on cortical activation/arousal after lesions of LC neurons [18]. The LC can be viewed as a central sympathetic system that enhances the activation of the brain and increases arousal especially during times of increased stress [6].

Ventral mesencephalic dopaminergic neurons
The majority of these ventral mesencephalic dopaminergic synthesizing neurons are located in the ventral tegmental area (VTA) and substantia nigra (SN). Projection areas from these regions include dorsal and ventral striatum, BF, and cerebral cortex [19,20]. Clinical [21,22] and experimental [23,24] observations support the importance of dopamine in maintaining wakefulness and an alert state particularly in association with situations involving positive reward [6]. However, because studies have not demonstrated changes in discharge rates of dopaminergic neurons across the sleep–wake cycle, the precise way this is accomplished is not well understood [25,26].

Raphe serotonergic neurons
Raphe serotonergic neurons produce serotonin (5-HT) and include the midbrain dorsal raphe (DR) nuclei. This group of neurons is located bilaterally in the midline region of the brainstem. Ascending fibers from DR neurons project to many areas of the central nervous system (CNS), including cerebral cortex and forebrain (see Fig. 2) [27]. DR neuronal activity across the sleep–wake cycle is similar to that of LC noradrenergic neurons in that they fire maximally during wakefulness, fire minimally during REM sleep, and discharge at a rate somewhere between these two levels during SWS (see Table 1) [28,29]. Because of the many 5-HT receptor subtypes, understanding how changes in levels of 5-HT affect behavior is challenging. The majority of recent studies are consistent with an association between increasing 5-HT levels and an increase in a quiet or satiated waking state [30–32].

Thalamocortical activating system

All of the previously discussed brainstem neuronal systems send signals to thalamic nuclei, from which thalamocortical projections emanate. These nonspecific thalamocortical projections emanate from multiple groups of thalamic neurons, including the midline, medial, and intralaminar nuclei [13]. These widespread, excitatory thalamocortical projections are associated with cortical activation presumably through the release of glutamate [33] during wakefulness and REM sleep [34]. At sleep onset and during SWS, thalamocortical projection neurons are inhibited by GABAergic thalamic neurons (reticularis thalamic neurons) in response to a decrease in brainstem activation [35].

Hypothalamic arousal systems

These may be divided into three anatomic regions/neurochemical systems: (1) posterior hypothalamus, (2) histaminergic tuberomammillary neurons, and (3) orexinergic perifornical neurons.

Posterior hypothalamus

Cortical activation and wakefulness are associated with a maximal rate of discharge of neurons in the posterior hypothalamus and a decrease in activity during SWS [36,37]. Neurons in the posterior hypothalamus are also involved in activation of the sympathetic nervous system and hypothalamic pituitary axis during the awake state [6]. The multifaceted, redundant, and complex aspects of the arousal systems are illustrated by the finding that experimental neurotoxic destruction of posterior hypothalamic neurons in the cat did not result in prolonged deficits in wakefulness [38].

Histaminergic tuberomammillary neurons

Histaminergic neurons in the tuberomammillary nucleus (TMN) of the posterior hypothalamus project diffusely throughout the CNS, including the cerebral cortex (see Fig. 2) [39]. Studies using stimulation and pharmacologic manipulations are consistent with the wake-activating properties of TMN histaminergic neurons (see Table 1). Clinical experience with antihistamines is consistent with histamine (HA) activating the cerebral cortex and increasing wakefulness [6]. Recent data suggests HA is of particular importance in promoting wakefulness during exposure to novel environments, which require higher behavioral arousal and initially after waking [40].

Orexinergic posterior/lateral hypothalamic neurons

Orexin (ORX) is a peptide, also known as *hypocretin*. ORX-producing neurons are located in the posterior and lateral aspects of the hypothalamus and project diffusely throughout the CNS [41,42]. In addition to cerebral cortical projections, there are significant excitatory connections with brainstem and hypothalamic nuclear groups associated with arousal, including PPT, LDT, DR, LC, VTA, and TMN (Fig. 3) [42–45]. Interneurons near orexinergic neurons likely release glutamate that activates the orexinergic neurons, which in turn further activate the interneurons, creating a positive feedback system that maintains an increase in the orexinergic activity/tone [46]. There is a great deal of evidence consistent with ORX being important in maintaining the waking state. In addition, ORX may be a stabilizer/modulator of sleep (see Table 1) [41–43, 47,48]. This hypothesis is consistent with the findings that there is a lack of ORX signaling/activity in approximately 90% of patients who have narcolepsy associated with cataplexy [49], and a significant reduction in the number of orexinergic neurons in brains of those who have narcolepsy [50,51].

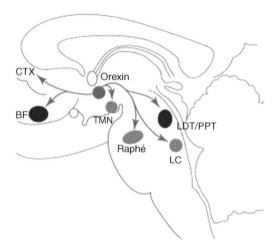

Fig. 3. ORX neurons in the lateral hypothalamic area innervate all of the components of the ascending arousal system and the cerebral cortex (CTX) itself. Blue circles indicate cholinergic neurons of the BF cholinergic nuclei, LDT, and PPT; green circles indicate monoaminergic nuclei. (*From* Saper CB, Chou TC, Scammell TE. The sleep switch: hypothalamic control of sleep and wakefulness. Trends Neurosci 2001;24:726–31; with permission.)

Orexinergic neurons in the posterior hypothalamus are in a strategic position to influence appetite/eating, metabolism/energy regulation, and autonomic and neuroendocrine function, in addition to sleep/wake behavior [41,43,48,52]. Thus, this group of neurons contributes to an appropriate level of arousal for a particular behavioral state (eg, being alert when eating). Also, the ORX level is highest at the end of the day, which suggests it may be of particular importance in maintaining wakefulness as the sleep drive increases [53,54].

Basal forebrain arousal system

The BF includes the area between the hypothalamus and orbital cortex, superficially from the anterior perforated substance it extends upward to the region of the rostrum of the corpus callosum [55]. This region includes the septal area and substantia innominata [55]. Cholinergic neurons located in the BF receive input from all of the hypothalamic and brainstem arousal projections previously discussed (ie, TMN, ORX, RF, PPT, LDT, DR, LC, and VTA) [6]. These neurons project diffusely to the cerebral cortex, hippocampus, and amygdala [56]. As with the brainstem cholinergic neurons (ie, PPT and LDT), the discharge of these neurons results in cortical activation and is most active during wakefulness and REM sleep [57]. Other BF neuronal groups include GABAergic and glutamatergic neurons. As with the cholinergic BF neurons, these neuronal groups may also be active during wakefulness and REM sleep

---

Box 1. Circumstances in which arousal systems are most active

- Cholinergic neurons (brainstem and basal forebrain) are particularly active during wakefulness associated with increased attention/motivation and during REM sleep [6].
- Dopaminergic neurons in VTA and SN are most active during wakefulness associated with highly rewarding/pleasurable situations and during REM sleep [6].
- NE-producing neurons in the LC are active during an awake state associated with highly stressful situations [6].
- Serotonergic neurons in the DR are active during a relaxed, contented waking state [30–32].
- Histaminergic neurons in the TMN of the hypothalamus are particularly active on awakening and when dealing with novel situations [40,62].
- Orexinergic neurons in the posterior and lateral hypothalamus may be particularly important in the complex process of maintaining wakefulness as the sleep drive (ie, sleep pressure) increases [53,54].

[58,59]. However, certain discrete areas of the BF may be active during SWS [60,61].

Behavioral states and activation of specific alerting regions

The various arousal systems described above interact in complex ways to maximize wakefulness/cortical activation during a variety of behavioral states. However, many of the arousal systems are most active during distinctive circumstances that depend on internal and external stimuli, such as those listed in Box 1.

The significant redundancy and multiple interconnections of the arousal systems may afford an evolutionary advantage. For example, an injury or malfunction of one activating system could be compensated for by other systems. However, for optimal performance across the sleep–wake cycle during many different circumstances, all of the arousal systems will be necessary.

Sleep-promoting regions

As mentioned, sleep is not just a state determined by the absence or decline of arousal systems activity. NREM and REM sleep are associated with an increased firing rate of neurons in the preoptic area and adjacent areas of the anterior hypothalamus and the BF [63–68] A discrete region within the preoptic area, referred to as the *ventrolateral preoptic area* (VLPO), and a more diffuse extension medially and dorsally (ie, the extended VLPO) [69,70] contain sleep-active cells (see Table 1).

Non–rapid eye movement sleep

VLPO cells are particularly active during deep NREM sleep (see Table 1) [70–72]. These neurons, by way of the inhibitory neurotransmitters γ-amino-butyric acid (GABA) and galanin, decrease activity of wake-promoting regions in the hypothalamus (eg, TMN, lateral hypothalamus) and brainstem (eg, PPT/LDT, DR, LC) [70,73].

Thus, multiple arousal systems are inhibited when VLPO cells are active (Fig. 4). The importance of the VLPO nucleus in the production of sleep is demonstrated by the fact that lesions of this region result in significant reduction in total sleep [74]. There are also neuronal groups in the BF that are most active during NREM sleep and are likely functionally similar to the adjacent VLPO neurons [75,76].

Rapid eye movement sleep

During REM sleep and wakefulness there is activation of thalamocortical projections and cortex. The difference between these two states is determined by the interaction between aminergic (eg, NE, 5-HT, HA) and cholinergic brainstem

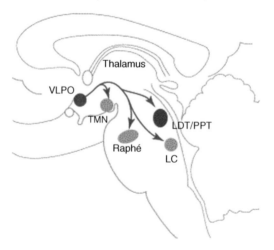

Fig. 4. The projections from the VLPO to the main components of the ascending arousal system. Axons from the VLPO directly innervate the cell bodies and proximal dendrites of neurons in the major monoamine arousal groups. Within the major cholinergic groups, axons from VLPO mainly innervate the interneurons rather than the principal cholinergic cells. The blue circle indicates neurons of the LDT and PPT; green circles indicate aminergic nuclei; and red circle indicates the VLPO. (*From* Saper CB, Chou TC, Scammell TE. The sleep switch: hypothalamic control of sleep and wakefulness. Trends Neurosci 2001;24:726–31; with permission.)

neurons (see Table 1). Within and near the PPT/LDT is a group of REM-active cholinergic cells [11,12,77,78]. These cells are highly active during REM sleep and, through activation of thalamocortical projections, result in the cortical activation (also referred to as *cortical desynchrony*) of REM sleep. This distinctive group of REM active cholinergic neurons of the PPT/LDT are tonically inhibited during wakefulness and NREM sleep by NE, 5-HT, and HA [79–81]. During REM sleep these aminergic neurons stop firing, which results in disinhibition of the REM active PPT/LDT neurons. During REM sleep, there is muscle atonia (excluding muscles required for breathing) in addition to rapid eye movements, [78,82]. The muscle atonia is produced through descending projections from PPT/LDT to the medial medulla. Activation of these neurons in the medial medulla results in loss of muscle tone resulting from a direct effect on motor neurons (through the release of glycine) [83] and inhibition of excitatory pathways from LC and the red nucleus (Fig. 5) [84]. Because of the location of these neuronal groups it is not surprising that animals that have experimental lesions between the dorsal pons and medial medulla experience REM sleep without loss of muscle tone and that these animals apparently manifest a behavior similar to patients who have REM-sleep behavior disorder [62].

Functional neuroanatomy of Sleep Stages

Deactivation of thalamic nuclei (particularly medial thalamus) is a consistent finding in neuroimaging studies of Stage 2 NREM sleep and SWS [85]. At the onset and continuation of sleep, a subgroup of thalamic neurons (reticularis

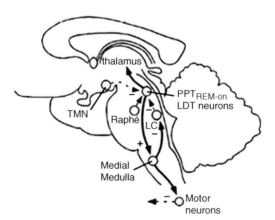

Fig. 5. REM sleep pathways. REM sleep is driven by a distinct population of cholinergic PPT/LDT neurons. During wakefulness and NREM sleep, these cells are inhibited by NE, 5-HT, and histamine, but during REM sleep, the aminergic neurons fall silent, thus disinhibiting the PPT/LDT REM-generating neurons. These cholinergic neurons also produce the atonia of REM sleep by activating the medial medulla, which inhibits motor neurons. The medial medulla also reduces excitatory signals from the LC that normally increase motor tone. (*From* Espana RA, Scammell TE. Sleep neurobiology for the clinician. Sleep 2004;27(4):811–20; with permission.)

thalamic neurons) become hyperpolarized as the result of decreased activation from brainstem arousal systems [86]. Subsequent to this, because of its special membrane properties, the reticularis thalamic neurons discharge in a phasic mode that results in the release of GABA, which in turn inhibits the thalamocortical neurons [35,85]. Depending on the frequency of this phasic activity, either spindles (12–14 Hz) during Stage 2 sleep or slow waves during SWS will be propagated through the interaction with thalamocortical projections and then cortex [35]. Thus, the spindles of Stage 2 sleep and delta activity of SWS are generated by the same mechanism of rhythmically bursting thalamic neurons interacting with cortical neurons. Functional imaging during SWS reveals low cerebral blood flow in many regions, including brainstem, thalamus, BF, cerebellum, and several cortical regions including frontal, parietal, and mesocortical [85].

As opposed to SWS, which is associated with a significant reduction in cerebral activity, during REM sleep there are increased neuronal discharges [10,11], increased cerebral blood flow [87–89], and increased brain-energy requirements [90]. Areas with increased activation on functional imaging during REM sleep include the mesopontine tegmentum, thalamus, limbic/paralimbic structures, and posterior cortical regions [85]. Areas with a relative decrease in activation include the frontal and parietal cortical regions [85]. The distribution of cortical activity during REM sleep is heterogeneous and different from that of NREM sleep and the waking state. The meaning of these findings is an open topic [85,91].

The sleep–wake cycle

We have examined wakefulness and sleep separately, but an ongoing interaction between several processes is necessary to account for the human sleep–wake cycle. Useful models in analyzing the sleep–wake cycle, first described by Borbely [92], usually refer to an interaction between the circadian pacemaker (process C) and an appetitive process referred to as *sleep homeostasis* (process S) [93,94].

Process S is the homeostatic factor

Process S involves a sleep homeostat that regulates the average amount of sleep debt, which increases during wakefulness and decreases rapidly during sleep [95]. The homeostatic signal is likely mediated through the neuromodulator adenosine and other sleep-inducing substances which activate sleep-generating neurons of the VLPO and BF [62,95]. Caffeine, an adenosine antagonist, is commonly used to increase alertness. The mechanisms controlling sleep and wakefulness interact in such a way as to avoid an intermediate state between sleep and wakefulness (Fig. 6) [96]. This is accomplished by a system of mutual inhibition between the sleep-active regions, such as VLPO and the major arousal systems of the brain (eg, monoaminergic neurons). VLPO neurons are inhibited

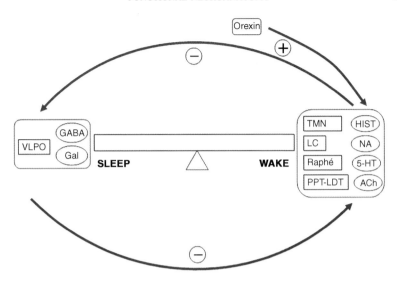

Fig. 6. This is a simplified model (not differentiating between REM and NREM sleep) that illustrates reciprocal interactions between sleep- (*blue*) and wake-promoting (*red*) regions, which result in a flip-flop switch (simplified model). Aminergic regions such as the TMN, LC, and DR promote wakefulness by direct excitatory effects on the cortex and by inhibition of sleep-promoting neurons of the VLPO. During sleep, the VLPO inhibits amine-mediated arousal regions through GABAergic and galaninergic projections. This inhibition of the amine-mediated arousal system disinhibits VLPO neurons, further stabilizing the production of sleep. ORX in the lateral hypothalamic area further stabilizes behavioral state by increasing the activity of aminergic neurons, thus maintaining consistent inhibition of sleep-promoting neurons in the VLPO. (*Adapted from* Saper CB, Chou TC, Scammell TE. The sleep switch: hypothalamic control of sleep and wakefulness. Trends Neurosci 2001;24:726–31.)

by monoaminergic cells during wakefulness. This in turn results in loss of inhibition of the monoaminergic neurons by VLPO, which further stabilizes the waking state. Likewise, when VLPO cells are active during sleep they inhibit arousal regions, which then result in loss of inhibition of the VLPO by these same neurons.

This circumstance (ie, strong reciprocal inhibition) allows for what is referred to in electrical engineering as a "flip-flop circuit" [97]. When this occurs there is a bistable feedback loop with two stable patterns of firing and avoidance of intermediate states (see Fig. 6). It will take a large or significant influence to change the behavioral state, but when it occurs it is compelling (eg, a significantly increased homeostatic pressure from sleep deprivation) [96]. The evolutionary importance of this is obvious in that it reinforces either being awake or asleep and will help to avoid the potentially dangerous state of being half awake.

Narcolepsy, which is associated with loss of ORX-producing cells [98–100], is manifested by inappropriate episodes of sleep and difficulty in maintaining sleep. This disorder can be viewed as an instability of the bistable circuit. The loss of ORX results in decreased activity of the monoaminergic arousal systems

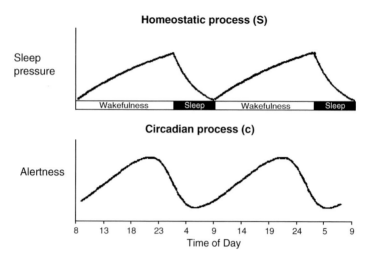

Fig. 7. Interaction of process S and process C. The homeostatic pressure for sleep builds up during wakefulness and dissipates rapidly during sleep. The circadian process is related to the time of day, is independent of the amount of previous sleep and opposes the homeostatic process. (*Modified from* Borbély AA. A two process model of sleep regulation. Hum Neurobiol 1982;1(3):195:204.)

(under normal circumstances, ORX would activate this system), which would result in a decrease in the amount of reciprocal inhibition of sleep-inducing VLPO neurons and a less stable "switch." This reaction would result in a risk of small changes in homeostatic sleep pressure leading to inappropriate episodes of sleep.

Process C is the circadian factor

Process C generates a signal of wakefulness that increases during the biological day and decreases during the biological night (see Fig. 7, bottom). The circadian system, which is discussed later, is also involved with the timing of sleep, particularly during the second half of a sleep occurrence and the entry into REM sleep [94,101]. The circadian effect on the sleep–wake cycle is mediated by the suprachiasmatic nucleus (SCN), also referred to as the *master clock*, through local connections in the hypothalamus. This local information signaling is accomplished through the SCN-derived peptides prokineticin 2 or transforming growth factor-α (TGF-α) [76,102]. Specifically, the SCN releases peptides into the subparaventricular zone from where a signal is sent to the dorsomedial nucleus of the hypothalamus, which is an important area for integration with endocrine and behavioral influences [103]. This region in turn sends excitatory projections to arousal centers of the brain, including lateral hypothalamus, LC, DR, and TMN, and inhibitory projections to the sleep-active VLPO region, thus promoting wakefulness [74,104–106]. Circadian influences on sleep and wakefulness are significantly reduced by lesions of either the subparaventricular or dorsomedial nucleus region of the hypothalamus [103,106].

Interaction of process S and process C

The homeostatic factor is an accumulating drive to sleep that becomes greater the longer one stays awake and rapidly dissipates as one falls asleep (see Fig. 7, *top*), and may be mediated through somnogens such as adenosine and is reflected in the EEG by the degree of slow-wave activity [107].

This homeostatic factor is superimposed on a separate circadian process (through the SCN and its connections) that is related to the time of day, is independent of the amount of prior sleep, and opposes the homeostatic drive for sleep (see Fig. 7, *bottom*). Process C may be deciphered by recording physiologic parameters, such as core temperature or melatonin secretion [108]. Under normal circumstances, the interaction between the sleep homeostat and the circadian signal results in a sleep–wake cycle that is appropriate for optimal functioning.

The functional neuroanatomy of circadian rhythms

Terminology and definitions of circadian rhythms

Before discussing the functional neuroanatomy of circadian rhythm, it is useful to clarify terminology and provide a more detailed explanation of entrainment and phase-response curves (PRC), which are key concepts in chronobiology.

Circadian rhythm refers to oscillations in physiologic parameters with a period of approximately 24 hours. The neural system that generates and regulates circadian rhythms is referred to as the *circadian timing system*. In humans, a rhythm with a period slightly greater than 24 hours is "free running" and is generated internally by an endogenous pacemaker or biological clock. The endogenous pacemaker or clock produces these rhythms through genetic mechanisms of the clock genes. Entrainment refers to the adjustment or resetting of the circadian rhythm by an environmental stimulus, such as light, to a 24-hour day. *Zeitgeber*, or "time giver," refers to major environmental variables that can reset the clock (eg, light, time of food availability, exercise). Subjective day is an internal physiologic state corresponding to the time when an organism has been regularly exposed to daylight, and subjective night refers to an internal physiologic state corresponding to the time when an organism has been regularly exposed to dark (Fig. 8).

Entrainment and the phase-response curve

Although it was once believed that social cues were more important than light as the Zeitgeber for humans, it is now known that as with other mammals light is the principal time giver and establishes the period and phase of the circadian pacemaker (Fig. 9) [109]. How light effects the pacemaker is determined by the

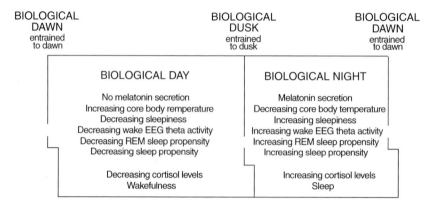

Fig. 8. Physiologic variables which define biological day and night. These states alternate with a rapid transition (biological dusk and dawn) between them. They are generated within the organism, and mirror and anticipate features of the solar day to which they correspond and with which they are synchronized. (*From* Wehr TA, Aeschbach D, Duncan Jr WC. Evidence for a biological dawn and dusk in the human circadian timing system. J Physiol 2001;535(Pt 3):937–51; with permission.)

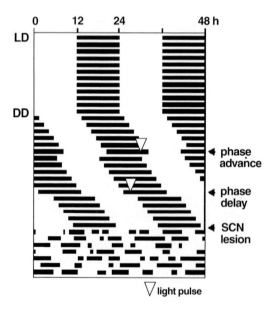

Fig. 9. Schematic representation of a circadian rhythm as normally entrained to a 24-hour light–dark cycle (LD), as free-running pattern in constant darkness (DD), and SCN lesion condition. The dark bars indicate the active (movement, drinking, eating for rodents) periods on successive days (the onset of activity is arbitrarily chosen), presented in a so-called double-plotted actogram. The free-running rhythm is phase-delayed by a light pulse at the beginning of the active period (CT12–18), and phase-advanced by a light pulse at the end of the active period (CT18–23). Note in particular the point where there is a lesion of the SCN. This results in a dramatic change in circadian rhythm (ie, a fragmented activity pattern) and is consistent with the loss of master pacemaker function of the SCN. (*From* van Esseveldt KE, Lehman MN, Boer GJ. The suprachiasmatic nucleus and the circadian time-keeping system revisited. Brain Res Brain Res Rev 2000;33(1):34–77; with permission.)

time of day that exposure takes place (ie, at what phase of the cycle the light is encountered) as well as the intensity and wavelength of the light, and can be described by a PRC. Specifically, light during the subjective day causes little shift, as described by Postolache and Oren elsewhere in this issue, whereas light in the early part of the subjective night causes a phase delay (shift to a later time), and light in the late subjective night results in a phase advance (shift to an earlier time).

Suprachiasmatic nucleus (pacemaker or master clock)

van Esseveldt et al [110] provide an extensive review of the anatomy and neurophysiology of the SCN. Although individual organs may have their own circadian oscillators, referred to as *peripheral oscillators*, their rhythms are coordinated by a master circadian pacemaker or clock [111]. Multiple lines of evidence, including ablation [112,113], transplantation [114,115], and in vivo [116] and in vitro experiments [117] involving isolation of SCN from the rest of brain, establish the SCN as the site of the master circadian pacemaker (Fig. 9). However, recent evidence points to the BF as possibly being a "co-master circadian pacemaker," necessary for many nonphotic influences. Thus, for normal entrainment, the forebrain and SCN likely work together [111,118].

The SCN is a very small region located bilaterally in the anterior hypo-thalamus above the optic chiasm and abutting the third ventricle [110]. It is made up of less than 10,000 neurons on each side [55], and in mammals is divided into a core and shell [109]. The shell is in the dorsal SCN and is sometimes referred to as the *dmSCN*. The core is located primarily in the ventral SCN and is sometimes called the *vlSCN* [119]. The core and shell differ with respect to the afferents they receive and their neurotransmitter/neuromodulator contents. The core receives mainly visual input from the retinohypothalamic tract (RHT), as discussed later, and its neurons contain vasoactive intestinal polypeptide (VIP), gastrin-releasing peptide, and GABA [110,119]. The shell receives nonphotic input and its neurons contain arginine vasopressin, calretinin, and GABA [110,119]. Also, the output connections of these two subdivisions differ to some degree [119]. The ability of SCN neurons to generate circadian rhythms is apparently intrinsic, in that defined subgroups of SCN neurons, when isolated, continue to manifest circadian rhyth-micity [120].

Three main afferent projections to the suprachiasmatic nucleus

Retinohypothalamic tract

Because light entrainment occurs in animals who lack rods and cones [121], the presence of other photoreceptors was initially postulated and subsequently demonstrated to include a subset of retinal ganglion cells, many of which express the photo pigment melanopsin [122,123]. For further discussion of this issue, see the article by Postolache and Oren elsewhere in this issue.

The RHT is distinct from the visual pathway. It projects directly from these specialized retinal ganglion cells to the SCN [124] and uses glutamate (binding to N-methyl-D-aspartate [NMDA] and non-NMDA receptors) and pituitary adenylate-activating cyclase polypeptide as neurotransmitters [125,126]. Because interruption of the RHT eliminates photic entrainment [124] and transection of all other retinal pathways (excluding the RHT) has no effect on photic entrainment [109], it is clear that light entrainment is mediated through the RHT.

Geniculohypothalamic tract

The same class of retinal ganglion cells that give rise to the RHT has projections to the intergeniculate leaflet, which is an area within the lateral geniculate body of the thalamus [128,129]. The intergeniculate leaflet sends projections back to the SCN by way of the geniculohypothalamic tract, which uses GABA and neuropeptide Y as neurotransmitters [129]. The geniculohypothalamic tract is likely important in integrating photic and nonphotic information (eg, locomotion, availability of food) used in entrainment by the SCN [130–132].

Raphe serotonergic neuronal projections to the suprachiasmatic nucleus

Serotonergic afferents from midbrain raphe neurons also contribute to the modulation of SCN through postsynaptic SCN receptors of 5-HT and synaptic connections with RHT terminals [127,132]. For instance, there is a 50% increase in the phase delay induced by a time-appropriate light pulse during subjective night in mice whose serotonergic systems have been destroyed [133], and activation of the 5-HT system results in a decrease in light-induced phase shifts [127,134,135].

Suprachiasmatic nucleus efferent pathways

Output from the SCN is primarily directed to the hypothalamus, including the medial preoptic nucleus, paraventricular nucleus, dorsomedial nucleus, and subparaventricular zone [136], and to a lesser extent the midline thalamus and BF [137]. Secondary projections from these regions are widespread, enabling the SCN to influence many physiologic and behavioral functions (Fig. 10) [137]. Prokineticin 2 and TGF-α have been implicated as SCN output neurotransmitters/neuromodulators in circadian locomotor rhythms [76,102] and, in the absence

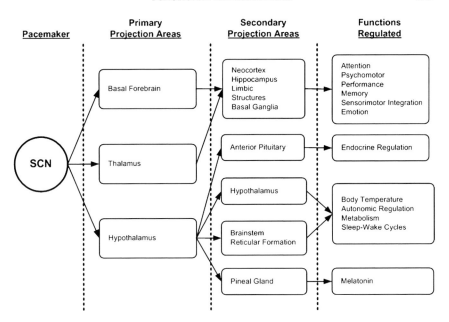

Fig. 10. Efferent projections of the SCN and functional correlations. The SCN has limited primary projections but widespread secondary projections to areas involved in control of the many functions regulated by the circadian system. (*From* Moore RY. Circadian rhythms: basic neurobiology and clinical applications. Annu Rev Med 1997;48:253–66; with permission.)

of synaptic transmission, diffusible molecules can control circadian locomotor rhythms at least in part [138].

Suprachiasmatic nucleus (master clock) at the molecular level

A fascinating feature of the circadian system is that the rhythmicity present at the molecular level of gene transcription is somehow coupled and ultimately manifested at a physiologic system (eg, hormonal, temperature, locomotion) and behavioral level. On a molecular level, the SCN functions through positive and negative intracellular feedback loops at the level of DNA transcription and translation that ultimately results in circadian oscillations (Fig. 11).

The importance of these rhythms, at the level of the clock genes, for the proper functioning of the SCN as the circadian timekeeper is demonstrated by the aberrant effect of clock-gene mutations on circadian rhythms [119]. For instance, a serine to glycine mutation in the Period2 gene on chromosome 2q causes familial advanced sleep-phase syndrome (FASPS), an inherited disorder characterized by early morning awakening and early sleep onset [119]. Specifically, the mutation results in a decrease in the phosphorylation of PER2 protein and thus less degradation of the PER protein, resulting in an increased concentration of nuclear PER which affects the negative-feedback loop timing [139,140]. Thus,

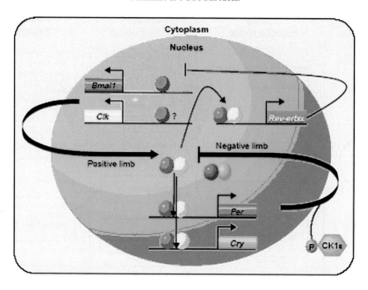

Fig. 11. Diagram of the mammalian circadian clock mechanism. Clk (*yellow*) and Bmal1 (*pink*) proteins (positive limb) drive the expression of Per, Cry, and Rev-*erbα* genes in the nucleus. Per (*red*) and Cry (*light green*) proteins in the nucleus inhibit Clk/Bmal1 action by a yet unknown mechanism and thereby down-regulate their own expression and that of Rev-*erbα* (*dark green*). When Rev-*erbα* protein is absent, Bmal1 (and possibly also Clk) genes are derepressed and hence transcribed to produce new Clk/Bmal1 transcription factors that reinitiate a new circadian cycle. Clk proteins are posttranslationally modified; casein kinase Ie (CK1e), for example, phosphorylates PER2. Hyperphosphorylation of PER2 decreases its stability and thus promotes its degradation. A typical circadian cycle would begin with activation of Per (and Cry) transcription by Clk/Bmal1 in the early morning. Transcript levels peak around noon and protein levels in the cytoplasm reach the zenith 2 hours later. PER shuttles between the cytoplasm and the nucleus. In the cytoplasm, it is degraded following hyperphosphorylation and in the nucleus it is complexed with Cry and thereby blocks Clk/Bmal1 function resulting in termination of Per and Cry transcription. At some point, when much Per is degraded in the cytoplasm, Per concentration in the nucleus is too low to keep up negative feedback and the cycle reinitiates. (*From* Albrecht U, Eichele G. The mammalian circadian clock. Curr Opin Genet Dev 2003;13(3):271–7; with permission.)

FASPS is a cogent example of how a change in rhythm at the molecular level can lead to a significant physiologic (sleep–wake cycle) circadian disorder. Another genetic disorder associated with an extreme form of advanced sleep-phase syndrome (ASPS) is the Smith-Magenis Syndrome (SMS). SMS is caused by a deletion of a portion of chromosome 17 (17p11.2), which results in an inversion of the circadian rhythm of melatonin and an ASPS [141].

Interaction between peripheral oscillators and suprachiasmatic nucleus

Peripheral circadian oscillators (clocks) are present in many tissues (eg, liver, lung, skeletal muscle) and are important in the timing of the functions related to these tissues. As opposed to the SCN, these peripheral oscillators tend to dampen rapidly in vitro and ultimately need to interact with the SCN to optimally maintain function. The SCN likely entrains these peripheral circadian oscillators to an appropriate adaptive phase control in response to changes in the environmental light cycle [110]. However, circumstances that cause large rapid shifts in the light–dark cycle (ie, intercontinental travel) may result in a "lag phase" where there is a temporary mismatch between the phase shift of the SCN and the peripheral oscillator. Practically, this phenomenon may be central to the explanation of jet lag and suboptimal athletic performance associated with travel.

The functional neuroanatomy of the menstrual rhythm

First let us correct a commonly used misnomer: the menstrual cycle is not a cycle but a rhythm. Cycles are quantitative undulatory oscillations whereas rhythms are qualitative alternations between different, distinct states (Fig. 12). The menstrual rhythm includes four distinct phases: menstrual, follicular, periovulatory, and luteal. For an in depth discussion of the menstrual rhythm, see the article by Constantini et al elsewhere in this issue.

Menstrual rhythm

On the first day of the menstrual rhythm (day 1 of menstruation) there is a pulsatile secretion of gonadotropin-releasing hormone (GnRH) that causes an increase in follicle-stimulating hormone (FSH) from the pituitary, which in turn causes increased estrogen from the ovarian follicle. There is feedback inhibition of FSH release by ovarian hormones, and at the end of the first week of the cycle an individual follicle begins to mature with increased estrogen production. During the second week of the menstrual rhythm, there is an increase in the frequency, and to a lesser extent the amplitude, of the pulsatile release of GnRH. The increasing frequency of GnRH pulses leads to a surge of luteinizing hormone (LH) secretion which causes ovulation 35 to 44 hours after the LH surge. The reason that the GnRH pulse reaches a critical level sufficient to cause the LH surge is that the effect of estrogen on GnRH suddenly and inexplicably changes

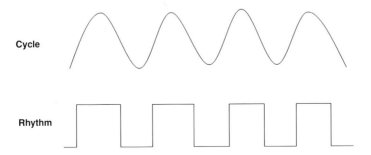

Fig. 12. Cycles (*above*) versus rhythms (*below*).

from a negative-feedback influence to a positive one. The follicular phase ends with ovulation and the luteal phase begins. During the luteal phase the amplitude of GnRH pulsations decreases, and under the influence of endogenous opioids the frequency markedly decreases. If fertilization does not take place, menstruation occurs within 12 to 16 days of ovulation. The decline of estradiol during the end of the luteal phase results in an increase in FSH and the start of another cycle [142].

Hypothalamic-pituitary-ovarian axis

GnRH is a 10-amino-acid peptide synthesized in parvocellular neurons of the arcuate nucleus located in the tuberal region of the medial hypothalamus. The axons project a short distance along the tuberoinfundibular tract, where GnRH is released into the fenestrated capillary bed of the median eminence and travels through the hypophyseal portal system to the anterior pituitary where it regulates FSH and LH. FSH and LH, by way of the systemic circulation, subsequently stimulate the ovaries and the release of gonadal steroids (eg, estradiol, progesterone). There is feedback regulation of GnRH by ovarian and pituitary hormones (Fig. 13). Neuromodulators such as corticotrophin-releasing hormone and endogenous opioids contribute to the complex regulation of GnRH [142].

Functional neuroanatomy of seasonal rhythms

It is not uncommon for individuals to notice mild changes in the way they feel and act during different seasons, such as having a little less energy or

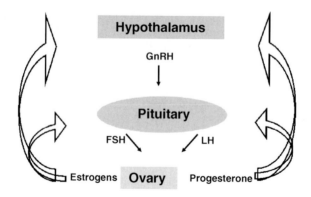

Fig. 13. Hypothalamic-pituitary-ovarian axis. There is feedback regulation of gonadotropin-releasing hormone (GnRH) by ovarian and pituitary hormones. (*From* Rubinow DR, Schmidt PJ. Psychoneuroendocrinology. In: Kaplan I, Sadock D, editors. Comprehensive textbook of psychiatry. 6th edition. Baltimore, MD: Williams & Wilkins; 1995. p. 104–12; with permission.)

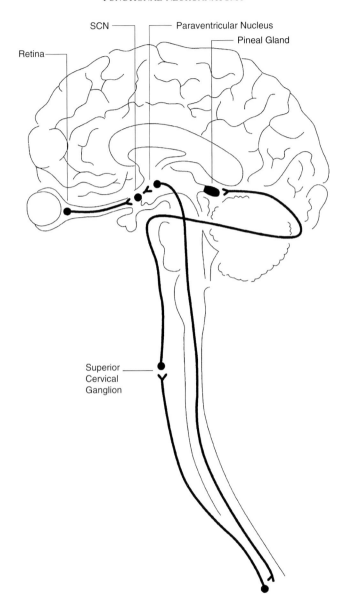

Fig. 14. If uninhibited, the paraventricular neurons stimulate (by way of multisynaptic pathways) the secretion of melatonin by the pineal glad. The SCN firing results in inhibition of paraventricular neurons, which will in turn result in an inhibition of melatonin secretion. Thus, the duration of the environmental night is encoded in the duration of decreased SCN firing and then in the duration of nocturnal melatonin secretion (ie, internal or biological night), which in turn conveys seasonal information to other hypothalamic hormonal systems, and to other organs and tissues. (*From* Wehr TA, Duncan Jr WC, Sher L, et al. A circadian signal of change of season in patients with seasonal affective disorder. Arch Gen Psychiatry 2001;58:1108–14; with permission.)

increased appetite in the fall/winter. However, some individuals experience marked seasonal changes that are similar to the behavioral changes observed in photoperiodic mammals (ie, those that have marked changes in behavior in response to changes in day length). These individuals may develop many symptoms during fall/winter, such as lack of initiative; changes in weight, appetite, and sleep pattern; and decreased interest in sex. Some develop full-blown episodes of major depression in fall/winter that improve with the administration of bright light and spontaneously remit during spring/summer. These individuals may be diagnosed with seasonal affective disorder (SAD) [149]. See the article by Postolache and Oren elsewhere in this issue for further discussion of SAD.

As with circadian rhythms, the SCN is also the central neuronal structure controlling seasonal rhythms [112,113], which is consistent with the report of a lack of photoperiodic responses following SCN destruction [143]. SCN neurons discharge at a high rate during daytime and less intensely at night, and there is a sharp transition in firing rate at dusk and dawn. This pattern persists in isolated hypothalamic tissue slices and dissociated cell cultures under constant conditions [143]. The duration of diurnal firing under constant conditions in vitro is related to the length of the previous day that the animal experienced. The longer the previous day, the longer the diurnal discharge the following day, and vice versa for shorter day lengths [144], suggesting that SCN cells "remember" the previous photoperiod exposure [145]. The duration of light exposure influences the SCN through the RHT and modifies the duration of SCN neuronal firing. SCN efferents project to the paraventricular neurons in the hypothalamus which, by way of a multisynaptic pathway, inhibits secretion of melatonin from the pineal gland (Fig. 14).

In photoperiodic animals, many seasonal changes are mediated through the duration of melatonin secretion. Similar to animals that manifest complex and robust seasonal rhythms, Wehr and colleagues [146] showed that patients who had SAD, but not matched controls, had a longer duration of active melatonin secretion in winter compared with summer. This confirms that the neuroanatomic and photoperiodic elements that mediate seasonality in mammals are preserved in humans [147,148].

Summary

The level of understanding of the functional neuroanatomy of biological rhythms has advanced exponentially. Now we must narrow the gaps in our knowledge between molecular and clinical domains. Hopefully, this will lead to a better understanding of the importance of sleep and biological rhythms for practicing and performing at one's peak, when most needed, and to the development of novel prophylactic and therapeutic approaches to preserve human abilities, health, safety, and well-being.

References

[1] von Economo C. Sleep as a problem of localization. J Nerv Ment Dis 1930;71:249–59.

[2] Carskadon MA, Dement WC. Normal human sleep: an overview. In: Kryger MH, Roth T, Dement WC, editors. Principles and practice of sleep medicine. 3rd edition. London: W.B. Saunders; 2000. p. 15–25.

[3] McCarley RW. Neurophysiology of sleep: basic mechanisms underlying control of wakefulness and sleep. In: Chokroverty S, Daroff RB, editors. Sleep disorders medicine: basic science, technical considerations, and clinical aspects. 2nd edition. Boston: Butterworth-Heinemann; 1999. p. 21–50.

[4] Stevens S, Comella CL, Walters AS, Hening WA. Sleep and wakefulness. In: Goetz CG, editor. Textbook of clinical neurology. 2nd edition. Philadelphia: W.B. Saunders; 2003. p. 19–20.

[5] Rechtschaffen A, Kales AA. A manual of standardized terminology, techniques, and scoring system for sleep stages of human subjects. Los Angeles, CA: UCLA: Brain Information Service/Brain Research Institute; 1968.

[6] Jones BE. Arousal systems. Front Biosci 2003;8:s438–51.

[7] Moruzzi G, Magoun HW. Brain stem reticular formation activation of the EEG. 1949. J Neuropsychiatry Clin Neurosci 1995;7:251–67.

[8] Jones BE. Reticular formation. Cytoarchitecture, transmitters and projections. In: Paxinos G, editor. The rat nervous system. Australia New South Wales: Academic Press; 1995. p. 155–71.

[9] Kaneko T, Itoh K, Shigemoto R, et al. Glutaminase-like immunoreactivity in the lower brainstem and cerebellum of the adult rat. Neuroscience 1989;32:79–98.

[10] Jones BE. Immunohistochemical study of choline acetyltransferase-immunoreactive processes and cells innervating the pontomedullary reticular formation in the rat. J Comp Neurol 1990; 295:485–514.

[11] Steriade M, Datta S, Pare D, et al. Neuronal activities in brain-stem cholinergic nuclei related to tonic activation processes in thalamocortical systems. J Neurosci 1990;10:2541–59.

[12] el Mansari M, Sakai K, Jouvet M. Unitary characteristics of presumptive cholinergic tegmental neurons during the sleep-waking cycle in freely moving cats. Exp Brain Res 1989;76: 519–29.

[13] Jones BE, Yang TZ. The efferent projections from the reticular formation and the locus coeruleus studied by anterograde and retrograde axonal transport in the rat. J Comp Neurol 1985;242:56–92.

[14] Jones BE, Moore RY. Ascending projections of the locus coeruleus in the rat. II. Autoradiographic study. Brain Res 1977;127:25–53.

[15] Aston-Jones G, Bloom FE. Activity of norepinephrine-containing locus coeruleus neurons in behaving rats anticipates fluctuations in the sleep-waking cycle. J Neurosci 1981;1:876–86.

[16] Foote SL, Aston-Jones G, Bloom FE. Impulse activity of locus coeruleus neurons in awake rats and monkeys is a function of sensory stimulation and arousal. Proc Natl Acad Sci USA 1980; 77:3033–7.

[17] Hobson JA, McCarley RW, Wyzinski PW. Sleep cycle oscillation: reciprocal discharge by two brainstem neuronal groups. Science 1975;189:55–8.

[18] Jones BE, Harper ST, Halaris AE. Effects of locus coeruleus lesions upon cerebral monoamine content, sleep-wakefulness states and the response to amphetamine in the cat. Brain Res 1977; 124:473–96.

[19] Hillarp NA, Fuxe K, Dahlstrom A. Demonstration and mapping of central neurons containing dopamine, noradrenaline, and 5-hydroxytryptamine and their reactions to psychopharmaca. Pharmacol Rev 1966;18:727–41.

[20] Freeman A, Ciliax B, Bakay R, et al. Nigrostriatal collaterals to thalamus degenerate in parkinsonian animal models. Ann Neurol 2001;50:321–9.

[21] Neylan TC, van Kammen DP, Kelley ME, et al. Sleep in schizophrenic patients on and off haloperidol therapy. Clinically stable vs relapsed patients. Arch Gen Psychiatry 1992;49: 643–9.

[22] Roth T, Rye DB, Borchert LD, et al. Assessment of sleepiness and unintended sleep in Parkinson's disease patients taking dopamine agonists. Sleep Med 2003;4:275–80.

[23] Wisor JP, Nishino S, Sora I, et al. Dopaminergic role in stimulant-induced wakefulness. J Neurosci 2001;21:1787–94.

[24] Ongini E, Bonizzoni E, Ferri N, et al. Differential effects of dopamine D-1 and D-2 receptor antagonist antipsychotics on sleep-wake patterns in the rat. J Pharmacol Exp Ther 1993;266: 726–31.

[25] Trulson ME, Preussler DW, Howell GA. Activity of substantia nigra units across the sleep-waking cycle in freely moving cats. Neurosci Lett 1981;26:183–8.

[26] Trulson ME, Preussler DW. Dopamine-containing ventral tegmental area neurons in freely moving cats: activity during the sleep-waking cycle and effects of stress. Exp Neurol 1984; 83:367–77.

[27] Tork I. Anatomy of the serotonergic system. Ann N Y Acad Sci 1990;600:9–34 [discussion 34–5].

[28] Trulson ME, Jacobs BL. Raphe unit activity in freely moving cats: correlation with level of behavioral arousal. Brain Res 1979;163:135–50.

[29] Portas CM, Bjorvatn B, Fagerland S, et al. On-line detection of extracellular levels of serotonin in dorsal raphe nucleus and frontal cortex over the sleep/wake cycle in the freely moving rat. Neuroscience 1998;83:807–14.

[30] Ursin R. The effects of 5-hydroxytryptophan and L-tryptophan on wakefulness and sleep patterns in the cat. Brain Res 1976;106:105–15.

[31] Wojcik WJ, Fornal C, Radulovacki M. Effect of tryptophan on sleep in the rat. Neuro-pharmacology 1980;19:163–7.

[32] Bjorvatn B, Ursin R. Effects of zimeldine, a selective 5-HT reuptake inhibitor, combined with ritanserin, a selective 5–HT2 antagonist, on waking and sleep stages in rats. Behav Brain Res 1990;40:239–46.

[33] Kaneko T, Mizuno N. Immunohistochemical study of glutaminase-containing neurons in the cerebral cortex and thalamus of the rat. J Comp Neurol 1988;267:590–602.

[34] Glenn LL, Steriade M. Discharge rate and excitability of cortically projecting intralaminar thalamic neurons during waking and sleep states. J Neurosci 1982;2:1387–404.

[35] Steriade M, Llinas RR. The functional states of the thalamus and the associated neuronal interplay. Physiol Rev 1988;68:649–742.

[36] Sakai K, El Mansari M, Lin JS, et al. The posterior hypothalamus in the regulation of wakefulness and paradoxical sleep. In: Mancia M, Marini G, editors. The diencephalon and sleep. New York: Raven Press; 1990. p. 171–98.

[37] Steininger TL, Alam MN, Gong H, et al. Sleep-waking discharge of neurons in the posterior lateral hypothalamus of the albino rat. Brain Res 1999;840:138–47.

[38] Denoyer M, Sallanon M, Buda C, et al. Neurotoxic lesion of the mesencephalic reticular formation and/or the posterior hypothalamus does not alter waking in the cat. Brain Res 1991; 539:287–303.

[39] Panula P, Pirvola U, Auvinen S, et al. Histamine-immunoreactive nerve fibers in the rat brain. Neuroscience 1989;28:585–610.

[40] Parmentier R, Ohtsu H, Djebbara-Hannas Z, et al. Anatomical, physiological, and phar-macological characteristics of histidine decarboxylase knock-out mice: evidence for the role of brain histamine in behavioral and sleep-wake control. J Neurosci 2002;22:7695–711.

[41] de Lecea L, Kilduff TS, Peyron C, et al. The hypocretins: hypothalamus-specific peptides with neuroexcitatory activity. Proc Natl Acad Sci USA 1998;95:322–7.

[42] Peyron C, Tighe DK, van den Pol AN, et al. Neurons containing hypocretin (orexin) project to multiple neuronal systems. J Neurosci 1998;18:9996–10015.

[43] Sakurai T, Amemiya A, Ishii M, et al. Orexins and orexin receptors: a family of hypothalamic neuropeptides and G protein-coupled receptors that regulate feeding behavior. Cell 1998;92: 573–85.

[44] Taheri S, Mahmoodi M, Opacka-Juffry J, et al. Distribution and quantification of immu-noreactive orexin A in rat tissues. FEBS Lett 1999;457:157–61.

[45] Nambu T, Sakurai T, Mizukami K, et al. Distribution of orexin neurons in the adult rat brain. Brain Res 1999;827:243–60.

[46] Li Y, Gao XB, Sakurai T, et al. Hypocretin/Orexin excites hypocretin neurons via a local glutamate neuron-A potential mechanism for orchestrating the hypothalamic arousal system. Neuron 2002;36:1169–81.

[47] Chemelli RM, Willie JT, Sinton CM, et al. Narcolepsy in orexin knockout mice: molecular genetics of sleep regulation. Cell 1999;98:437–51.

[48] Date Y, Ueta Y, Yamashita H, et al. Orexins, orexigenic hypothalamic peptides, interact with autonomic, neuroendocrine and neuroregulatory systems. Proc Natl Acad Sci USA 1999;96: 748–53.

[49] Mignot E, Lammers GJ, Ripley B, et al. The role of cerebrospinal fluid hypocretin measurement in the diagnosis of narcolepsy and other hypersomnias. Arch Neurol 2002;59:1553–62.

[50] Peyron C, Faraco J, Rogers W, et al. A mutation in a case of early onset narcolepsy and a generalized absence of hypocretin peptides in human narcoleptic brains. Nat Med 2000;6: 991–7.

[51] Thannickal TC, Moore RY, Nienhuis R, et al. Reduced number of hypocretin neurons in human narcolepsy. Neuron 2000;27:469–74.

[52] Hara J, Beuckmann CT, Nambu T, et al. Genetic ablation of orexin neurons in mice results in narcolepsy, hypophagia, and obesity. Neuron 2001;30:345–54.

[53] Zeitzer JM, Buckmaster CL, Parker KJ, et al. Circadian and homeostatic regulation of hypocretin in a primate model: implications for the consolidation of wakefulness. J Neurosci 2003;23:3555–60.

[54] Piper DC, Upton N, Smith MI, et al. The novel brain neuropeptide, orexin-A, modulates the sleep-wake cycle of rats. Eur J Neurosci 2000;12:726–30.

[55] Nolte J. The human brain. 5th edition. St. Louis: Mosby; 2002.

[56] Mesulam MM, Mufson EJ, Wainer BH, et al. Central cholinergic pathways in the rat: an overview based on an alternative nomenclature (Ch1-Ch6). Neuroscience 1983;10:1185–201.

[57] Lee MG, Henny P, Jones B. Sleep-wake discharge properties of juxtacellularly labeled and immunohistochemically identified cholinergic basal forebrain neurons in head-restrained rats. Presented at the Society for Neuroscience 33rd Annual Meeting. New Orleans, November 8–12, 2003.

[58] Gritti I, Mainville L, Mancia M, et al. GABAergic and other noncholinergic basal forebrain neurons, together with cholinergic neurons, project to the mesocortex and isocortex in the rat. J Comp Neurol 1997;383:163–77.

[59] Manns ID, Mainville L, Jones BE. Evidence for glutamate, in addition to acetylcholine and GABA, neurotransmitter synthesis in basal forebrain neurons projecting to the entorhinal cortex. Neuroscience 2001;107:249–63.

[60] Sterman MB, Clemente CD. Forebrain inhibitory mechanisms: sleep patterns induced by basal forebrain stimulation in the behaving cat. Exp Neurol 1962;6:103–17.

[61] Sterman MB, Clemente CD. Forebrain inhibitory mechanisms: cortical synchronization induced by basal forebrain stimulation. Exp Neurol 1962;6:91–102.

[62] Espana RA, Scammell TE. Sleep neurobiology for the clinician. Sleep 2004;27:811–20.

[63] Kaitin KI. Preoptic area unit activity during sleep and wakefulness in the cat. Exp Neurol 1984;83:347–57.

[64] Burikov AA, Suntsova NV. The neuronal impulse activity of the preoptic area in the rabbit during electrocorticographic correlates of wakefulness and slow-wave sleep. Zh Vyssh Nerv Deiat Im I P Pavlova 1989;39:1146–8 [in Russian].

[65] Koyama Y, Hayaishi O. Firing of neurons in the preoptic/anterior hypothalamic areas in rat: its possible involvement in slow wave sleep and paradoxical sleep. Neurosci Res 1994;19:31–8.

[66] Alam MN, McGinty D, Szymusiak R. Neuronal discharge of preoptic/anterior hypothalamic thermosensitive neurons: relation to NREM sleep. Am J Physiol 1995;269:R1240–9.

[67] Suntsova NV, Burikov AA. The restructuring of the neuronal activity of the lateral hypothalamic preoptic area during the development of sleep. Zh Vyssh Nerv Deiat Im I P Pavlova 1995;45:948–56 [in Russian].

[68] Gong H, Szymusiak R, King J, et al. Sleep-related c-Fos protein expression in the preoptic hypothalamus: effects of ambient warming. Am J Physiol Regul Integr Comp Physiol 2000; 279:R2079–88.

[69] Sherin JE, Shiromani PJ, McCarley RW, et al. Activation of ventrolateral preoptic neurons during sleep. Science 1996;271:216–9.

[70] Sherin JE, Elmquist JK, Torrealba F, et al. Innervation of histaminergic tuberomammillary neurons by GABAergic and galaninergic neurons in the ventrolateral preoptic nucleus of the rat. J Neurosci 1998;18:4705–21.

[71] Szymusiak R, Alam N, Steininger TL, et al. Sleep-waking discharge patterns of ventrolateral preoptic/anterior hypothalamic neurons in rats. Brain Res 1998;803:178–88.

[72] Steininger TL, Gong H, McGinty D, et al. Subregional organization of preoptic area/anterior hypothalamic projections to arousal-related monoaminergic cell groups. J Comp Neurol 2001; 429:638–53.

[73] Gaus SE, Strecker RE, Tate BA, et al. Ventrolateral preoptic nucleus contains sleep-active, galaninergic neurons in multiple mammalian species. Neuroscience 2002;115:285–94.

[74] Lu J, Greco MA, Shiromani P, et al. Effect of lesions of the ventrolateral preoptic nucleus on NREM and REM sleep. J Neurosci 2000;20:3830–42.

[75] Szymusiak R, McGinty D. Sleep-related neuronal discharge in the basal forebrain of cats. Brain Res 1986;370:82–92.

[76] Cheng MY, Bullock CM, Li C, et al. Prokineticin 2 transmits the behavioural circadian rhythm of the suprachiasmatic nucleus. Nature 2002;417:405–10.

[77] Jasper HH, Tessier J. Acetylcholine liberation from cerebral cortex during paradoxical (REM) sleep. Science 1971;172:601–2.

[78] Boissard R, Gervasoni D, Schmidt MH, et al. The rat ponto-medullary network responsible for paradoxical sleep onset and maintenance: a combined microinjection and functional neuro-anatomical study. Eur J Neurosci 2002;16:1959–73.

[79] Nitz D, Siegel J. GABA release in the dorsal raphe nucleus: role in the control of REM sleep. Am J Physiol 1997;273:R451–5.

[80] Gervasoni D, Darracq L, Fort P, et al. Electrophysiological evidence that noradrenergic neurons of the rat locus coeruleus are tonically inhibited by GABA during sleep. Eur J Neurosci 1998;10:964–70.

[81] Crochet S, Sakai K. Effects of microdialysis application of monoamines on the EEG and behavioural states in the cat mesopontine tegmentum. Eur J Neurosci 1999;11:3738–52.

[82] Morales FR, Engelhardt JK, Soja PJ, et al. Motoneuron properties during motor inhibition produced by microinjection of carbachol into the pontine reticular formation of the decerebrate cat. J Neurophysiol 1987;57:1118–29.

[83] Curtis DR, Hosli L, Johnston GA, et al. The hyperpolarization of spinal motoneurones by glycine and related amino acids. Exp Brain Res 1968;5:235–58.

[84] Mileykovskiy BY, Kiyashchenko LI, Siegel JM. Cessation of activity in red nucleus neurons during stimulation of the medial medulla in decerebrate rats. J Physiol 2002;545:997–1006.

[85] Maquet P. Functional neuroimaging of normal human sleep by positron emission tomography. J Sleep Res 2000;9:207–31.

[86] McCormick DA. Neurotransmitter actions in the thalamus and cerebral cortex and their role in neuromodulation of thalamocortical activity. Prog Neurobiol 1992;39:337–88.

[87] Madsen PL, Holm S, Vorstrup S, et al. Human regional cerebral blood flow during rapid-eye-movement sleep. J Cereb Blood Flow Metab 1991;11:502–7.

[88] Madsen PL, Vorstrup S. Cerebral blood flow and metabolism during sleep. Cerebrovasc Brain Metab Rev 1991;3:281–96.

[89] Franzini C. Brain metabolism and blood flow during sleep. J Sleep Res 1992;1:3–16.

[90] Maquet P, Dive D, Salmon E, et al. Cerebral glucose utilization during sleep-wake cycle in man determined by positron emission tomography and [18F]2-fluoro-2-deoxy-D-glucose method. Brain Res 1990;513:136–43.

[91] Aggleton JP. The contribution of the amygdala to normal and abnormal emotional states. Trends Neurosci 1993;16:328–33.

[92] Borbely AA. A two process model of sleep regulation. Hum Neurobiol 1982;1:195–204.
[93] Borbely AA, Achermann P. Concepts and models of sleep regulation: an overview. J Sleep Res 1992;1:63–79.
[94] Wurts SW, Edgar DM. Circadian and homeostatic control of rapid eye movement (REM) sleep: promotion of REM tendency by the suprachiasmatic nucleus. J Neurosci 2000;20:4300–10.
[95] Dijk DJ, Lockley SW. Integration of human sleep-wake regulation and circadian rhythmicity. J Appl Physiol 2002;92:852–62.
[96] Saper CB, Chou TC, Scammell TE. The sleep switch: hypothalamic control of sleep and wakefulness. Trends Neurosci 2001;24:726–31.
[97] Horowitz P, Hill W. Devices with memory: flip flops. In: Horowitz P, Hill W, editors. The art of electronics. 2nd edition. Cambridge, UK: Cambridge University Press; 1986. p. 506.
[98] Nishino S, Ripley B, Overeem S, et al. Hypocretin (orexin) deficiency in human narcolepsy. Lancet 2000;355:39–40.
[99] Peyron C, Faraco J, Rogers W, et al. A mutation in a case of early onset narcolepsy and a generalized absence of hypocretin peptides in human narcoleptic brains. Nat Med 2000;6: 991–7.
[100] Thannickal TC, Moore RY, Nienhuis R, et al. Reduced number of hypocretin neurons in human narcolepsy. Neuron 2000;27:469–74.
[101] Dijk DJ, Duffy JF, Riel E, et al. Ageing and the circadian and homeostatic regulation of human sleep during forced desynchrony of rest, melatonin and temperature rhythms. J Physiol 1999; 516(Pt 2):611–27.
[102] Kramer A, Yang FC, Snodgrass P, et al. Regulation of daily locomotor activity and sleep by hypothalamic EGF receptor signaling. Science 2001;294:2511–5.
[103] Chou TC, Scammell TE, Gooley JJ, et al. Critical role of dorsomedial hypothalamic nucleus in a wide range of behavioral circadian rhythms. J Neurosci 2003;23:10691–702.
[104] Abrahamson EE, Leak RK, Moore RY. The suprachiasmatic nucleus projects to posterior hypothalamic arousal systems. Neuroreport 2001;12:435–40.
[105] Aston-Jones G, Chen S, Zhu Y, et al. A neural circuit for circadian regulation of arousal. Nat Neurosci 2001;4:732–8.
[106] Lu J, Zhang YH, Chou TC, et al. Contrasting effects of ibotenate lesions of the paraventricular nucleus and subparaventricular zone on sleep-wake cycle and temperature regulation. J Neurosci 2001;21:4864–74.
[107] Dijk DJ, Shanahan TL, Duffy JF, et al. Variation of electroencephalographic activity during non-rapid eye movement and rapid eye movement sleep with phase of circadian melatonin rhythm in humans. J Physiol 1997;505(Pt 3):851–8.
[108] Duffy JF, Dijk DJ, Klerman EB, et al. Later endogenous circadian temperature nadir relative to an earlier wake time in older people. Am J Physiol 1998;275:R1478–87.
[109] Moore RY. Circadian rhythms: basic neurobiology and clinical applications. Annu Rev Med 1997;48:253–66.
[110] van Esseveldt KE, Lehman MN, Boer GJ. The suprachiasmatic nucleus and the circadian time-keeping system revisited. Brain Res Brain Res Rev 2000;33:34–77.
[111] Green CB, Menaker M. Circadian rhythms. Clocks on the brain. Science 2003;301:319–20.
[112] Moore RY. Neural control of the pineal gland. Behav Brain Res 1996;73:125–30.
[113] Meijer JH, Rietveld WJ. Neurophysiology of the suprachiasmatic circadian pacemaker in rodents. Physiol Rev 1989;69:671–707.
[114] Lehman MN, Silver R, Gladstone WR, et al. Circadian rhythmicity restored by neural transplant. Immunocytochemical characterization of the graft and its integration with the host brain. J Neurosci 1987;7:1626–38.
[115] Ralph MR, Foster RG, Davis FC, et al. Transplanted suprachiasmatic nucleus determines circadian period. Science 1990;247:975–8.
[116] Inouye ST, Kawamura H. Persistence of circadian rhythmicity in a mammalian hypothalamic "island" containing the suprachiasmatic nucleus. Proc Natl Acad Sci USA 1979;76:5962–6.
[117] Shibata S, Moore RY. Electrical and metabolic activity of suprachiasmatic nucleus neurons in hamster hypothalamic slices. Brain Res 1988;438:374–8.

[118] Dudley CA, Erbel-Sieler C, Estill SJ, et al. Altered patterns of sleep and behavioral adaptability in NPAS2-deficient mice. Science 2003;301:379–83.

[119] Van Gelder RN. Recent insights into mammalian circadian rhythms. Sleep 2004;27:166–71.

[120] Welsh DK, Logothetis DE, Meister M, et al. Individual neurons dissociated from rat suprachiasmatic nucleus express independently phased circadian firing rhythms. Neuron 1995;14:697–706.

[121] Freedman MS, Lucas RJ, Soni B, et al. Regulation of mammalian circadian behavior by non-rod, non-cone, ocular photoreceptors. Science 1999;284:502–4.

[122] Hattar S, Liao HW, Takao M, et al. Melanopsin-containing retinal ganglion cells: architecture, projections, and intrinsic photosensitivity. Science 2002;295:1065–70.

[123] Provencio I, Rodriguez IR, Jiang G, et al. A novel human opsin in the inner retina. J Neurosci 2000;20:600–5.

[124] Johnson RF, Moore RY, Morin LP. Loss of entrainment and anatomical plasticity after lesions of the hamster retinohypothalamic tract. Brain Res 1988;460:297–313.

[125] Hannibal J, Moller M, Ottersen OP, et al. PACAP and glutamate are co-stored in the retinohypothalamic tract. J Comp Neurol 2000;418:147–55.

[126] Hannibal J, Ding JM, Chen D, et al. Pituitary adenylate cyclase-activating peptide (PACAP) in the retinohypothalamic tract: a potential daytime regulator of the biological clock. J Neurosci 1997;17:2637–44.

[127] Pickard GE, Rea MA. TFMPP, a 5HT1B receptor agonist, inhibits light-induced phase shifts of the circadian activity rhythm and c-Fos expression in the mouse suprachiasmatic nucleus. Neurosci Lett 1997;231:95–8.

[128] Treep JA, Abe H, Rusak B, et al. Two distinct retinal projections to the hamster suprachiasmatic nucleus. J Biol Rhythms 1995;10:299–307.

[129] Moore RY, Card JP. Intergeniculate leaflet: an anatomically and functionally distinct subdivision of the lateral geniculate complex. J Comp Neurol 1994;344:403–30.

[130] Reebs SG, Mrosovsky N. Large phase-shifts of circadian rhythms caused by induced running in a re-entrainment paradigm: the role of pulse duration and light. J Comp Physiol [A] 1989; 165:819–25.

[131] Turek FW. Effects of stimulated physical activity on the circadian pacemaker of vertebrates. J Biol Rhythms 1989;4:135–47.

[132] Pickard GE, Rea MA. Serotonergic innervation of the hypothalamic suprachiasmatic nucleus and photic regulation of circadian rhythms. Biol Cell 1997;89:513–23.

[133] Bradbury MJ, Dement WC, Edgar DM. Serotonin-containing fibers in the suprachiasmatic hypothalamus attenuate light-induced phase delays in mice. Brain Res 1997;768:125–34.

[134] Pickard GE, Weber ET, Scott PA, et al. 5HT1B receptor agonists inhibit light-induced phase shifts of behavioral circadian rhythms and expression of the immediate-early gene c-fos in the suprachiasmatic nucleus. J Neurosci 1996;16:8208–20.

[135] Weber ET, Gannon RL, Rea MA. Local administration of serotonin agonists blocks light-induced phase advances of the circadian activity rhythm in the hamster. J Biol Rhythms 1998;13:209–18.

[136] Kalsbeek A, Teclemariam-Mesbah R, Pevet P. Efferent projections of the suprachiasmatic nucleus in the golden hamster (Mesocricetus auratus). J Comp Neurol 1993;332:293–314.

[137] Watts AG. The efferent projections of the suprachiasmatic nucleus: anatomical insights into the control of circadian rhythms. In: Klein DC, Moore RY, Reppert ST, editors. The suprachiasmatic nucleus: the mind's clock. New York: Oxford; 1991. p. 77–106.

[138] Silver R, LeSauter J, Tresco PA, et al. A diffusible coupling signal from the transplanted suprachiasmatic nucleus controlling circadian locomotor rhythms. Nature 1996;382:810–3.

[139] Jones CR, Campbell SS, Zone SE, et al. Familial advanced sleep-phase syndrome: A short-period circadian rhythm variant in humans. Nat Med 1999;5:1062–5.

[140] Toh KL, Jones CR, He Y, et al. An hPer2 phosphorylation site mutation in familial advanced sleep phase syndrome. Science 2001;291:1040–3.

[141] De Leersnyder H, De Blois MC, Claustrat B, et al. Inversion of the circadian rhythm of melatonin in the Smith-Magenis syndrome. J Pediatr 2001;139:111–6.

[142] Yen SSC, Jaffe RB, Barbieri RL. Reproductive endocrinology: physiology, pathophysiology, and clinical management. 4th edition. Philadelphia: W.B. Saunders; 1999.

[143] Schwartz WJ, de la Iglesia HO, Zlomanczuk P, et al. Encoding le quattro stagioni within the mammalian brain: photoperiodic orchestration through the suprachiasmatic nucleus. J Biol Rhythms 2001;16:302–11.

[144] Mrugala M, Zlomanczuk P, Jagota A, et al. Rhythmic multiunit neural activity in slices of hamster suprachiasmatic nucleus reflect prior photoperiod. Am J Physiol Regul Integr Comp Physiol 2000;278:R987–94.

[145] Jac M, Kiss A, Sumova A, et al. Daily profiles of arginine vasopressin mRNA in the suprachiasmatic, supraoptic and paraventricular nuclei of the rat hypothalamus under various photoperiods. Brain Res 2000;887:472–6.

[146] Wehr TA, Duncan Jr WC, Sher L, et al. A circadian signal of change of season in patients with seasonal affective disorder. Arch Gen Psychiatry 2001;58:1108–14.

[147] Wehr T. Photoperiodism in humans and other primates: evidence and implications. J Biol Rhythms 2001;16:348–64.

[148] Jac M, Sumova A, Illnerova H. c-Fos rhythm in subdivisions of the rat suprachiasmatic nucleus under artificial and natural photoperiods. Am J Physiol Regul Integr Comp Physiol 2000; 279:R2270–6.

[149] Rosenthal NE, Sack DA, Gillin JC, et al. Seasonal affective disorder. A description of the syndrome and preliminary findings with light therapy. Arch Gen Psychiatry 1984;41:72–80.

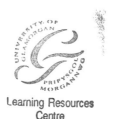

ELSEVIER
SAUNDERS

CLINICS
IN SPORTS
MEDICINE

Clin Sports Med 24 (2005) 237–249

Sleep, Circadian Rhythms, and Psychomotor Vigilance

Hans P.A. Van Dongen, PhD*, David F. Dinges, PhD

*Division of Sleep and Chronobiology, Department of Psychiatry,
University of Pennsylvania School of Medicine, 10 Blockley Hall, 423 Guardian Drive, Philadelphia,
PA 19104, USA*

There is no doubt that sleep is important for cognitive performance. Although the functions of sleep are not yet fully understood, its relationship to performance is evident through the deterioration of cognitive functioning under conditions of sleep deprivation and the recuperation provided by subsequent sleep [1,2]. The alternation of sleep and wakefulness is driven by a complex neurobiology that has only partially been unraveled [3]. Nevertheless, two primary processes of sleep/wake regulation have been putatively distinguished [4].

The first process, referred to as the *sleep homeostat*, seeks to balance time spent awake and time spent asleep. It can be conceptualized as the buildup of homeostatic pressure for sleep during periods of wakefulness, and the dissipation of this pressure during periods of sleep. The second process is the endogenous circadian rhythm, which is driven by the biological clock in the suprachiasmatic nuclei of the hypothalamus in the brain. This "internal clock" keeps track of the time of day (the term *circadian* refers to a near–24-hour cycle). Given that humans are a diurnal species, the circadian process seeks to place wakefulness during the day and sleep during the night. The circadian process can be envisaged as providing pressure for wakefulness [5,6] that is strongest during

This work was supported by grants NR04281 and HL70154 from the National Institutes of Health, grants F49620-95-1-0388 and F49620-00-1-0266 from the Air Force Office of Scientific Research, grant NAG9-1161 from the National Aeronautics and Space Administration, and NASA cooperative agreement NCC 9-58 with the National Space Biomedical Research Institute.

* Corresponding author.

E-mail address: vdongen@mail.med.upenn.edu (H.P.A. Van Dongen).

the early evening hours and weakest in the early morning. The sleep homeostatic process and the circadian process interact with each other neurobiologically.

During the day, the homeostatic and circadian processes act in opposition to promote wakefulness [7]. In the morning hours just after awakening from a sleep period, not much homeostatic pressure for sleep is present, and there is also relatively little compensatory circadian pressure for wakefulness. (The awakening process itself is characterized by a brief period of "sleep inertia," which is discussed later.) As the day progresses, the homeostatic pressure for sleep builds up, and at the same time, the circadian pressure for wakefulness increases. The net effect is stable waking pressure throughout the day, which in healthy individuals results in a consolidated period of wakefulness.

At night, the homeostatic and circadian processes act synergistically to promote sleep [7]. In the beginning of the night before falling asleep, the circadian pressure for wakefulness gradually withdraws, whereas the homeostatic pressure for sleep continues to accumulate. As a result, there is a notable net increase in pressure for sleep and, under appropriate circumstances (eg, lying supine), the sleep state is initiated. During sleep, the homeostatic pressure for sleep dissipates. The circadian pressure for wakefulness further diminishes as well. Thus, there is little net waking pressure throughout the night, which in healthy individuals results in a consolidated period of sleep.

In the morning, the circadian pressure for wakefulness gradually rises again and exceeds the largely dissipated homeostatic pressure for sleep. Consequently, spontaneous awakening occurs, and the cycle starts again with the homeostatic and circadian processes acting in opposition to promote wakefulness. These interactions of sleep homeostatic and circadian neurobiology have been studied extensively [8] and have been instantiated in contemporary theoretical and mathematical models [9,10].

Even though the alternation of sleep and wakefulness is regulated fairly precisely, giving rise to the term *sleep/wake cycle*, humans are a rather unique species in that they can voluntarily choose to temporarily ignore the homeostatic and circadian-mediated signals for sleep [11]. When humans stay awake to pursue other activities, though, this is not without consequence, which will be discussed later.

Homeostatic and circadian influences on performance

To systematically examine the effects of the homeostatic pressure for sleep and the circadian pressure for wakefulness on cognitive performance, studies have been conducted in laboratories set up specifically to monitor and control sleep and wakefulness, circadian rhythms, and neurobehavioral functions [1,12,13]. This article focuses on psychomotor vigilance performance, because it involves reaction time and sustained attention, which are elemental features of a wide range of human performance.

Psychomotor vigilance performance can be measured with the psychomotor vigilance task (PVT) [14], a portable, easily usable reaction-time test with a high stimulus load (visual or auditory) that can yield rapid (ie, in 10 minutes) and reliable assessments of psychomotor vigilance impairment [15,16]. The PVT has been used in the laboratory to precisely measure, at brief intervals (typically every 2 hours of wakefulness), the changes in psychomotor vigilance performance caused by sleep loss and circadian rhythmicity [16].

The changes in psychomotor vigilance performance over time in a laboratory study involving 88 hours of extended wakefulness (ie, three nights without sleep) [15] are shown in Fig. 1. In Fig. 1A, lapses of attention (ie, reaction

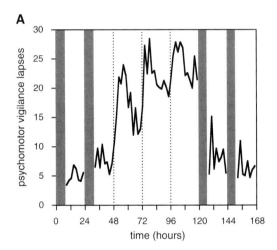

Fig. 1. Performance data from 13 healthy young adult males (mean age ± SD: 27.3 ± 4.6 years) who spent 10 days in the controlled environment of a laboratory. After one adaptation day and two baseline days with 8 hours time in bed (23:30–07:30), they were assigned to a condition involving 88 hours of extended wakefulness. Thereafter, during the last 3 days of the experiment, they received recovery sleep each night. A subset of 7 subjects were allowed 7 hours time in bed (23:30–06:30) on the first 2 recovery days and 14 hours time in bed (23:30–13:30) on the last recovery day, whereas the other 6 subjects were allowed 14 hours time in bed on all 3 recovery days. Throughout scheduled wakefulness, subjects underwent cognitive testing every 2 hours. The cognitive test battery included a 10-minute psychomotor vigilance task (PVT). (A) The number of lapses (reaction times ≥ 500 ms) on the PVT. (B) The average of the 10% fastest reaction times (in ms) on the PVT. In both cases, group averages are plotted against cumulative clock time. Gray bars indicate scheduled sleep periods—the 2 baseline nights and the first 2 recovery nights (7 hours time in bed) are shown. Dotted lines in the 88-hour sleep deprivation period indicate midnight. On the last baseline day (before the last baseline sleep period) and on the first day of sleep deprivation, psychomotor vigilance lapses were relatively rare and fastest reaction times were relatively short. However, both psychomotor vigilance lapses and fastest reaction times increased significantly during the rest of the 88 hours of wakefulness. The progressive increases over days of sleep deprivation were modulated by a circadian rhythm: the number of lapses and the fastest reaction times were reduced during the diurnal hours compared with the nocturnal hours even after 3 days without sleep. Recovery sleep rapidly reduced the level of impairment; after 2 nights with 7 hours in bed, performance was almost back to the baseline level (for the recovery days, averages are shown for the 7 subjects who received 7 hours time in bed only).

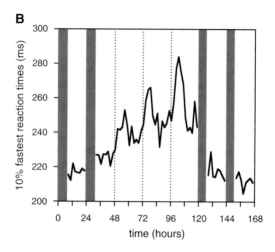

Fig. 1 (*continued*).

times ≥ 500 milliseconds) on the PVT can be seen, whereas Fig. 1B shows the 10% fastest reaction times on the PVT. The changes in fastest reaction times showed the same temporal pattern as the changes in psychomotor vigilance lapses. With every day of sleep deprivation, the average number of psychomotor vigilance lapses and the average duration of the fastest reaction times increased. In addition, nighttime performance was consistently worse than daytime performance.

This temporal pattern can be readily interpreted as the interaction between the homeostatic and circadian processes of sleep/wake regulation. The two processes are considered to have a combined effect on waking cognitive performance, which can be approximated by subtracting the homeostatic pressure for sleep from the circadian pressure for wakefulness [17]. The net pressure for sleep determines the degree of cognitive performance impairment. This explains why in the study of Fig. 1, psychomotor vigilance lapses and fastest reaction times increased over days of sleep deprivation, since the homeostatic pressure for sleep continued to accumulate in the absence of sleep. Furthermore, it explains why daytime performance was consistently better than nighttime performance, for the circadian pressure for wakefulness was greatest during the diurnal portion of each day.

The interaction of the homeostatic and circadian processes can also be observed in the phenomenon of jet lag. This is the transient period of impairment following rapid travel to a different time zone. On arrival in the new time zone, the circadian pressure for wakefulness is initially not timed appropriately relative to the time of day, which has an adverse effect on daytime cognitive performance. The circadian pressure for wakefulness is also not withdrawn at the right time to promote nighttime sleep. This may cause problems with the timing and consolidation of sleep, resulting in reduced dissipation of the homeostatic pressure for sleep. The remaining pressure for sleep may further compromise cognitive performance. Depending on the direction of travel and the number of time zones crossed, it can take several days for the circadian process to align properly with the new time zone and for the homeostatic process to restore the balance between sleep and wakefulness [18].

Effects of napping on performance

The dissipation of homeostatic pressure during sleep is thought to be an exponential process [9], where the greater the level of homeostatic pressure reached during wakefulness, the faster the dissipation during subsequent sleep. This implies that recuperation from performance deficits caused by prior sleep loss should occur rapidly even if time available for sleep is relatively short. The data in Fig. 1 (see right-hand side of Figs. 1A and 1B), which show that a single episode of 7 hours time in bed markedly reduced psychomotor vigilance lapses and fastest reaction times after the 88 hours of total sleep deprivation, confirm this.

Based on the disproportionate recovery potential of relatively short sleep periods, naps ("power naps") have been investigated as a strategy to attenuate performance deficits during and following periods of sleep deprivation [19,20]. Fig. 2 illustrates the effects of nap sleep on psychomotor vigilance lapses during

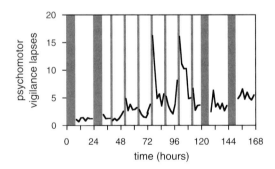

Fig. 2. Performance data from 13 healthy young adult males (mean age ± SD: 28.2 ± 8.9 years) who participated in the same experiment as those of Fig. 1, but were randomized to a condition involving 2-hour nap opportunities every 12 hours (14:45–16:45 and 02:45–04:45) during 88 hours of otherwise continuous wakefulness. Details of the figure are the same as for Fig. 1A, but there is a difference in the range of the ordinate scale. Thin gray bars indicate the scheduled 2-hour nap periods. A subset of 8 subjects were allowed 7 hours time in bed on the first 2 recovery days, whereas the other 5 subjects were allowed 14 hours time in bed. For these recovery days, averages are shown for the 8 subjects who received 7 hours time in bed only. Compared with 88 hours of total sleep deprivation (Fig. 1A), the 2-hour nap opportunities considerably attenuated the magnitude of psychomotor vigilance deficits from sleep loss, although a minor buildup of performance impairment still occurred across the 88-hour experimental period. Nap sleep resulted in vigilance performance deficits immediately on awakening, however. This "sleep inertia" effect intensified with progressive sleep loss, especially at night.

otherwise continuous wakefulness. The experimental condition depicted in this figure was comparable to the 88 hours of extended wakefulness shown in Fig. 1, but in this case the 88 hours were interrupted by 2-hour nap opportunities occurring every 12 hours [15,21]. As a consequence, the buildup of psychomotor vigilance impairment over the 88-hour period was considerably attenuated, which highlights the recuperative potential of nap sleep.

Unfortunately, the napping strategy has an adverse effect called *sleep inertia*, which is the cognitive performance impairment commonly experienced immediately after awakening [22]. As evident in Fig. 2, sleep inertia is particularly noticeable under conditions of sleep loss and during the circadian night [23–25]. Thus, the magnitude of sleep inertia appears to be a function of increased homeostatic pressure for sleep and decreased circadian pressure for wakefulness. In situations where optimal performance capability right after awakening is not required, napping may still be useful to mitigate the effects of sleep loss. Also, very short naps (approximately 10 minutes) may offer some recuperative benefit without noticeable levels of sleep inertia [26]. Even so, strategic napping cannot be considered a universal substitute for obtaining sufficient amounts of sleep.

Effects of chronic sleep restriction

Even though brief sleep periods can limit the cognitive deficits from cumulative sleep loss in the short-term (see Fig. 2), they fail to preserve optimal cognitive functioning in the long-term. This has been demonstrated in recent experiments of chronic sleep restriction [13,27,28]. In one of these studies [13], subjects were randomized to 14 days of restriction to 4-, 6-, or 8-hours time in bed per day. Fig. 3 shows results of this study for psychomotor vigilance lapses as measured with the PVT, averaged within days. Because of this averaging, changes within days resulting from the interaction of the homeostatic process and the circadian process are not visible in the figure, but more long-term changes in cognitive performance are clearly exposed. Compared with the control condition of 8 hours time in bed per day (in which subjects actually obtained approximately 7 hours of physiologic sleep), the sleep restriction conditions of 4 and 6 hours time in bed per day (dotted and thin curves, respectively) displayed progressive increases in psychomotor vigilance impairment. After 14 days of sleep restriction, the magnitude of impairment in the condition with 4 hours time in bed actually approached the daytime level of impairment observed during 88 hours of total sleep deprivation (see Fig. 1A).

These findings cannot be understood solely in terms of homeostatic pressure for sleep [13,29]. Based on the exponential nature of the homeostatic process, a new equilibrium would have been predicted to set in within a few days, when the dissipation of homeostatic pressure during restricted sleep should have become so much swifter (ie, exponentially faster) that it could compensate for the additional increase of homeostatic pressure during extended wakefulness each day. The results of chronic sleep restriction studies [13,27] have not

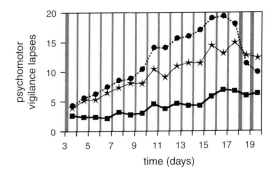

Fig. 3. Performance data from 34 healthy young adults (mean age ± SD: 27.7 ± 5.0 years; 6 females) who spent 20 days in the controlled environment of a laboratory. After 1 adaptation day and 2 baseline days with 8 hours time in bed (23:30–07:30), sleep was restricted for 14 days. Subjects were randomized to 14 days with 4 hours time in bed (13 subjects), 6 hours time in bed (13 subjects), or 8 hours time in bed (control group, 8 subjects); each bedtime period ended at 07:30. At the end of the sleep restriction period, subjects received 3 recovery days with 8 hours time in bed (23:30–07:30). Throughout scheduled wakefulness, subjects underwent cognitive testing every 2 hours. The figure shows lapses (reaction times ≥ 500 ms) on a 10-minute psychomotor vigilance task that was part of the cognitive test battery, plotted as daily means (07:30–23:30) for each of the three sleep restriction conditions (averaged over subjects within each condition). Solid lines (■) correspond to the control condition with 8 hours time in bed; thin lines (★) to the condition with 6 hours time in bed; and dotted lines (●) to the condition with 4 hours time in bed. Gray bars indicate scheduled sleep periods—the last baseline night, the 14 restricted nights (illustrated for the condition with 4 hours time in bed per night), and the first 2 recovery nights are shown. On the first condition day (before the first restricted sleep period), psychomotor vigilance lapses were relatively rare in all conditions. In the control condition, lapses continued to be rare (there was a small increase over days but this was not statistically significant). In the condition with 6 hours time in bed, however, and especially in the condition with 4 hours time in bed, cumulative increases in psychomotor vigilance impairment were observed across the sleep restriction days. Following recovery sleep at the end of the study, lapses were reduced substantially, but 2 days of recovery with 8 hours time in bed seemed to be insufficient to eliminate the cumulative deficits from chronic sleep restriction completely. More research is needed, however, to establish the precise relationship between recovery sleep duration and psychomotor vigilance recuperation.

supported this prediction, as performance impairment continued to accumulate over days of sleep restriction. Two alternative models have been proposed: one in which the effects of sleep deprivation are described in terms of cumulative time of wake extension instead of a sleep homeostatic process [13], and one in which long-term changes in sensitivity to sleep loss are postulated [27,30]. New experiments are needed to determine which of these models best reflects the true nature of cognitive impairment from chronic sleep restriction.

It has been pointed out that the recuperation of performance capability appears to be slower after chronic sleep restriction (Fig. 3) than after acute total sleep deprivation (see Fig. 1) [27]. As can be seen in Fig. 3 (*right side*), two nights with 8 hours time in bed for recovery sleep appeared to only partially reduce the psychomotor vigilance lapses from the prior 14 days of sleep restriction (6 hours or 4 hours time in bed per day). The subjects in the condition with

6 hours time in bed (*thin curve*) seemed to recuperate less than those in the condition with 4 hours time in bed (*dotted curve*), although the difference between conditions was not significant on the first recovery day ($F_{1,24} = 0.10$, $P = 0.76$) or on the second recovery day ($F_{1,24} = 0.32$; $P = 0.58$). However, the data shown are averages over subjects, so it is possible that only a few subjects with heightened vulnerability to sleep loss (as discussed later) created the appearance of incomplete recovery. Available data sets [13,27] have not resolved this issue definitively, and further studies are underway.

The performance-impairing effects of chronic sleep restriction can also be seen in a variety of cognitive functions other than psychomotor vigilance, but many of the performance tasks used to measure these other cognitive functions exhibit practice effects. An example is given in Fig. 4, which shows performance on a serial addition/subtraction task (SAST) [31] in the same study as depicted in Fig. 3 [13]. The extent of the practice effect is exposed in Fig. 4 by the considerable performance improvement over days (ie, upward trend) for the control condition (8 hours time in bed per day). The performance improvement was moderated in the conditions with less than 8 hours time in bed per day (Fig. 4, *thin* and *dotted curves*) because of the effect of cumulative sleep loss, but performance on the SAST did not decrease over days even in the condition with 4 hours time in bed per day. Thus, if performance changes resulting from the practice effect had been overlooked, and a control condition (8 hours time in bed per day) had not been included in the study, a false conclusion could have

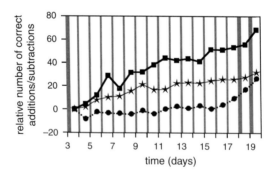

Fig. 4. Data from the same experiment as shown in Fig. 3, but for a different measure of cognitive function. The number of correct responses on a serial addition/subtraction task is displayed (as daily means), expressed relative to baseline performance on day 3 (ie, on the first condition day, before the first restricted sleep period). In this figure, upwards on the ordinate corresponds to performance improvement (not impairment as in the other figures). In the control condition with 8 hours time in bed per day, performance improved steadily over days because of the practice effect associated with the serial addition/subtraction task. In the condition with 6 hours time in bed, the improvement over days was attenuated because of the cumulative sleep loss, and in the condition with 4 hours time in bed, almost no improvement was observed—until after the first recovery sleep. Even after two recovery sleep periods at the end of the study, both sleep restriction conditions exhibited reduced task performance relative to the control condition.

been drawn from these data, suggesting that chronic sleep restriction did not adversely affect cognitive functioning, although in reality it did.

It has not yet been established whether chronic sleep restriction merely affects performance output; and/or for cognitive tasks with a practice effect, whether chronic sleep loss interferes with the actual learning of the task. It could be argued that if the data in Fig. 4 simply reflected a reduction in performance output that masked the underlying practice effect (which by itself continued unaltered regardless of sleep loss), then at the end of the study, after recovery sleep, cognitive performance levels in the two sleep restriction conditions should have approached those in the control condition. No evidence of this is displayed in Fig. 4; the difference among the three conditions in SAST performance (expressed relative to each subject's baseline performance) was significant on the first recovery day ($F_{2,31}$ = 5.35, P = 0.010) and the second recovery day ($F_{2,31}$ = 3.70, P = 0.036). This suggests that chronic sleep loss may have interfered with the practice effect proper.

Such an adverse effect of sleep loss on the cognitive benefit of practice would be in line with recent discoveries that sleep deprivation may reduce the brain's ability to learn performance tasks [32]. Yet, some further evidence has indicated that even brief sleep periods could suffice for learning [33]. This matter may be dependent on the structure of sleep and on the nature of the performance task [34]. Psychomotor vigilance performance as measured with the PVT does not show any significant practice effect [13], and therefore task learning was not a notable factor for the psychomotor vigilance results shown in Figs. 1–3.

Individual differences in vulnerability to sleep loss

Humans have been found to differ substantially in the degree of cognitive performance impairment they suffer from sleep loss [35–37], whether under conditions of acute total sleep deprivation or chronic partial sleep deprivation [13]. This is illustrated in Fig. 5, which shows PVT lapse data from a study in which subjects repeatedly underwent 36 hours of continuous wakefulness, that is, on two separate occasions [37]. Let us consider the group-average performance profiles in this study first.

The two thick, solid curves in Fig. 5 represent the group-average changes in psychomotor vigilance lapses during the two exposures to sleep deprivation. As expected, the shape of these curves resembles the first part of the 88-hour sleep deprivation curve shown in Fig. 1A (up to approximately hour 70 on the abscissa). Nevertheless, the average number of lapses after any given duration of wakefulness was much greater in the repeated 36-hour sleep deprivation study (see Fig. 5) than in the 88-hour sleep deprivation study (see Fig. 1A), because of the difference in task duration between the studies (20 minutes versus 10 minutes, respectively). Lapses on the PVT increase progressively with time on task [15], so that the number of lapses that may occur in a 20-minute PVT bout is much greater than twice the number occurring in a 10-minute PVT

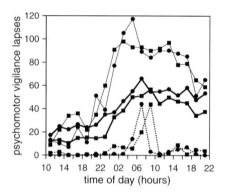

Fig. 5. Performance data from 19 healthy young adults (mean age ± SD: 29.4 ± 5.5 years; 8 females) who each participated in two identical sleep deprivation experiments in the controlled environment of a laboratory. Before each of the experiments, they extended their daily time in bed to 12 hours (22:00–10:00) for 7 days (the first 6 days they slept at home, and the seventh day they slept inside the laboratory). Subsequently, they were kept awake for 36 hours, from 10:00 until 22:00 the next day. They then spent 12 hours time in bed for recovery sleep, and went home. A period of 2 to 4 weeks passed between the two exposures to sleep deprivation. During the two sleep deprivations, subjects underwent cognitive testing every 2 hours. The figure shows lapses (reaction times ≥500 ms) on a 20-minute psychomotor vigilance task that was part of the cognitive test battery. The solid curves represent group-average performance during the first sleep deprivation (■) and the second sleep deprivation (●), plotted against clock time. The dotted curves show performance data for a single individual who was relatively resistant, and the thin curves show performance data for a single individual who was relatively vulnerable to performance impairment—during the first (■) and second (●) sleep deprivations. For each of these individuals, and for all others in the group, the temporal profile of performance changes was highly replicable from the first to the second exposure to sleep deprivation; but differences among individuals were considerable.

bout (under otherwise identical circumstances). Regardless of this difference in the absolute number of performance lapses, however, the normal interaction of the homeostatic process with the circadian process was observed in the profile of performance changes during the repeated 36-hour sleep deprivation study, and this profile was very similar between the two sleep deprivations (see Fig. 5, solid curves).

Fig. 5 also shows the profiles of performance changes in two individual subjects participating in the repeated sleep deprivation study. One subject, indicated with the dotted curves, was relatively resistant to the 36 hours of sleep deprivation, showing only a small dip in performance in the early morning hours (ie, when the circadian pressure for wakefulness should have been low). This same pattern was observed during both sleep deprivations, indicating that it was not a chance observation but a characteristic of the individual at hand. Another subject, indicated with the thin curves, was relatively vulnerable to the effects of sleep deprivation. This was seen at all times of wakefulness past the normal waking day, and for both exposures to sleep deprivation. This same phenomenon was observed across all subjects involved in the study; compared with each other, they varied substantially in the magnitude of performance impairment during sleep deprivation, but the performance profile was highly replicable within each individual. In fact, as much as 67.5% of the variance in the psychomotor vigilance data was explained by consistent individual differences [37].

Each 36-hour sleep deprivation session was preceded by seven consecutive days with time in bed extended to 12 hours per night. Thus, the differences among individuals observed during sleep deprivation could not have been caused by uncontrolled differences in prior amounts of sleep (or sleep insufficiency) [37]. The issue of prior sleep amounts (ie, "sleep history") was investigated further by having each of the subjects undergo a third 36-hour sleep deprivation, which was preceded by seven consecutive days with time in bed restricted to 6 hours per night. As implied by the data in Fig. 3 (days 4–10), this chronic sleep restriction would have been expected to induce marked susceptibility to performance impairment even before the 36-hour sleep deprivation began. It turned out, however, that the effect of the seven prior days of sleep restriction (at 6 hours time in bed per day) on psychomotor vigilance impairment during total sleep deprivation was small compared with the considerable individual differences consistently observed during the other two sleep deprivation sessions (and again noticed during the third). This finding indicates that individual differences in psychomotor vigilance impairment from sleep loss are a robust trait, which has been dubbed *differential vulnerability* [37].

The origin of the trait individual differences in performance impairment from sleep loss has remained unclear. The individual subjects' data in Fig. 5 would suggest that differences in psychomotor vigilance performance at baseline (ie, during the first 12 hours of continuous wakefulness) might predict the performance response to sleep deprivation (ie, during the last 24 hours of continuous wakefulness). However, less than 25% of the between-subjects variance in PVT performance during sleep deprivation was actually explained by individual differences at baseline; the correlation between baseline performance (the average over the first 12 hours of wakefulness) and the response to sleep deprivation (the average over the last 24 hours of wakefulness) for subjects' first exposure to sleep deprivation (preceded by 7 days of sleep extension to 12 hours time in bed) was $r = 0.486$ ($P = 0.025$). A search for better predictors of differential vulnerability to sleep loss is ongoing.

Individual differences in performance impairment during sleep deprivation were also noticed in other cognitive functions such as working memory, but when individuals were ranked by their degree of vulnerability, their rank order was found to be different for psychomotor vigilance performance than for other performance measures investigated thus far. It appears, therefore, that psychomotor vigilance is a distinct aspect of cognitive functioning, possibly subserved by specific neurocognitive pathways in the brain. These pathways appear to clearly reflect the interaction of sleep homeostatic and circadian neurobiology. As such, they are of relevance to more complex tasks [16], such as motor vehicle operation and athletic performance.

References

[1] Dinges DF, Kribbs NB. Performing while sleepy: effects of experimentally-induced sleepiness. In: Monk TH, editor. Sleep, sleepiness and performance. Chichester, England: John Wiley & Sons; 1991. p. 97–128.

[2] Durmer JS, Dinges DF. Neurocognitive consequences of sleep deprivation. Semin Neurol 2005;25(1):117–29.

[3] Saper CB, Chou TC, Scammell TE. The sleep switch: hypothalamic control of sleep and wakefulness. Trends Neurosci 2001;24(12):726–31.

[4] Borbély AA. A two process model of sleep regulation. Hum Neurobiol 1982;1(3):195–204.

[5] Edgar DM, Dement WC, Fuller CA. Effect of SCN lesions on sleep in squirrel monkeys: evidence for opponent processes in sleep-wake regulation. J Neurosci 1993;13(3):1065–79.

[6] Easton A, Meerlo P, Bergmann B, et al. The suprachiasmatic nucleus regulates sleep timing and amount in mice. Sleep 2004;27(7):1307–18.

[7] Dijk DJ, Czeisler CA. Paradoxical timing of the circadian rhythm of sleep propensity serves to consolidate sleep and wakefulness in humans. Neurosci Lett 1994;166:63–8.

[8] Dijk DJ, Lockley SW. Integration of human sleep-wake regulation and circadian rhythmicity. J Appl Physiol 2002;92:852–62.

[9] Borbély AA, Achermann P. Sleep homeostasis and models of sleep regulation. J Biol Rhythms 1999;14(6):557–68.

[10] Mallis MM, Mejdal S, Nguyen TT, et al. Summary of the key features of seven biomathematical models of human fatigue and performance. Aviat Space Environ Med 2004;75(3): A4–14.

[11] Van Dongen HPA, Kerkhof GA, Dinges DF. Human circadian rhythms. In: Sehgal A, editor. Molecular biology of circadian rhythms. Hoboken, NJ: John Wiley & Sons; 2004. p. 255–69.

[12] Dijk DJ, Duffy JF, Czeisler CA. Circadian and sleep/wake dependent aspects of subjective alertness and cognitive performance. J Sleep Res 1992;1(2):112–7.

[13] Van Dongen HPA, Maislin G, Mullington JM, et al. The cumulative cost of additional wakefulness: dose-response effects on neurobehavioral functions and sleep physiology from chronic sleep restriction and total sleep deprivation. Sleep 2003;26(2):117–28.

[14] Dinges DF, Powell JW. Microcomputer analyses of performance on a portable, simple visual RT task during sustained operations. Behav Res Meth Instr Comp 1985;17(6):652–5.

[15] Doran SM, Van Dongen HPA, Dinges DF. Sustained attention performance during sleep deprivation: Evidence of state instability. Arch Ital Biol 2001;139:253–67.

[16] Dorrian J, Rogers NL, Dinges DF. Psychomotor vigilance performance: a neurocognitive assay sensitive to sleep loss. In: Kushida C, editor. Sleep deprivation. New York: Marcel Dekker; in press.

[17] Achermann P, Borbély AA. Simulation of daytime vigilance by the additive interaction of a homeostatic and a circadian process. Biol Cybern 1994;71:115–21.

[18] Reilly T, Waterhouse J. Jet lag and air travel: implications for performance. Clin Sports Med 2005;24:367–80.

[19] Dinges DF, Whitehouse WG, Orne EC, Orne MT. The benefits of a nap during prolonged work and wakefulness. Work Stress 1988;2(2):139–53.

[20] Gillberg M, Kecklund G, Axelsson J, et al. The effects of a short daytime nap after restricted night sleep. Sleep 1996;19(7):570–5.

[21] Van Dongen HPA, Price NJ, Mullington JM, et al. Caffeine eliminates psychomotor vigilance deficits from sleep inertia. Sleep 2001;24(7):813–9.

[22] Dinges DF. Are you awake? Cognitive performance and reverie during the hypnopompic state. In: Bootzin RR, Kihlstrom JF, Schacter D, editors. Sleep and cognition. Washington, DC: American Psychological Association; 1990. p. 159–75.

[23] Naitoh P. Circadian cycles and restorative power of naps. In: Johnson LC, Tepas DI, Colquhoun WP, Colligan MJ, editors. Biological rhythms, sleep and shift work. New York: Spectrum; 1981. p. 553–80.

[24] Dinges DF, Orne MT, Orne EC. Assessing performance upon abrupt awakening from naps during quasi-continuous operations. Behav Res Meth Instr Comp 1985;17(1):37–45.

[25] Balkin TJ, Badia P. Relationship between sleep inertia and sleepiness: Cumulative effects of four nights of sleep disruption/restriction on performance following abrupt nocturnal awakenings. Biol Psychol 1988;27(3):245–58.

[26] Tietzel AJ, Lack LC. The short-term benefits of brief and long naps following nocturnal sleep restriction. Sleep 2001;24(3):293–300.

[27] Belenky G, Wesensten NJ, Thorne DR, et al. Patterns of performance degradation and restoration during sleep restriction and subsequent recovery: A sleep dose-response study. J Sleep Res 2003;12(1):1–12.

[28] Vgontzas AN, Zoumakis E, Bixler EO, et al. Adverse effects of modest sleep restriction on sleepiness, performance, and inflammatory cytokines. J Clin Endocrinol Metab 2004;89(5): 2119–26.

[29] Van Dongen HPA, Rogers NL, Dinges DF. Sleep debt: Theoretical and empirical issues. Sleep Biol Rhythms 2003;1(1):5–13.

[30] Johnson ML, Belenky G, Redmond DP, et al. Modulating the homeostatic process to predict performance during chronic sleep restriction. Aviat Space Environ Med 2004;75(3):A141–6.

[31] Thorne DR, Genser SG, Sing HC, et al. The Walter Reed performance assessment battery. Neurobehav Toxicol Teratol 1985;7(4):415–8.

[32] Walker P, Stickgold R. It's practice, with sleep, that makes perfect: implications of sleep-dependent learning and plasticity for skill performance. Clin Sports Med 2005;24:301–17.

[33] Mednick S, Nakayama K, Stickgold R. Sleep-dependent learning: a nap is as good as a night. Nat Neurosci 2003;6(7):697–8.

[34] Walker P, Stickgold R. Sleep-dependent learning and memory consolidation. Neuron 2004;44: 121–33.

[35] Morgan Jr BB, Winne PS, Dugan J. The range and consistency of individual differences in continuous work. Hum Factors 1980;22:331–40.

[36] Leproult R, Colecchia EF, Berardi AM, et al. Individual differences in subjective and objective alertness during sleep deprivation are stable and unrelated. Am J Physiol Regul Integr Comp Physiol 2003;284(2):R280–90.

[37] Van Dongen HPA, Baynard MD, Maislin G, et al. Systematic interindividual differences in neurobehavioral impairment from sleep loss: evidence of trait-like differential vulnerability. Sleep 2004;27(3):423–33.

ELSEVIER
SAUNDERS

CLINICS
IN SPORTS
MEDICINE

Clin Sports Med 24 (2005) 251–268

Sleep Extension: Getting as Much Extra Sleep as Possible

William C. Dement, MD, PhD

*The Stanford Sleep Disorders Clinic and Research Center, Stanford University, 701 Welch Road,
Suite 2226, Stanford, CA 94304, USA*

In the early days of sleep research, before the discovery of rapid eye movement (REM) sleep, studies of total sleep deprivation in humans and animals were directed mainly at discovering the fundamental purpose of sleep. These earlier studies did not use electroencephalogram (EEG) readings nor did researchers have the knowledge to understand that subjects were actually being simultaneously deprived of two entirely different kinds of sleep. In recent years, the most persistent and comprehensive attempts to discover the biological purposes of sleep were performed by Rechtschaffen and his group [1] at the University of Chicago. Although they formulated a number of hypotheses from their results, the one completely consistent finding was that total sleep prevention was eventually fatal for all experimental animals (rodents).

Countless observations of the effect of sleep loss in humans and animals have conclusively established that sleep is regulated homeostatically [2]. This simply means that when the daily amount of sleep is reduced, the tendency for sleep to occur in the waking organism is increased, and when it does occur, sleep tends to be deeper. Conversely, when the daily amount of sleep is increased, the tendency to fall asleep while awake is lessened and sleep itself is lighter. A strong sleep tendency interfering with waking performance is assumed to be the cause of most of the ill effects of sleep loss.

E-mail address: dement@stanford.edu

Quantifying sleep tendency

The development of methods to quantify sleep tendencies and infer subjective sleepiness levels from these tendencies was mainly in response to clinical needs; for example, if certain compounds were beneficial in reducing daytime sleepiness in patients who experienced narcolepsy. The first attempt to measure levels of sleepiness was the Stanford Sleepiness Scale. The scale had seven levels and was a plausible way to quantify sleepiness. However, this scale was often unreliable and in middle 1970s, Carskadon et al [3] developed and introduced the Multiple Sleep Latency Test (MSLT) as an objective measure of daytime sleepiness. This test has been of immense value in basic research and clinical practice.

The MSLT measures the speed of falling asleep in the daytime. As a desperately thirsty person will gulp down a glass of water in a few seconds, a person who is very sleep deprived will fall asleep very quickly, often in less than a minute. As it is possible to identify the moment of sleep onset with great precision using continuous brain-wave recordings, the strength of the physiologic tendency to fall asleep can be evaluated directly by measuring the length of time it takes a person to go from full wakefulness to the moment of sleep. This value is called the *sleep latency*. Sleep latency values are typically reported to the nearest half-minute. In many individuals, the onset of sleep can be pinpointed within a second or two. However, identifying the moment of sleep to the nearest half-minute is entirely adequate for the objective measurement of sleep tendency in almost every instance and for almost every purpose.

Clearly, the presence of noise and other disturbing factors will delay the onset of sleep. Therefore, a valid measurement of sleep latency can only be made in the absence of stimulation and activity. For all practical purposes, lying quietly on a comfortable bed in a sound-attenuated, darkened room with an empty bladder, wearing comfortable loose clothing, and being neither hungry nor thirsty will sufficiently remove disturbing stimuli. In these conditions, measuring the speed of falling asleep by means of brainwave patterns becomes a completely accurate and reproducible representation of the underlying physiologic sleep tendency at that particular moment.

Details of the Multiple Sleep Latency Test

Precision and reliability in characterizing daytime sleep tendency requires rigid adherence to a standardized protocol. In the standard version of the MSLT, the speed of falling asleep is measured every 2 hours. The first measurement is usually taken at 10 AM, with sleep latency measurements then taken precisely at noon, 2 PM, 4 PM, and 6 PM. The sleep latency measurements are typically performed in a sleep laboratory bedroom.

Brainwave patterns are scored in 30-second epochs, and the sleep latency is defined as the duration of the interval from the beginning of the test to the first 30-second epoch scored as sleep. Almost without exception, the first epoch is NREM stage 1. When awake with eyes closed, most individuals' brainwave

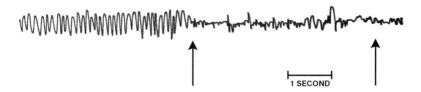

Fig. 1. The transition from wakefulness to stage 1 sleep. The obvious signal of the nearly instantaneous transition is the abrupt cessation of rhythmic alpha activity (8–12 cps) followed by a low-amplitude, mixed-frequency pattern. The change in EEG patterns to stage 1 as illustrated here is designated the onset of sleep. Therefore, the moment of sleep occurs at the arrow. The second arrow represents the moment the test should be terminated.

patterns show unambiguous occipital alpha rhythm. The moment of sleep onset is associated with the abrupt disappearance of this alpha rhythm. Fig. 1 shows the brainwave changes that characterize the moment of sleep onset.

When the MSLT is used in scientific studies that seek to understand the effect of sleep reduction on daytime sleep tendency and to illuminate the formal properties of sleep homeostasis, the ongoing test is terminated as soon as the brainwave changes that indicate the occurrence of sleep onset are recognized (see Fig. 1, *second arrow*). The intent is to prevent sleep from occurring. The subject is aroused and required to get out of bed and remain awake by reading, watching television, or engaging in other relatively quiet activities until the next test.

It is important to understand the purpose of this methodology. If much more than a few seconds of sleep were allowed, the accumulation of extra sleep over the course of the five individual tests could independently change the test results as the day progressed and invalidate the measurement. Using the MSLT protocol, the total duration of each individual test should only be a few seconds more than each individual sleep latency. In addition, if sleep onset does not occur within 20 minutes, the individual test should be terminated. This duration allows for a sufficiently wide range of sleep latency values and avoids the extreme boredom and restlessness that may occur if an individual is required to lie awake in the dark for much longer periods of time.

Sleep disorders clinics use a modified MSLT protocol for diagnostic purposes, performed according to the same 2-hour schedule. However, the individual tests are not terminated at sleep onset. Rather, the patient is allowed to remain asleep for 10 to 15 minutes to demonstrate the presence or absence of a pathologic sleep sequence in which the transition is from wakefulness immediately into REM sleep (ie, sleep-onset REM periods). The sleep disorder called narcolepsy is diagnosed if such sleep-onset REM periods are seen in two or more of the five individual tests.

Reporting multiple sleep latency test results

The conventional method of displaying results from an MSLT is shown in Fig. 2. Longer sleep latency values are plotted in the upward direction.

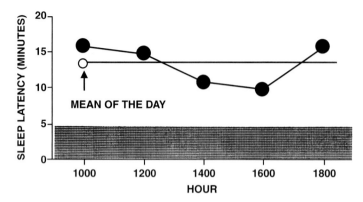

Fig. 2. The results of an idealized MSLT. The speed of falling asleep is related to the amount of sleep on prior nights. A standard series of calibrations are performed while the subject is awake that require about a minute. Then the subject is given the instruction, "close your eyes and try to go to sleep." The precise second the lights are out, the sleep latency measure begins. The five individual test results connected by a line comprise a "sleep latency profile." Examining the profile can give an overall sense of daytime sleep tendency. Alternatively, the mean of the five individual tests can also be used as a descriptor of the overall strength of the daytime sleep tendency on this particular day. It must always be kept in mind that the individual test is terminated within seconds after the onset of sleep. It is extremely rare that it takes more than 30 seconds for an observer to make this decision. Each test is always terminated if the subject does not fall asleep in 20 minutes.

Thus, decreased sleep latencies indicate an increased physiologic daytime sleep tendency, and increased sleep latencies represent a decreased physiologic sleep tendency.

When physiologic alertness/sleepiness needs to be described over several days, the five values of individual tests are typically collapsed into the mean for the day and the daily means are plotted. Otherwise, plotting the individual results of the five sleep latency measures displays the MSLT profile and the overall sleep tendency for that particular day in that particular person. The MSLT profile is widely regarded as the gold standard indicator of the ongoing sleep tendency throughout the day.

Relating multiple sleep latency test scores to real life

The levels of the sleep latency profiles are given interpretive labels in Fig. 3. The "twilight zone" designates the range of very short sleep latencies and indicates a very strong sleep tendency that is associated with impaired mental function and inability to maintain attentiveness. When patients with sleep apnea and narcolepsy (ie, sleep disorders characterized by persistent excessive daytime sleepiness) are tested, the MSLT scores are almost always within this twilight zone range. Persons whose MSLT profiles are in the top range of the graph have extremely good alertness. They will never fall asleep inappropriately while working, studying, driving long distances, watching television, in a class or conference, or in any other circumstance.

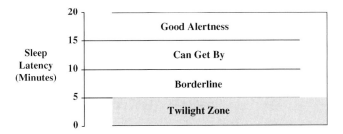

Fig. 3. There is a general correspondence between the MSLT mean score and the overall level or degree of daytime alertness. If an individual falls asleep in less than 5 minutes on every test (sometimes less than a minute), this indicates a very strong sleep tendency and a very strong sleep drive. The label "twilight zone" is meaningful in this respect because memory and clarity of thinking is usually substantially impaired in individuals whose MSLT score is less than 5.

In summary, under standard conditions when the presence of any contaminating stimulation are reduced to an absolute minimum, the sleep latency (ie, the speed of falling asleep) is an objective measure of the internal strength of the physiologic tendency to fall asleep at that particular moment of the day or night.

Relation of daytime physiologic sleep tendency to different amounts of sleep at night

The relationship of sleep tendency during the day to the amount of sleep at night has been thoroughly studied. The relationship for young adults is illustrated in Fig. 4, which shows the daytime sleep latency profiles that follow

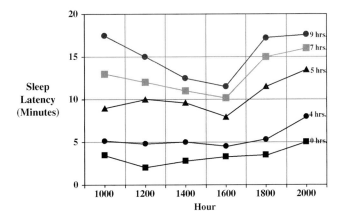

Fig. 4. MSLT profiles after varying amounts of nocturnal sleep. This figure is based on a very large amount of data. The MSLT profiles and mean scores are directly related to the amount of sleep at night. In these tests, the scheduled time in bed varied from 10 hours to zero. Generally, with 10 hours in bed, total sleep time was 9 hours or more. With the lower values, total sleep time closely approached total time in bed.

various amounts of sleep the night before. As the amount of sleep at night decreases, the strength of sleep tendency in the daytime increases. The relationship, however, is not linear. The effect is somewhat greater at less than 5 hours of sleep. The profiles in Fig. 4 demonstrate another important phenomenon. Sleep tendency increases in the middle of the day and decreases toward the end of the day in the absence of daytime sleep or napping.

The studies that generated these results were all performed by measuring physiologic sleep tendency through the day following a nocturnal sleep period of varying amounts ranging from over 9 hours to zero. The nocturnal sleep period was reduced by delaying the bedtime or getting up early or a combination of both. The sleep latency profiles following different amounts of sleep at night illustrated in Fig. 4 are the average results for groups of young adult subjects.

Chronic partial sleep loss: the most important cause of increased daytime sleep tendency

The most important aspect of the homeostatic regulation of sleep is that sleep loss is cumulative. When total nightly sleep is reduced by exactly the same amount each night for several consecutive nights, the tendency to fall asleep in

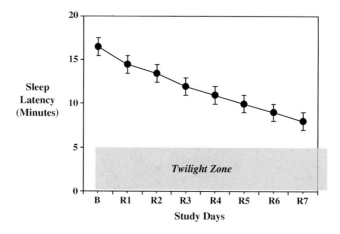

Fig. 5. Cumulative effects of sleep deprivation. This figure summarizes the first experiment demonstrating that sleep loss accumulates. Ten young adults participated. After three baseline measurements with 9 hours in bed for three consecutive nights, the MSLT was performed on each successive day. Because time out of bed increased each day by 4 hours, an additional sleep latency test (total 6) was added. Each point in the graph is the grand mean of ten daily mean MSLT scores, or a grand total of 50 measurements each day during baseline, and 60 measurements each day during restriction. As can be clearly seen there is a progressive decrease in the overall sleep latency, indicating a progressive increase in daytime sleep tendency. The vertical bars indicate the standard deviation. These results led directly to the very important concept of sleep debt. Other researchers have since replicated and confirmed the findings. Although there is often considerable individual variation, no one has reported a single instance of the failure of sleep tendency to increase with accumulating sleep debt.

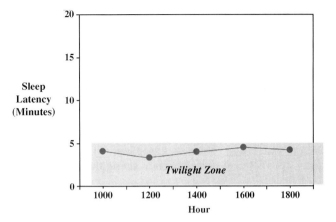

Fig. 6. This graph illustrates the results in a single individual during the baseline MSLT. The sleep latency values are in the area of good alertness.

the daytime becomes progressively stronger each day. Carskadon and Dement [4] first demonstrated this effect in 1977, in their study of a sample of ten young adults over ten consecutive days. The subjects slept in laboratory bedrooms where all-night sleep recordings were performed every night. Subjects were in bed from 10 PM to 8 AM on three baseline nights, sleeping about 9 hours on the average. After baseline measurements, sleep in the laboratory was restricted to 5 hours a night for seven consecutive nights. Throughout each day, the standard MSLT was administered to each subject and no napping was allowed at any time.

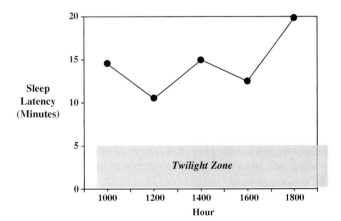

Fig. 7. This graph illustrates the results in a single individual on Friday after only five nights of sleep restriction. The MSLT profile on Friday is well within the twilight zone even though the baseline score is at the level of good alertness. Most of the subjects did not show a rapid decrease in sleep latency scores but all showed a significant decrease.

With an identical 5 hours of sleep each night, the mean MSLT scores of the subjects progressively decreased on each successive day. The pooled results for the entire group are displayed in Fig. 5. Fig. 6 shows the MSLT profile from the baseline period. Fig. 7 is the MSLT profile from the day after the fifth night of moderately restricted sleep. Fig. 6, which is the MSLT profile from the day after the fifth night of moderately restricted sleep, shows a sleep latency profile from the baseline period. Comparing the profile in Fig. 6 to the profile in Fig. 7 demonstrates an ambiguous buildup of physiologic sleep in the subject after only 5 nights of restricted sleep. Without exception, all subjects showed a progressively increasing daytime sleep tendency during the 7 days of reduced sleep.

The maintenance of wakefulness test

Examining Figs. 4 and 5, it is clear that the MSLT has a limitation. Once an individual begins falling asleep in less than a minute on every test, there can be little additional change, although the underlying sleep drive and sleep tendency can continue to increase. One way to solve this problem is to make the MSLT situation less soporific, perhaps by having it performed while the subjects are sitting in a chair rather than lying on a bed; or by instructing subjects to stay awake rather than go to sleep. This type of maneuver has been standardized as the Maintenance of Wakefulness Test (MWT), about which Doghramji et al [5] have published informative data.

Recently, partial sleep loss has been studied for longer durations by Dinges et al [6] and Van Dongen et al [7] at the University of Pennsylvania, where subjects were restricted to 4 hours of sleep each night for 2 weeks. As in the Carskadon and Dement study, the subjects' tendency to fall asleep became progressively stronger. On the fourteenth day after the last night of restricted sleep, the impairment of the subjects had not leveled off. The effect of nightly sleep loss was presumably continuing to accumulate. The subjects were at their worst level of psychomotor impairment.

Although laboratory studies of large numbers of consecutive nights of sleep restriction (eg, 30 or more) have not been conducted, it is likely that the sleep tendency builds up to great strength as the amount of accumulated sleep loss gets larger and larger. In the real world, many people (eg, hospital interns and residents) may exhibit severe impairment and make grotesque errors after prolonged partial sleep deprivation resulting from excessive work hours. Because individuals sometimes do not feel sleepy even when they have accumulated a very large sleep debt, they have a very high risk of making a sleep-related error or having an accident.

Sleep debt

The concept of sleep debt is recent and refers to an individual's total amount of lost sleep. Every hour of sleep that is less than an individual's nightly requirement appears to be carefully registered by the brain as a debt, and this debt appears to precisely add up over time. It is possible that the debt includes an hour of sleep that was lost a month or a week ago, in addition to an hour that was lost the previous night.

The concept of sleep debt presumes that for each individual there is a specific amount of sleep that, if obtained on a nightly basis, will maintain the same level of daytime physiologic alertness over successive days. It also presumes that the daily sleep need may vary somewhat from individual to individual.

A large sleep debt does not go away spontaneously. It does not diffuse out of the nervous system; it can only be reduced by extra sleep. Sleep loss of only an hour or two over a number of nights can eventually lead to serious physiologic sleepiness that manifests as a very strong tendency to fall asleep in lectures, on automobile trips, and other soporific activities.

A breakthrough experiment

A study by Barbato et al [8] at the National Institutes of Health examined the effect of different photoperiods (duration of time spent in the light each 24-hour day) on human mood and emotion. The nocturnal portion of the experiment was performed in a laboratory setting. Sleep parameters were recorded while subjects remained continuously in bed in the dark. When they were out of bed in the light, they were allowed to go about their daily routines. The sleep of each subject was monitored 7 nights a week for 35 consecutive nights.

During the first seven baseline days, the daily photoperiod during which subjects were out of bed in the light was the conventional 16 hours, and each night they were in bed in the dark from 11 PM to 7 AM (a total of 8 hours). After the baseline week, the photoperiod during which the subjects were out of bed in the light was decreased to 10 hours. They were consequently in bed in the dark for 14 hours every night (9 PM to 11 AM) for 28 consecutive nights. During the 5-week period, daily mood scales and a variety of other tests were administered to the subjects.

The subjects' average nightly baseline sleep time was 7 hours and 36 minutes. When the subjects were switched to the 10-hour photoperiod followed by 14 hours in bed in the dark, their total daily sleep times jumped to amounts above 12 hours on the first night and then gradually declined. During the fourth week of the 10-hour photoperiod schedule, total sleep time for the group was level at a nightly average of 8 hours and 15 minutes even though they continued to be in bed in the dark for 14 hours every night. Their mean time lying awake in the dark doing nothing was 5 hours and 45 minutes.

The interpretation of these results is that the subjects entered the protocol carrying sizeable individual sleep debts. Of course, neither the subjects nor the researchers were aware of such a possibility. The baseline period of 8 hours in bed certainly did little to reduce the subjects' sleep debts, and may even have resulted in a small increase. When the opportunity to sleep was greatly increased, their large sleep debts caused a very large increase in total daily sleep time. As the subjects' sleep debts decreased, total sleep time per day declined proportionally.

If the 8 hour 15 minute "steady state" value in the last week of the 10-hour photoperiod schedule (14 hours in bed in the dark) represents the real daily sleep need for this group of subjects, it may be concluded that all amounts of sleep above these values represented extra or make-up sleep. Accordingly, the mean payback of sleep debt for this group of volunteers averaged about 30 hours.

Another very important result of this experiment was a dramatic improvement in the subjects' mood, energy level, and sense of well being as indicated by daily check lists and questionnaires. Fig. 8 shows the nightly amounts of sleep for one typical subject during the 14-hour in-bed schedule.

Individual homeostatic sleep requirement

The homeostatic formulation stated at the beginning of this article should include a clearer and more precise description of what is meant by reducing sleep or obtaining extra sleep. The basic assumption is that every individual requires a specific and characteristic amount of sleep that, if obtained each night on the

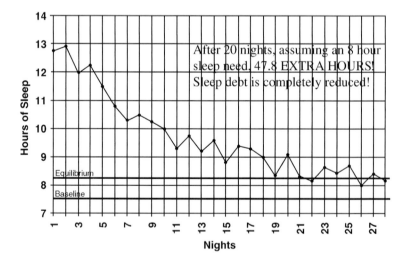

Fig. 8. Typical subject in the 14 hours in bed study. The last 7 nights of the experimental period are not shown because there was no further change in total sleep time. Total sleep time on the first 4 nights of the 14-hour schedule is 12 hours or more. There is an asymptotic decline in total sleep time which levels off at about night 21. For the next 2 weeks the nightly total sleep time hovered around the mean for the group (8 hours 15 minutes). The sleep debt figure is on the low side because the 8 hour and 15 minute amount is obtained in a very inefficient manner and is probably fragmented and light as a result of the 14 hours in bed. The major point is that when the sleep debt is completely repaid no extra sleep can be obtained, and even having to lie in the dark awake for 5 hours and 45 minutes does not enable extra sleep to occur. The 8 hours and 15 minutes could be considered this individual's daily sleep requirement, although it should be set somewhat lower in a real world situation.

average, will be associated with an identical or near-identical sleep propensity during each successive day. This is best illustrated by MSLT studies performed by Carskadon over two decades ago in the Stanford University Summer Sleep Camp.

In this particular set of observations, subjects had a standard nocturnal time in bed (8 to 9 hours) for seven consecutive nights. After each of the 7 nights, subjects had six daytime sleep latency measures at 2-hour intervals (first test at 9:30 AM), using the standard approach of terminating the test as soon as sleep onset occurred or terminating after 20 minutes if sleep onset did not occur. With the same amount of sleep each night (±10–15 minutes), some subjects had essentially the same MSLT score during each of the 7 days. For other subjects, the same amount of sleep each night was associated with a gradual shortening of daily mean sleep latency or a gradual lengthening of the mean sleep latency. These results indicate that subjects in the first group are exactly fulfilling their daily needs, whereas the other two groups are either getting a little less or a little more sleep than their daily requirement. Thus, it is clear that there is an amount of sleep below which daytime sleep tendency will increase and above which daytime sleep tendency will decrease. This amount represents the individual's specific and characteristic sleep requirement. The rate of decreasing or increasing daytime sleep tendency would be determined by whether the amount of lost or extra nightly sleep was large or small.

Sleep/wake homeostasis may be regarded as a very finely tuned mechanism that operates over time. The high level of tracking precision is illustrated by the study of Wright et al [9]. These investigators required young adults to spend exactly 8 hours in bed for 25 consecutive nights, sleeping as much as possible. Each day their reaction times were measured by means of the widely used standardized Psychomotor Vigilance Task (PVT). The results showed a very small increase in reaction time on each successive day, but were nonetheless sufficient. The results on the day after the 25th night were significantly worse compared with the day after the first night. It appeared that 8 hours in bed every night did not allow enough sleep for the subjects to avoid the slow development of impairment. However, the nightly sleep loss may have been as little as 15 to 30 minutes.

Sleep debt or excess wakefulness

In their landmark studies mentioned earlier, Dinges et al [6] and Van Dongen et al [7] showed a near-linear increase of neurocognitive impairment during 14 consecutive days of sleep restricted to 4 hours per day. They also demonstrated that the best way to interpret their results is by totaling the extra time awake. This makes the rapidly developing neurocognitive impairment associated with total sleep deprivation comparable to the slower developing neurocognitive impairment associated with partial sleep loss.

Another approach to understanding the impairment of sleep loss is the 28-hour forced desynchronization studies of Dijk and colleagues [10]. In this protocol, the period length of the sleep–wake cycle (28 hours) and the period length of the circadian temperature cycle (slightly more than 24 hours) are very different, in that the two cycles go in and out of alignment during the course of many days in the laboratory. This allows the neurocognitive impact of the circadian fluctuation and the neurocognitive impact of continuing wakefulness to be evaluated independently. The results show that fatigue and neurocognitive impairment increase progressively as a direct function of time awake. This is tantamount to saying that all wakefulness is sleep deprivation. Another way of defining sleep debt is the amount of sleep that will be required to reverse the effect of extra wakefulness.

Recovery

Although there are numerous studies of total and partial sleep deprivation, careful evaluations of the recovery process are rare. This shortage is mainly because the primary focus of interest is almost always on the effect of losing sleep. For example, in 1964, high school senior Randy Gardner stayed awake for 11 days. This episode still holds the record for professionally monitored sleep deprivation [11]. However, only the first period of recovery sleep was recorded in the sleep laboratory. A second sleep recording was performed a week later. Although it would have been of great interest in light of today's knowledge to determine the amount extra of sleep required for Randy Gardner to recover completely after his heroic wakefulness marathon, this was not done.

Sleep extension

Carskadon and Dement [12] reported the first sleep extension study using the MSLT in 1979 and showed a highly significant improvement in alertness after subjects spent 10 hours in bed during four consecutive nights. Other studies of sleep extension have yielded less conclusive results. For example, Taub et al [13] showed decrements in performance on a pinball task following extended sleep. Harrison and Horne [14] reported little change in auditory vigilance and in MSLT scores during 2 weeks of moderately extended sleep. Finally, the large-scale dose-response study of sleep loss recently reported by Belenky et al [15] included a subgroup that spent 9 hours in bed for 7 nights. This subgroup showed no improvement in performance, although they may not have been achieving substantial extra sleep.

Conversely, there are studies showing that sleep extension has beneficial effects. Although originally intended as a sleep extension study, Barbato and colleagues [8] reported large improvements in energy and mood in subjects spending 14 hours in bed for 4 weeks. In their study of sleep extension mentioned earlier, Carskadon and Dement [12] found significant improvements in MSLT scores and nonsignificant improvements in performance with 4 nights of extended sleep. They attributed the improvement to the reversal of the sleep debt caused by prior partial sleep loss. Roehrs et al [16] found that extending time in bed to 10 hours a night for 6 days led to increased MSLT scores and improved reaction times, especially for sleepy (baseline MSLT score ≤ 6 minutes) subjects. A subsequent study by the same investigators [17] found increases in MSLT scores of up to 6 minutes in sleepy (MSLT score ≤ 6 minutes) subjects who maintained a 10-hour time in bed schedule for 2 weeks. These researchers concluded that the short sleep latencies found at baseline were related to chronic undersleeping. Howard et al [18] showed that anesthesia residents who extended their nightly sleep were less likely to fall asleep on the job. One night of extended sleep has been shown to significantly improve MSLT scores [19] and even small increases in total sleep can improve mood and vigilance levels [20,21].

Obtaining as much extra sleep as possible

For a number of years at Stanford University, the author has required students in his large undergraduate class, "Sleep and Dreams," to keep sleep logs and obtain as much extra sleep as possible. Extra sleep was not an absolute requirement, and the success of obtaining large amounts of extra sleep was largely related to the class load the students were carrying and number of extracurricular commitments that competed for their time. Nonetheless, some students, assuming a baseline sleep requirement of 8 to 9 hours, obtained up to 50 hours of extra sleep over the course of the 10-week quarter, according to their sleep logs. The large amounts of extra sleep were typically associated with reports of feeling less tired, more energetic, disappearance of drowsiness in afternoon classes, and so forth.

The landmark 14 hours in the study of Barbato et al [8] strongly supports the principles and conclusions of Carskadon and Dement [12]. During the final nights of the study the subjects could not obtain extra sleep even though they had to lie awake in bed in the dark for an average of 5 hours and 45 minutes per night. The interpretation is that they had obtained sufficient extra sleep (depending on how the baseline was calculated) to reduce their carryover sleep debt to zero or very close to zero. In other words, getting up and spending 10 hours out of bed (ie, 10 hours of wakefulness) did not provide enough waking sleep deprivation to foster a continuous occurrence of their constitutional nightly requirement during the 14 hours in bed. This supports the principle that all wakefulness is sleep deprivation and that without sleep debt, it is not possible to sleep continuously through the night. This principle is further supported by animal studies in which high doses of sedatives could not induce sleep in sleep-satiated rats [22], but were able to induce sleep after periods of sleep deprivation [23].

Although measures of performance and cognitive functions were not part of Wehr's 14-hour in-bed study, the investigators did carry out surveys of fatigue, energy levels, well being, alertness, and so forth. All of the subjects in the study were substantially less fatigued and more energetic and had a marked improvement in mood. The substantial reduction in light exposure (10-hour photoperiod) was not at all depressing, contrary to what some might have hypothesized. The positive increase in mood in the Wehr study was almost certainly related to sleep-debt reduction.

Zero sleep debt study

Over the years, the author has observed that students who obtained substantial amounts of extra sleep usually reached a point where extra sleep was no longer possible and in some cases, students actually reported insomnia (ie, being unable to fall asleep at their usual bed time). At this point, it is necessary to differentiate two categories of sleep debt: the carryover sleep debt that would be present in the morning immediately after a night of sleep, and the normal sleep debt accumulated during the usual daily hours of wakefulness that is presumably adequate to foster sleeping through the night.

In the summer of 2002, a scientific study was initiated in which the goal would be to get as close to zero carryover sleep dept as possible by requiring subjects to obtain as much extra sleep as possible [24]. This "zero sleep debt" project studied 15 healthy college students who reported minimal or no experience of daytime sleepiness and had no symptoms suggesting a sleep disorder. The mean age was 20 years (range of 18 to 23 years) and the group included four women. The study was organized into three phases: a baseline phase (7 days total), early sleep-extension phase (days one through seven), and late-sleep extension phase (days eight to the last day, whatever it was) with day one marking the first day of the extension period. To minimize the cost of polysomnographic recordings, sleep was monitored by means of daily sleep logs and wrist actigraphy. During the baseline phase, subjects were encouraged to maintain their habitual sleep schedule, but within the limits of no less than 6 hours and no more than 9.

Each subject had three complete MSLTs: the first on the day after the end of the baseline phase, the second on the day after the last night of extension phase one, and the third on the day after the final night of the study. Performance testing used the PVT, which was administered every day at the same time and 10 minutes after each sleep latency test on the three MSLT testing days. The Profile of Moods States (POMS) questionnaire was administered at three separate times on MSLT days. The endpoint of the study was when subjects completed the 7 days of phase two, or when it was clear that a subject was still able to obtain extra sleep and stay in the study longer. For these individuals, the study endpoint was when they were unable to exceed their baseline amount of sleep.

All of the subjects obtained substantial extra sleep compared with a presumed daily requirement of 8.5 hours. The mean of the subject's baseline MSLT scores was 7.4. By the end of the sleep extension, seven of the subjects achieved a fully alert score on the MSLT (mean 20 minutes) and were classified "sleep satiated." The end extension MSLT score for the eight subjects who did not reach 20 ranged from 10.3 to 17.6. The MSLT improved during sleep extension in 14 subjects. The baseline MSLT score was 10.3 for the single subject who did not improve and his end extension was also 10.3.

There was a statistically significant improvement in mean reaction time on PVT testing and significant improvement in the fastest 10%. For the seven satiated subjects, there was a dramatic difference in baseline and end extension reaction time (271 ms versus 204 ms). For the unsatiated subjects, there was a trend toward faster reaction times, but the difference between baseline and end extension was not statistically significant. For all subjects, the fatigue scales on the POMS was reduced to nearly zero, a highly significant result. Vigor was statistically significantly increased in the satiated group and showed a non-significant trend in the unsatiated group.

A number of paper and pencil tests were performed whose results have not yet been scored and tabulated. Spot checking on such things as the Bushke Selective Reminding test has suggested improvement of cognitive performance. Finally, there is no question that the subjects felt much better and reported feeling much more energetic on their daily sleepiness and fatigue ratings; feelings of tiredness almost entirely disappeared. It has been postulated that tiredness alone may indicate a large sleep debt [25,26].

Overall, it is clear that nearly all people, whether they consider themselves sleep deprived or not, can initially obtain extra sleep. However, as accumulating extra sleep reduces carryover sleep debt, a point is reached where it is no longer possible to obtain extra sleep. If there were a practical method to make a precise measurement of a person's daily sleep requirement, it may be possible to show that most individuals are carrying a very large sleep debt. All subjects in the sleep extension study felt they were not sleep deprived, and they denied any problems with daytime sleepiness.

Sleep extension and its potential for enhanced athletic performance

There is no question that laboratory performance is impaired by sleep deprivation, and therefore it can be assumed that athletic performance is also impaired. However, there is very little scientific evidence that either sleep deprivation or sleep extension in ordinary individuals affects athletic performance. There is probably a general feeling throughout the athletic community that getting enough sleep is important. However, a precise definition of *enough* does not exist in this community. Therefore, the big question is whether the best performance of any athlete can be improved by sleep extension. Some types of athletic performance involve a single best time or highest jump, whereas other measures of athletic performance would sum over time (ie, a season's batting average).

All that can be offered at this time regarding sleep extension and athletic performance are anecdotes. For example, several members of the Stanford University varsity swimming team took part in a sleep extension study and claimed that their best performance in sprints was improved during the period of sleep extension. One swimmer claimed a 6 second improvement in his 100m freestyle time. Two high jumpers claimed that they were able to jump an inch or two higher. Several subjects claimed to be more accurate in shooting baskets in casual pick-up basketball games. However, it will be necessary to develop acceptable scientific methods for evaluating improvements in athletic performance. For example, batting machines and baseline testing may be used at the same time each day for a period of days and then similar testing carried out after substantial sleep extension. The stakes are too high in most intercollegiate competitions to see what happens if, for example, a football team stays up all night (ie, gets no sleep) before a big game. Even though it might be dramatic, such a result would not really be conclusive. Although it is believed that the stimulation and excitement of a hotly contested sports event will easily overwhelm any sleep-related fatigue that might be present, there is also no evidence that this is a completely valid assumption.

Too much sleep

Finally, there it is believed by many, including coaches, that an individual can obtain too much sleep. That is, if someone were to sleep 10 to 12 hours a night before a game, his or her performance would be sluggish. This issue was rigorously studied by Carskadon et al [19]. After 1 night of extra sleep, they found that MSLT scores and performance were significantly improved. Only the way subjects felt did not improve, and there are good explanations for this that are not related to obtaining extra sleep.

Summary

Several observations and studies demonstrate that almost everyone is sleep deprived and carries some amount of sleep debt. How long such an indebtedness will persist without change if no extra sleep is obtained is not known. However, the 14-hours in-bed, multi-week study shows that the ability to sleep 30 extra hours and the accumulation of such a debt in small increments means that sleep indebtedness must persist for substantial amounts of time—weeks or months at the very least.

Furthermore, getting extra sleep until it is no longer possible to obtain extra sleep improves neurocognitive performance and eliminates feelings of fatigue during the day. Eliminating sleep debt is an important issue and should receive much more scientific attention. It cannot be concluded that sleep extension will improve athletic performance, but it is an exciting possibility. A final thought is that, in the same way the clandestine use of drugs by athletes is taboo, if only one side in a contest obtained extra sleep, could this secret advantage be deemed unfair?

References

[1] Rechtschaffen A. Current perspectives on the function of sleep. Perspect Biol Med 1998; 41:359–90.

[2] Dement W, Vaughn C. The Promise of Sleep. New York: Delacorte Press; 1999.

[3] Carskadon MA, Dement WC. Daytime sleepiness: quantification of a behavioral state. Neurosci Biobehav Rev 1987;11:307–17.

[4] Carskadon M, Dement W. Cumulative effects of sleep restriction on daytime sleepiness. Psychophysiology 1981;18(2):107–13.

[5] Doghramji K, Mitler M, Sangal R, et al. A normative study of the maintenance of wakefulness test (MWT). Electroencephalogr Clin Neurophysiol 1997;103:554–62.

[6] Dinges D, Pack A, Williams K, et al. Cumulative sleepiness, mood disturbance, and psychomotor vigilance performance decrements during a week of sleep restricted to 4–5 hours per night. Sleep 1997;20(4):267–77.

[7] Van Dongen HP, Maislin G, Mullington JM, et al. The cumulative cost of additional wakefulness: dose-response effects on neurobehavioral functions and sleep physiology from chronic sleep restriction and total sleep deprivation. Sleep 2003;26(2):117–26.

[8] Barbato G, Barker C, Bender C, et al. Extended sleep in humans in 14 hour nights (LD 10:14): relationship between REM density and spontaneous awakening. Electroencephalogr Clin Neurophysiol 1994;90:291–7.

[9] Wright Jr K, Hughes R, Hull J, et al. Cumulative neurobehavioral performance deficits on a 24-hr day with 8-hr of scheduled sleep. Sleep 2000;23(Suppl):A21.

[10] Dijk D, Duffy J, Riel E, et al. Ageing and the circadian and homeostatic regulation of human sleep during scheduled desynchrony of rest, melatonin and temperature rhythms. J Phys 1999;516:611–27.

[11] Johnson L, Slye E, Dement W. Electroencephalographic and autonomic activity during and after prolonged sleep deprivation. Psychosom Med 1965;27:415–23.

[12] Carskadon M, Dement W. Sleep tendency during extension of nocturnal sleep. Sleep Res 1979; 8:147.

[13] Taub J, Globus G, Phoebus E, et al. Extended sleep and performance. Nature 1971;233: 142–3.

[14] Harrison Y, Horne J. Long term extension to sleep—are we really chronically sleep deprived? Psychophysiology 1996;33:22–30.

[15] Belenky G, Wesensten NJ, Thorne DR, et al. Patterns of performance degradation and restoration during sleep restriction and subsequent recovery: a sleep dose-response study. J Sleep Res 2003;12:1–12.

[16] Roehrs T, Timms V, Zwyghuizen-Doorenbos A, Roth T. Sleep extension in sleepy and alert normals. Sleep 1989;12(5):449–57.

[17] Roehrs T, Shore E, Papineau K, et al. A two-week sleep extension in sleepy normals. Sleep 1996;19(7):576–82.

[18] Howard S, Gaba D, Smith B, et al. Simulation study of rested versus sleep-deprived anesthesiologists. Anesthesiology 2003;98(6):1345–55.

[19] Carskadon M, Mancuso J, Keenan S, et al. Sleepiness following oversleeping. J Sleep Res 1986; 15:70.

[20] Hayashi M, Watanabe M, Hori T. The effects of a 20 min nap in the mid-afternoon on mood, performance and EEG activity. Clin Neurophysiol 1999;110:272–9.

[21] Dinges D, Orne M, Whitehouse W, et al. Temporal placement of a nap for alertness: contributions of circadian phase and prior wakefulness. Sleep 1987;10(4):313–29.

[22] Edgar D, Seidel W, Martin C, et al. Triazolam fails to induce sleep in suprachiasmatic nucleus-lesioned rats. Neurosci Lett 1991;125:125–8.

[23] Trachsel L, Edgar D, Seidel W, et al. Sleep homeostasis in suprachiasmatic nuclei-lesioned rats: effects of sleep deprivation and triazolam administration. Brain Res 1992;589:253–61.

[24] Kamdar B, Kaplan K, Kezirian E, et al. The impact of extended sleep on daytime alertness, vigilance, and mood. Sleep Med 2004;5:441–8.

[25] Dement W, Hall J, Walsh J. Tiredness versus sleepiness: semantics or a target for public education? Sleep 2003;26(4):485–6.

[26] Dement W. More on feeling tired. Sleep 2003;26:764.

CLINICS IN SPORTS MEDICINE

Clin Sports Med 24 (2005) 269–285

Insomnia and Sleep Disruption: Relevance for Athletic Performance

Damien Leger, MD, Biol D[a,b],*, Arnaud Metlaine, MD[a], Dominique Choudat, MD[b]

[a]*Centre du Sommeil, Hotel Dieu de Paris, 1, Place du Parvis Notre Dame, 75181 Paris Cedex 04, France*
[b]*Department of Occupational Medicine, Hopital Cochin, University of Paris V, School of Medicine, 27 Rue du faubourg Saint Jacques, 75679 Paris Cedex 14, France*

Insomnia is a very common complaint among adults around the world [1,2]. Despite its high occurrence, insomnia may be unrecognized as a serious problem by health professionals. One reason is that insomnia is frequently considered a symptom rather than a true disease; practitioners are not clear if it should be considered a symptom and a disease. Another challenge is that it is often difficult for patients and health professionals to understand when insomnia is severe enough to require treatment. Furthermore, there is still insufficient knowledge about the management of insomnia. Several consensus meetings have convened in the last decade to address the recognition, diagnosis, and treatment of insomnia [3–7]. This paper's aim is to resume the major aspects of these discussions to help sports doctors and scientists manage insomnia in athletes.

Recognition and diagnosis of insomnia

Definition of insomnia: criteria

In terms of clinical practice and epidemiology, chronic insomnia is usually defined based on the criteria of the *Diagnostic and Statistical Manual of Mental*

---

* Corresponding author. Centre du Sommeil, Hotel Dieu de Paris, 1, Place du Parvis Notre Dame, 75181 Paris Cedex 04, France.

E-mail address: damien.leger@htd.aphp.fr (D. Leger).

doi:10.1016/j.csm.2004.12.011   *sportsmed.theclinics.com*

Disorders (DSM-IV) [8] or the *International Classification of Sleep Disorders* (ICSD) [9]. These may include

- Difficulty falling asleep (sleep-initiating insomnia), the occurrence of nocturnal awakenings with difficulties getting back to sleep (sleep-maintenance insomnia), an early morning awakening (sleep-offset insomnia), or a nonrefreshing or nonrestorative sleep, and often a combination of all of these factors
- Symptoms occurring at least three times a week for a minimum of 1 month
- Clinically significant distress or impairment in social, occupational, or other important areas of daytime functioning

Insomnia may be primary or secondary to a variety of disorders, environmental factors, or comorbidities. Identifying and treating potential underlying conditions are priorities in the management of insomnia. Otherwise, insomnia will remain unresolved.

Primary insomnia

Primary insomnia is an intrinsic sleep disorder that is characterized by the presence of insomnia that

- Does not occur exclusively during the course of another sleep disorder (eg, sleep-disordered breathing, periodic limb movements, restless leg syndrome, or circadian rhythm disorder)
- Does not occur exclusively in the course of another mental disorder
- Is not caused by the direct physiologic effect of a general medical condition, substance or treatment, or physical environmental factor

A common mechanism of persistent insomnia is conditioned (ie, learned or psychophysiologic) insomnia. It begins usually by an episode of acute situational insomnia, secondary to insomnia-precipitating factors such as a stress, jet lag, pain, illness, or medication. The patient then begins to associate bed with non-sleeping, becomes hyperaroused at night, and develops strategies for coping that perpetuate insomnia (insomnia-perpetuating factors) [10]. Individual differences in vulnerability to sleep disturbances may constitute a continuum from transient or episodic insomnia through overt chronic primary insomnia [11]. Ruminating about not being able to sleep plays a major role in perpetuating insomnia.

Secondary insomnia

Insomnia is frequently associated with numerous other conditions, such as sleep disorders, mental or physical disorders, or toxicologic or environmental factors. The role of the practitioner is to carefully check all of these conditions before considering insomnia as a primary disorder.

Almost all other sleep disorders disturb sleep seriously enough to induce a complaint of insomnia or poor sleep, as Emsellem et al describe elsewhere in this issue. Sleep apnea affects 5% to 10% of the general population, increases with age and body mass index, and causes arousals and awakenings during all stages of sleep. Patients usually complain of nonrestorative sleep rather than real insomnia. Restless leg syndrome may also affect sleep initiation and sleep maintenance. Restless leg syndrome affects between 5% and 10% of the general population and may be associated with apnea. Circadian rhythm disorders are linked to a dysfunction of the biological clock, caused by an internal condition (delayed or advanced phase syndromes) that is secondary to the underexposure of the retina to light (eg, as with blind people) or a misalignment between external and endogenous rhythms (eg, caused by shift work or jet lag). Circadian rhythm disorders may induce sleep-onset insomnia, early morning awakening, frequent arousals, and daytime sleepiness.

Mental disorders or comorbidities are commonly associated with insomnia. One survey of the general population found that 30.1% of the subjects who suffered from insomnia reported prior consultations for anxiety symptoms, and 23% reported prior consultations for depression [12]. Similarly, in primary care patients who experienced severe insomnia, there was a high prevalence of psychiatric diagnoses: 21.7% of severe insomniacs suffered from depression, 7.2% had neurosis/personality disorders, 10.2% suffered acute psychologic distress, 4.6% reported alcohol or drug abuse, 5.6% had psychosomatic disorders, and 1% demonstrated psychosis [13].

A variety of medical disorders may impact on sleep and awaken patients, such as central nervous system disorders, cardiorespiratory troubles, musculoskeletal disorders, and pain. Studies of specific populations reveal a strong correlation between pain and complaints of sleep disturbances [14]. Several endocrine and gastrointestinal disorders are also associated with sleep disruption. For example, nocturnal gastrointestinal reflux episodes may arise during sleep and induce abrupt arousals [15]. A large number of medications and toxins (eg, alcohol, drugs) also impact sleep continuity.

Environmental factors may also induce sleep disruption and fragmentation, even in good sleepers. Noise is one of the most common factors. Recently, the World Health Organization European Centre for Environment and Health considered insomnia one of the major health effects of noise exposure [16]. Low or high temperature, altitude, and light also influence sleep continuity.

Transient or chronic insomnia

The duration of a patient's complaint has important implications. The ICSD defines acute or transient insomnia as persisting for no more than 1 week and subacute or short-term insomnia as lasting from 1 week to 3 months [9]. Both types of insomnia are considered adjustment sleep disorders that are associated with a reaction to an identifiable stressor. Transient insomnia usually disappears with the reduction of or adaptation to the stressor; however, it may also be the foundation of a long-term condition. The individual's emotional and behavioral responses to the first episodes of transient insomnia seem to play an important role in the course of the disease [10,11,17]. Therefore, early identification and management of insomnia may play a role in the prevention of long-term insomnia. Insomnia is considered chronic if it lasts more than 1 [8] to 3 months [9]. This article's investigators believe 1 month is a reasonable period to begin to talk of chronic insomnia. Retrospective studies indicate that about 80% of severe insomniacs have had the problem for more than 1 year, with approximately 40% reporting a duration of more than 5 years [12,18]. Longitudinal studies suggest that 30% to 80% of moderate to severe insomniacs show no significant remission over time [5,18,19].

Severity

There is no clear consensus on the definition of severe insomnia; it seems insufficient to base it on patient reports. Many studies have observed that a large number of so-called "severe insomniacs" did not consult any practitioner for years about their sleep problem. Chronic duration or nightly frequency may be criteria for severity. The magnitude of the impaired daytime functioning may also be used to assess severe insomnia. In several studies focused on the daytime consequences of insomnia, severe insomniacs were considered to be subjects reporting at least two symptoms of poor sleep according to the DSM-IV definition of insomnia [20,21].

Epidemiology

Many studies in the past decade have used the clinical criteria for insomnia to assess its prevalence in the general population and some subgroups of adults [1,2,5,12]. These studies found a median prevalence for all insomnia of about 15% with a range of 10% to 25%. The studies also revealed that insomnia is more common in women than in men and that prevalence increases with age. With few exceptions, these studies do not attempt to identify etiologies of insomnia.

Sleep disruption and insomnia

The terms *insomnia* and *sleep disruption* are sometimes confused. Sleep-maintenance insomnia is defined by the occurrence of sleep disruptions (eg, arousals, awakenings) during sleep. Sleep may be disrupted by other sleep disorders or organic diseases, such as sleep apnea, restless leg syndrome, pain, and cardiac arrhythmia, and also by environmental disturbances, such as noise and temperature. Sleep disruption is always associated with an increased wake after sleep onset (WASO) and a decreased sleep efficiency. It may also affect the percentage of slow-wave and rapid eye movement (REM) sleep.

Subjective and objective assessments

Several subjective and objective tools are used by sleep specialists to assess insomnia, attempt to find a cause, and encompass the severity of the syndrome.

Subjective

Sleep logs are widely used in practice. These logs include data about time in bed, rising time, sleep latency, number and duration of awakenings, and napping. They are also frequently completed by visual analogic scales that inquire about sleep quality, whether there is a refreshed feeling in the morning, and about daytime functioning. Studies evaluating sleep logs versus objective recordings have shown that patients have a tendency to underestimate their total sleep time and overestimate their sleep latency on sleep logs [22,23]. However, the sleep log is a very easy and convenient tool to assess sleep symptoms on a medium–long-term basis.

Sleep questionnaires are also frequently used to address characteristics of sleep complaints and behaviors and to find the causes of secondary insomnia. The most widely used questionnaire in research and clinical practice is the Pittsburgh Sleep Quality Index [24], which has been applied in many settings to evaluate sleep in the elderly and in patients with psychiatric disorders, and in evaluating treatment response [25–27].

Recognizing psychiatric diseases that cause insomnia or that coexist with insomnia is one major aspect of the diagnosis. Psychiatric conditions are highly prevalent in insomniacs. Therefore, patients should be carefully interviewed to determine their psychiatric history and their current psychiatric complaints and treatments. In research, and in the case of a chronic and unresolved complaint of insomnia, the self-administered Primary Care Evaluation of Mental Disorders [28], the Profile of Mood States (POMS), and the Minnesota Multiphasic Personality Inventory may help physicians recognize mental disorders, and have therefore been used extensively in insomnia [29–31].

Objective

Actigraphy is a very simple device that looks like a watch and is worn on the wrist to record the number and amplitude of movements in a medium–long-term period (at least 1 week). When used conjointly with a sleep log, it provides an estimate of total sleep time (TST), sleep latency, sleep efficiency, and the number of awakenings. It may also give an estimate of napping and bouts of sleepiness during the daytime. Sleep habits are also well assessed by actigraphy, especially when the lag time between workdays and weekends is observed. Actigraphy has been used extensively in studies on insomnia. It is not indicated as a primary endpoint tool, although it may be useful for patients who have chronic and severe insomnia, or if there is a suspicion of a circadian disorder caused by shift work, jet lag, phase delay, or free-running rhythms [32].

Actigraphy has also been used with success in combination with respiratory polygraphy to detect sleep apnea [33]. In a recent study comparing polysomnography, actigraphy, and use of a sleep diary in 17 insomniacs, Vallières and Morin [34] concluded that, compared with polysomnography, actigraphy and sleep-diary instruments underestimated TST and sleep efficiency and overestimated total wake time. Also, actigraphy underestimated sleep-onset latency, whereas the sleep diary overestimated it compared with polysomnography (PSG). Actigraphy data were more accurate than sleep-diary data when compared with polysomnography. Finally, actigraphy was sensitive in detecting the effects of treatment on several sleep parameters. The investigators concluded that "actigraphy is a useful device for measuring treatment response and that it should be used as a complement to sleep-diary evaluation" [34].

PSG consists of one all-night simultaneous recording of the electroencephalogram (EEG), electromyogram, and electro-oculogram, considered conjointly with other secondary variables (eg, cardiopulmonary measurements, temperature, body position, leg movements). PSG may be used for insomnia when a primary sleep disorder is suspected, such as sleep apnea syndrome or restless leg syndrome. PSG is usually performed in a sleep laboratory; however, ambulatory recordings are also easily performed on insomniacs. Edinger et al [35] have shown that 34% of one sample of 100 chronic insomniacs who conducted ambulatory home recordings had PSG-dependant diagnoses and that the home assessment provided useful information for 65% of the patients. Other studies have shown a high level of night-to-night variability in home PSG [36], and an important first-night effect that made the use of ambulatory PSG very controversial in the clinical assessment of insomnia by itself [37]. WASO, sleep latency, and TST are the commonly accepted criteria to describe the presence and severity of insomnia.

A very simple device, the Nightcap (Respironics, Inc., Cambridge, Massachusetts), which is based on head-movement actigraphy and the detection of eyelid movements using a piezoelectric film sensor attached to the upper lid, has been shown to be a highly reliable tool to assess sleep latency, REM sleep, and TST, comparable to PSG [38]. Compared with conventional EEG techniques, the Nightcap is unable to separate slow-wave sleep from stage 1 and 2, but more acceptable in real-life settings such as sport.

Consequences of insomnia

Insomnia and daytime functioning

Even if there is a large consensus that the daytime impact is a major criteria in the definition of insomnia [8,9], the nature of this impact is still controversial. Recent studies have underlined objective impairments in subjects with primary insomnia, such as a high level of cortisol [39] and higher heart rate variability [40]. However, these objective data do not implicate a demonstrated link between insomnia and fatigue, irritability, and impairment of daytime functioning. In their review on insomnia and daytime functioning, Riedel and Lichstein [41] proposed that a paucity of objective findings in the literature may have occurred either because attempts at objective verification have focused on variables that are not impaired rather than areas of actual impairment, or because methodological problems, such as between-subjects variability, have hidden actual differences between insomniacs and persons with no insomnia. Daytime sleepiness has received the most attention, but it is becoming clear that a large number of insomniacs are not sleepy during the day [42,43]. Using the Multiple Sleep Latency Test (MSLT), Bonnet and Arand [43] demonstrated that insomniacs were even more alert than good sleepers during the daytime.

Relevance for athletic performance

The impact of insomnia on athletic performance is a crucial issue. Many athletes consider competition stressful enough to impact their sleep the night before the event and may fear the influence of poor sleep on performance. There are few studies, if any, devoted to the impact of insomnia on athletic performance. Optimum performance requires a combination of physical and cognitive excellence, so it is important to understand how insomnia may affect both aspects. Travel and jet lag are also sleep disruptive and frequently experienced by athletes before competition, as discussed by Reilly et al elsewhere in this issue.

On the physical aspect, some experimental work has been made recently on sleep deprivation and physical activity in healthy volunteers. Mougin et al [44] tested the effect of a voluntary partial sleep deprivation (3 hours) in seven athletes. Their findings showed a significant increase in heart rate and ventilation at submaximal exercise on the day after sleep deprivation, compared with the results obtained after a baseline night. Variables were also significantly enhanced at maximal exercise, although the peak of VO_2 dropped even though the maximum sustained exercise intensity was not different [44]. Meney et al [45] also observed the effect of one night's sleep deprivation on temperature, mood (assessed by POMS), and physical performance of 11 healthy men. The physical activity indicators included muscle strength, self-chosen work rate, perceived exertion, and heart rate. There was a significant negative effect of sleep deprivation on mood state the day after sleep deprivation, but no significant effect on other variables. The investigators commented that there were considerable interindividual variations in the responses to sleep loss among subjects and therefore it was difficult to give general advice about sport training capability after sleep loss.

Another study involved 13 healthy men who were sleep deprived for 1 night and tested the following day at 6 AM and 6 PM and the results compared with tests performed the day before [46]. The physical performance was assessed by the maximal power [P(max)], the peak power [P(peak)], and the mean power [P(mean)]. Blood lactate concentrations were measured at rest, at the end of the force-velocity test (F-V), and just after the Wingate test, and again 5 minutes later. Oral temperature was also measured every 2 hours. Analysis of variance revealed a significant (sleep × time of day of test) interaction effect on P(peak), P(mean), and P(max). These variables improved significantly from morning to afternoon during the baseline condition and after sleep deprivation. The reference night was followed by a greater improvement than the sleep deprivation night (SDN). Anaerobic power variables were not affected up to 24 hours after waking; however, they were impaired after 36 hours without sleep [46]. Analysis of variance revealed that blood lactate concentrations were unaffected by sleep loss, by time of day of testing, or by the interaction of the two. The investigators therefore concluded that sleep deprivation reduced the difference between morning and afternoon anaerobic power variables. A more recent study by these investigators on 19 young athletes showed the impact of circadian rhythms on performance during anaerobic cycle leg exercise, which was more easily assessed than the effect of sleep deprivation by itself [47].

In addition to physical performance, attention, concentration, and memory have major impacts in some sport competitions, and therefore insomnia may also impact these cognitive factors of performance excellence. However, it is not clear how insomnia affects next-day cognitive performance. In a review of 56 studies exploring the impact of poor sleep on cognitive dysfunction, Fulda and Schulz [48] found that neuropsychologic functions, such as attention, verbal immediate memory, and vigilance, were affected in only 22.8% of the studies. Impairment of memory performance was present in 20% of the studies on insomniacs compared with control subjects. Bonnet and Arand [49] also demonstrated that experimentally induced sleep disturbance, matched to the degree of disturbance in objective insomniacs, failed to produce significant performance decrements. Sateia et al [5] hypothesize that

> The absence of consistent deficits in this area suggests that either the current assessment methodology is not sensitive enough to detect impairments or that insomniacs amplify the adverse effects of disturbed sleep. Alternatively, it may also be the case that under mild sleep deprivation most individuals are able to sustain performance in a time-limited testing situation.

This discussion and the contradiction between the patient's feeling and the absence of objective performance deficits are illustrated in Fig. 1 and Fig. 2, where actigraphy was performed on athletes who were complaining of insomnia in our laboratory.

Fig. 1 illustrates the 21-day actigraphy of a 28-year-old woman, who was at the time of the recording the European champion in athletics and an Olympic gold medalist. She complained of insomnia the nights before important selections, especially when the race was early in the morning. The actigraphy showed regular and evening-oriented sleep schedules with an average bedtime of midnight and an average awakening time of 9 AM. Night awakenings were rare, the average sleep latency was 18 minutes, and the average TST was 7 to 8 hours. The peak of diurnal activity was around 11 AM, coinciding with the time of her regular training exercise. This subject's complaint of insomnia did not fit with

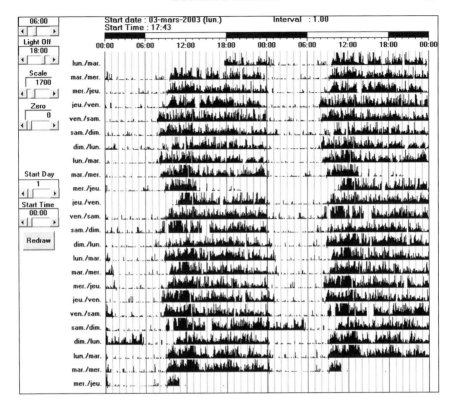

Fig. 1. 21-day actigraphy of a 28-year-old female athletic champion who complained of insomnia on the nights before important selections. Every line shows 48 hours of sleep/wake. The black parts of the lines represent daytime activity. The irregularity reflects the different levels of activity during the day, and the white part reflects the nights. Using the midnight line (00:00) as a reference, it is clear that the subject is rarely in bed before midnight. Referring to the end of the nights, the subject demonstrates irregular morning awakenings. However, there is almost no lag between workdays and weekends and no napping in the afternoon. Finally, the actigraphy shows regular and evening-oriented sleep schedules, with an average bedtime of midnight and an average awakening time of 9 AM. There were rare night awakenings, the average sleep latency was 18 minutes, and the average total sleep time was 7 to 8 hours. The peak of diurnal activity was around 11 AM (coincidental to the time of her regular training exercise) demonstrated by the black density, indicating that the daily pattern is higher at this time of day.

the objective assessment: she did not take any medication and had a rather good sleep at the actimetry. She received only cognitive behavioral therapy and won the European championship during the summer.

Fig. 2 is the 41-day actigraphy of a 38-year-old healthy man who was at the time the winner of a cross-oceanic sailing race. He complained of sleep-initiating and sleep-maintaining insomnia, exacerbated in the days preceding each race. The investigators performed an actigraphy during a selection race including 3 nights of sailing and four following days of 24-hour regattas, and then registered him during the next 34 days without competition. The investigators found

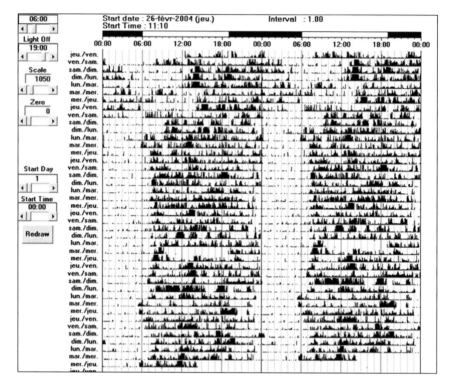

Fig. 2. 41-day actigraphy of a 38-year-old male sailor who was at this time the winner of a cross-oceanic sailing race. The subject complained of sleep-initiating insomnia and sleep-maintaining insomnia, exacerbated in the days preceding each race. An actigraphy was performed during a selection race including 3 nights of sailing and four following days of 24-hour regattas. Differences can be observed in the two parts of the figure. There are not regular patterns of sleep on the first days,. The subject is sleeping normally on the first line, but on the three following lines, it may be observed that he went to sleep around 6 AM after the afternoon and night regattas and his sleep is disturbed, with the thin lines representing night awakenings. The four following lines show that the subject was managing to stay awake as much as possible to stay alert during the race. He slept around 3 to 4 hours in 24 hours on a multiphasic pattern. Then, he went back to more regular patterns, going to bed around 11:30 PM and waking up around 7 AM during the 34 days after competition. However, the hour of awakening is irregular.

that he phase shifted pretty well on night shift during the first part of the competition, with an average TST of 6.4 hours between 6 AM and noon, and that he managed around 4 hours a day of polyphasic sleep (several phases of short sleep among the 24-hour cycle) during the 3 days after. He then returned to his regular schedule of going to sleep at midnight and getting up at 7 AM. He received advice on sleep hygiene, relaxation training, avoiding intense exercise and bright light before sleeping, and protection against noise. The use of hypnotics was discussed, but the athlete thought it unnecessary at the time.

Management of insomnia

There are several consensus publications about sleep management in insomnia [3–7], which involves educational, behavioral, and often pharmacologic intervention. There is ample evidence from this consensus that a multidisciplinary approach is required for the management of insomnia. Based on a review of 123 controlled medication studies (N = 9114 patients) and 33 controlled behavioral intervention studies (N = 1234 patients), Kupfer and Reynolds [6] concluded that

> Subjective symptoms and objective signs of chronic insomnia respond to short term behavioral and pharmacologic intervention. Although pharmacologic appear to act more reliably in the short term and behavioral interventions appear to produce more sustained effects, no direct comparisons with respect to long term efficiency are available. On the basis of these data, benzodiazepines, zolpidem, antidepressants and melatonin (one study) are effective pharmacologic agents. Stimulus control, sleep restriction, relaxation strategies, and cognitive behavioral therapy are effective behavioral interventions for short term management.

Treating the cause

When a secondary insomnia has been identified, it is first necessary to treat the cause and find an appropriate treatment for the medical, behavioral, or psychiatric diagnosis. However, multiple causes are the rule and not the exception. Additionally, although it is usually easier to find a precipitating factor and treat it in acute insomnia, it is more difficult to identify precipitating and perpetuating factors in chronic insomnia.

Educational and behavioral management

Educating patients is essential to reduce insomnia

Sleep hygiene consists of avoiding caffeine and stimulants and adopting regular sleep schedules. People should get out of bed at the same time regardless of how much they slept during the night, and those who have insomnia should avoid daytime napping. However, there might be circumstances when a well-timed short nap can restore daytime alertness and be beneficial for performance. Exercise during the day is recommended, but not too late in the evening. Particular attention should be given to stress reduction.

Stimulus control consists of limiting the time in bed and using the bedroom only for sleep and sexual relations. Patients should avoid reading or watching television in bed. When patients are unable to sleep for 15 or 20 minutes, they should get out of bed and go to another room. They can read, but should avoid bright light and watching television and should return to bed when sleepy. The goal of this method is to reestablish a link between the bed and sleeping [50].

Relaxation therapy has been used extensively in insomnia. It consists of using deep breathing and muscular relaxation. Several methods of approach have been used, although biofeedback is the most common.

Sleep restriction consists of curtailing the amount of time in bed to the evaluated time of sleeping assessed by the patient. This method produces a slight sleep debt that increases the patient's ability to fall asleep and sleep efficiency [51]. Then, the patient adds approximately 15 minutes in bed per day every week, as long as at least 85% of the time in bed is spent sleeping. This method should not be applied before important tests or competitions, or on a long-term basis.

Cognitive behavioral treatment (CBT) of insomnia, which focuses on psychologic and behavioral factors that play a role in maintaining sleep-related problems, has been shown to be of value in producing long-term benefits in primary insomniacs [52]. This treatment may represent an alternative to pharmacotherapy or be complementary during discontinuation of hypnotic medication. The CBT of insomnia may include different components, such as stimulus control, sleep restriction, relaxation, cognitive restructuring, and sleep hygiene [53]. For people who are dependent on benzodiazepines or other hypnotic medication, a supervised tapering based on attaining successive objectives is generally added to the CBT of insomnia. CBT has been used successfully in individual and group approaches. In a recent study, 45 adults suffering from primary insomnia received CBT implemented either in a group therapy format, in individual face-to-face therapy, or through individual telephone consultations. The results indicate that CBT was effective in improving sleep parameters with all three methods of treatment implementation, and there was no significant difference across methods of implementation. All three treatment modalities produced improvements in sleep that were maintained for 6 months after treatment completion [54]. These results suggest that group therapy and telephone consultations represent cost-effective alternatives to individual therapy for the management of insomnia.

The use of bright light may also be an effective treatment for insomnia resulting from circadian rhythm sleep disorders, as reported by Postolache and Oren elsewhere in this issue.

Pharmacologic treatment of insomnia

Hypnotics have a central role in the treatment of insomnia. In the western countries, approximately 20% of insomniacs and 40% of severe insomniacs are occasionally or regularly taking sleeping pills. The efficacy of the most commonly prescribed treatments in improving sleep latency and continuity has been shown by meta-analyses [6–55]. However, there is a public health concern about the potential abuse and misusage of hypnotics [4]. Thus, the pharmacologic approach of insomnia is generally framed by several consensual recommendations.

General recommendations on the prescription of hypnotics

1) Generally, prescribe hypnotics for short-term use (no more than 3 or 4 weeks). There are very few data assessing the efficacy of these treatments on a long-term pattern.
2) Inform patients about the recommended medication (and alternatives) and the duration of the treatment, and urge them to follow sleep hygiene techniques associated with the treatment.
3) Start low; the lowest dose should be tried first.
4) Intermittent dosing (several nights a week) has proven efficient for some treatments [56].
5) Discontinuation should be made gradually to avoid rebound insomnia.
6) Adverse effects on short-term memory and alertness should be considered before prescribing, and then must be monitored thereafter.

The hypnotics used in insomnia

The most commonly prescribed treatments for insomnia are γ-aminobutyric acid (GABA) agonists; specifically, receptor-selective-agonists such as zolpidem and zopiclone. These agents are selective compounds that interact preferentially with omega 1 receptors to produce sedative effects, whereas benzodiazepines interact with omega 2 receptors and produce adverse effects on cognitive performance and memory.

Zolpidem is a receptor-selective imidazopyridine GABA-agonist hypnotic with a short-term half-life of about 2.6 hours. The efficacy of zolpidem on sleep latency and sleep efficiency was assessed in 1997 by a meta-analysis on 16,944 subjects, and adverse effects were reported by only 1.1% [55]. Zolpidem has also been shown to be an effective treatment for insomnia when used intermittently (ie, on an as-needed basis) with no tendency to increase the dose prescribed [56].

Zopiclone is a cyclopyrolone short-acting GABA-specific agent with an elimination half-life of approximately 5 hours. Zopiclone has been shown to be efficient in short-term insomniacs (28 days) compared with triazolam, flunitrazepam, and placebo [57]. Sleep latency decreased and TST increased by 20% with zopiclone. There was also a decrease in the number of awakenings, a feeling of being more refreshed in the morning, and less daytime impairment. A long-term (8 weeks) study has also shown a good efficiency and lack of rebound after withdrawal [58]. Zaleplon is an ultrashort-acting agent (elimination half-life of 1.2 hours) and a pyrazolopyrimidine GABA receptor-selective agonist that is used in patients who experience nocturnal awakenings.

Older and less selective classic BZDs (eg, triazolam, flunitrazepam, lormetazepam, temazepam) are still used in many countries to treat insomnia. The efficacy of BZD on reducing night awakenings and inducing sleep has been repeatedly demonstrated. However, BZDs have side effects, including daytime sedating (depending of the half-life), alteration of short- and long-term memories, cognitive impairments, rebound insomnia, and dependence [3–7].

Other agents

Certain antidepressants, such as trazodone, nefazodone, mirtazipine, and paroxetine, decrease sleep disturbances associated with depression but they have not been tested for treatment of insomnia. Trazodone is often used for sleep independent of a depression diagnosis. The aim of antidepressant treatment is to avoid the side effects of BZD, including dependence in cases of continuous treatment for chronic insomniacs, and to try to prevent the appearance of depression. Antidepressants are prescribed at lower doses for insomnia than for depression. However, no controlled clinical trial could be found that assesses the efficacy of this method for use in insomnia. The longer half-life of these medications results in daytime sleepiness.

Melatonin is a hormone secreted at night by the pineal gland that can shift the circadian pacemaker in an opposite direction from light. In clinical trials, the indication of melatonin is more focused on circadian disorders (eg, caused by shift work, jet lag, phase delay) [59]. However, a recent study of 517 insomniacs showed that low nocturnal melatonin production is associated with insomnia in patients older than 55 years and identifies patients who are somewhat more likely to respond to melatonin replacement at the dose of 2 mg [60].

Sedating antihistamines (eg, diphenhydramine) are the main components in most over-the-counter sleeping pills. There are few studies of their effect on sleep architecture. Patients usually describe a better sleep continuity, but a residual sedation effect seems to be a common side effect.

How to use hypnotics in athletes who experience insomnia

If an athlete complains of regular insomnia before competition, a treatment should be tried days before competition, rather than the night before an important event. Athletes who have transient insomnia should be treated with zolpidem, or zopiclone may be first proposed. Zopiclone is preferred if a consolidated night of 6 to 8 hours of sleep is required, and zolpidem preferred if there is difficulty inducing sleep or a need for only 5 to 6 hours of sleep. Zaleplon may be indicated in cases involving night awakenings where there is difficulty going back to sleep. Stress management and sleep hygiene should be strongly recommended and explained.

Summary

Managing insomnia in athletes is not an easy task. As sleep is essential for a good performance, experiencing insomnia may affect an athlete's subjective feeling before competitions. Although pharmacologic management of insomnia is not the ideal solution, it is sometimes necessary. It is often difficult to apply nonpharmacologic recommendations in the context of competition, especially on a short-term basis. However, our experience indicates that sleep hygiene, sleep education, and relaxation may greatly help athletes, not only before competitions but also during the regular training periods. Sport physicians must interview young athletes about their sleep patterns to detect subjects who are vulnerable to insomnia [11], and should consult a specialist when insomnia persistently interferes with competition or training. This will help prevent episodes of insomnia during acute stress situations.

References

[1] Ohayon MM. Epidemiology of insomnia: what we know and what we still need to learn. Sleep Med Rev 2002;6:97–111.

[2] Leger D, Guilleminault C, Dreyfus JP, et al. Prevalence of insomnia in a survey of 12,778 adults in France. J Sleep Res 2000;9:35–42.

[3] Roth T, Hajak G, Ustun TB. Consensus for the pharmacological management of insomnia in the new millennium. Int J Clin Pract 2001;55:42–52.

[4] World Health Organization. Insomnia: report of an international consensus conference. Versailles, Paris: October 13–15, 1996. Geneva, Division of Mental Health and Prevention of Substance Abuse, WHO, 1998. Publication MSA/MND/98.2.

[5] Sateia MJ, Doghramji K, Hauri PJ, et al. Evaluation of chronic insomnia. An American Academy of Sleep Medicine review. Sleep 2000;23:243–308.

[6] Kupfer DJ, Reynolds 3rd CF. Management of insomnia. N Engl J Med 1997;336:341–6.

[7] Schenck CH, Mahowald MW, Sack RL. Assessment and management of insomnia. JAMA 2003;19:2475–9.

[8] American Psychiatric Association. Diagnostic and statistical manual of mental disorders. 4th edition. Washington, DC: American Psychiatric Association; 1994.

[9] Diagnostic Classification Steering Committee. International classification of sleep disorders: diagnostic and coding manual. Rochester, MN: American Sleep Disorders Association; 1990.

[10] Morin CM, Rodrigue S, Ivers H. Role of stress, arousal, and coping skills in primary insomnia. Psychosom Med 2003;65:259–67.

[11] Drake C, Richardson G, Roehrs T, et al. Vulnerability to stress-related sleep disturbance and hyperarousal. Sleep 2004;27:285–91.

[12] Ohayon MM, Caulet M, Priest RG, et al. DSM-IV and ICSD-90 insomnia symptoms and sleep dissatisfaction. Br J Psychiatry 1997;171:382–8.

[13] Hohagen F, Rink K, Kappler C, et al. Prevalence and treatment of insomnia in general practice. A longitudinal study. Eur Arch Psychiatry Clin Neurosci 1993;242:329–36.

[14] Pilowski I, Crettenden I, Townley M. Sleep disturbance in pain clinic patients. Pain 1985;23: 27–33.

[15] Shoenut JP, Yamashiro Y, Orr WC, et al. Effect of severe gastroesophageal reflux on sleep stage in patients with aperistaltic esophagus. Dig Dis Sci 1996;41:372–6.

[16] World Health Organization Regional Office for Europe. European technical meeting on sleep on health; January 22–24, 2004; Bonn, Germany.

[17] Edinger JD, Stout AL, Hoelscher TJ. Cluster analysis of insomniacs' MMPI profiles: relation of subtypes to sleep history and treatment outcome. Psychosom Med 1988;50:77–87.

[18] Hohagen F, Kappler C, Schramm E, et al. Sleep onset insomnia, sleep maintaining insomnia and insomnia with early morning awakening–temporal stability of subtypes in a longitudinal study on general practice attenders. Sleep 1994;17:551–4.

[19] Katz DA, McHorney CA. Clinical correlates of insomnia in patients with chronic illness. Arch Intern Med 1998;158:1099–107.

[20] Leger D, Guilleminault C, Bader G, et al. Medical and socio-professional impact of insomnia. Sleep 2002;25:625–9.

[21] Leger D, Scheuermaier K, Philip P, et al. SF-36: evaluation of quality of life in severe and mild insomniacs compared with good sleepers. Psychosom Med 2001;63:49–55.

[22] Brooks 3rd JO, Friedman L, Bliwise DL, et al. Use of the wrist actigraph to study insomnia in older adults. Sleep 1993;16:151–5.

[23] Krahn LE, Lin SC, Wisbey J, et al. Assessing sleep in psychiatric inpatients: nurse and patient reports versus wrist actigraphy. Ann Clin Psychiatry 1997;9:203–10.

[24] Buysse DJ, Reynolds CF, Monk TH, et al. The Pittsburgh Sleep Quality Index: a new instrument for psychiatric practice and research. Psychiatry Res 1989;28:193–213.

[25] Buysse DJ, Reynolds CF, Monk TH, et al. Quantification of subjective sleep quality in healthy elderly men and women using the Pittsburgh Sleep Quality Index (PSQI). Sleep 1991;14:331–8.

[26] Singh NA, Clements KM, Fiatarone MA. A randomized controlled trial of the effect of exercise on sleep. Sleep 1997;20:95–101.

[27] King AC, Oman RF, Brassington GS, et al. Moderate-intensity exercise and self-rated quality of sleep in older adults. A randomized controlled trial. JAMA 1997;277:32–7.

[28] Spitzer RL, Williams JB, Kroenke K, et al. Utility of a new procedure for diagnosing mental disorders in primary care. The PRIME-MD 1000 study. JAMA 1994;272:1749–56.

[29] Bonnet MH, Arand DL. Physiological activation in patients with Sleep State Misperception. Psychosom Med 1997;59:533–40.

[30] Piccione P, Tallarigo R, Zorick F, et al. Personality differences between insomniac and non-insomniac psychiatry outpatients. J Clin Psychiatry 1981;42:261–3.

[31] Stepanski EJ, Koshorek G, Zorick F, et al. Characteristics of individuals who do or do not seek treatment for chronic insomnia. Psychosomatics 1989;30:421–7.

[32] American Sleep Disorders Association. Practice parameters for the use of actigraphy in the clinical assessment of sleep disorders. American Sleep Disorders Association. Sleep 1995;18:285–7.

[33] Elbaz M, Roue GM, Lofaso F, et al. Utility of actigraphy in the diagnosis of obstructive sleep apnea. Sleep 2002;25(5):527–31.

[34] Vallieres A, Morin CM. Actigraphy in the assessment of insomnia. Sleep 2003;26:902–6.

[35] Edinger JD, Hoelscher TJ, Webb MD, et al. Polysomnographic assessment of DIMS: empirical evaluation of its diagnostic value. Sleep 1989;12:315–22.

[36] Edinger JD, Marsh GR, McCall WV, et al. Sleep variability across consecutive nights of home monitoring in older mixed DIMS patients. Sleep 1991;14:13–7.

[37] Wauquier A, van Sweden B, Kerkhof GA, et al. Ambulatory first night sleep effect recording in the elderly. Behav Brain Res 1991;42:7–11.

[38] Mamelak A, Hobson JA. Nightcap: a home-based sleep monitoring system. Sleep 1989;12:157–66.

[39] Partinen M, Putkonen PT, Kaprio J, et al. Sleep disorders in relation to coronary heart disease. Acta Med Scand Suppl 1982;660:69–83.

[40] Bonnet MH, Arand DL. Heart rate variability in insomniacs and matched normal sleepers. Psychosom Med 1998;60:610–5.

[41] Riedel BW, Lichstein KL. Insomnia and daytime functioning. Sleep Med Rev 2000;4:277–98.

[42] Stepanski E, Zorick F, Roehrs T, et al. Daytime alertness in patients with chronic insomnia compared with asymptomatic control subjects. Sleep 1988;11:54–60.

[43] Bonnet MH, Arand DL. Activity, arousal, and the MSLT in patients with insomnia. Sleep 2000;23:205–12.

[44] Mougin F, Simon-Rigaud ML, Davenne D, et al. Effects of sleep disturbances on subsequent physical performance. Eur J Appl Physiol Occup Physiol 1991;63:77–82.

[45] Meney I, Waterhouse J, Atkinson G, et al. The effect of one night's sleep deprivation on temperature, mood, and physical performance in subjects with different amounts of habitual physical activity. Chronobiol Int 1998;15:349–63.

[46] Souissi N, Sesboue B, Gauthier A, et al. Effects of one night's sleep deprivation on anaerobic performance the following day. Eur J Appl Physiol 2003;89:359–66.

[47] Souissi N, Gauthier A, Sesboue B, et al. Circadian rhythms in two types of anaerobic cycle leg exercise: force-velocity and 30-s Wingate tests. Int J Sports Med 2004;25:14–9.

[48] Fulda S, Schulz H. Cognitive dysfunction in sleep disorders. Sleep Med Rev 2001;5:423–45.

[49] Bonnet MH, Arand DL. The consequences of a week of insomnia. Sleep 1996;19:453–61.

[50] Hauri P. Treating psychophysiologic insomnia with biofeedback. Arch Gen Psychiatry 1981; 38:752–8.

[51] Spielman AJ, Saskin P, Thorpy MJ. Treatment of chronic insomnia by restriction of time in bed. Sleep 1987;10:45–56.

[52] Morin CM, Culbert JP, Schwartz SM. Nonpharmacological interventions for insomnia: a meta-analysis of treatment efficacy. Am J Psychiatry 1994;151:1172–80.

[53] Bastien CH, Morin CM, Ouellet MC, et al. Cognitive-behavioral therapy for insomnia: comparison of individual therapy, group therapy, and telephone consultations. J Consult Clin Psychol 2004;72:653–9.

[54] Belleville G, Belanger L, Morin CM. Traitement cognitivo-comportemental dans l'insomnie et son utilité dans le sevrage des hypnotiques [Cognitive-behavioral treatment of insomnia and its use during withdrawal of hypnotic medication]. Sante Ment Que 2003;28:87–101 [in French].

[55] Nowell PD, Mazumdar S, Buysse DJ, et al. Benzodiazepines and zolpidem for chronic insomnia: a meta-analysis of treatment efficacy. JAMA 1997;278:2170–7.

[56] Hajak G, Bandelow B, Zulley J, et al. "As needed" pharmacotherapy combined with stimulus control treatment in chronic insomnia–assessment of a novel intervention strategy in a primary care setting. Ann Clin Psychiatry 2002;14:1–7.

[57] Hajak G, Clarenbach P, Fischer W, et al. Zopiclone improves sleep quality and daytime well-being in insomniac patients: comparison with triazolam, flunitrazepam and placebo. Int Clin Psychopharmacol 1994;9(4):251–61.

[58] Terzano MG, Rossi M, Palomba V, et al. New drugs for insomnia: comparative tolerability of zopiclone, zolpidem and zaleplon. Drug Saf 2003;26:261–82.

[59] Sack RL, Lewy AJ, Hughes RJ. Use of melatonin for sleep and circadian rhythm disorders. Ann Med 1998;30:115–21.

[60] Leger D, Laudon M, Zisapel N. Nocturnal 6-sulfatoxymelatonin excretion in insomnia and its relation to the response to melatonin replacement therapy. Am J Med 2004;116:91–5.

ELSEVIER
SAUNDERS

CLINICS
IN SPORTS
MEDICINE

Clin Sports Med 24 (2005) 287–300

Thermophysiologic Aspects of the Three-Process-Model of Sleepiness Regulation

Kurt Kräuchi*, Christian Cajochen, PhD, Anna Wirz-Justice, PhD

Psychiatric University Clinic, Centre for Chronobiology, Wilhelm Klein Strasse 27, CH-4025 Basel, Switzerland

Sleepiness can be defined as a physiologic need for sleep and the behavioral measure of the subject's tendency to fall asleep at a certain time (sleep propensity) [1,2]. Sleepiness, and its converse alertness, are regulated and important determinants of vigilance and performance [3]. A better understanding of the mechanisms regulating sleepiness could lead to new strategies for sleepiness reduction and improved performance. Here we focus on the normal daily regulation of sleepiness and its relation to thermophysiologic processes.

In the last century, Kleitman [4] proposed that body temperature represents the underlying mechanism regulating performance. The speed of thinking and performance depends on the level of metabolic processes in neurons in the cerebral cortex. Raising the speed of performance through an increase in core body temperature (CBT) causes indirect acceleration of thought processes. In studies that have manipulated CBT through external means (eg, altering ambient temperature, cold water immersion), cognitive function improved by increasing CBT slightly above the normal temperature of approximately $37°C$, whereas decreasing CBT below normal induced a decline in cognitive function [5–7]. In a forced desynchrony protocol, in which the contributions of circadian phase and time awake can be assessed, a CBT increase of $0.15°C$ was associated with increased subjective alertness and improved neurobehavioral performance [8]. Alertness and vigilance are a prerequisite for good performance. Thus, when alertness and vigilance are increased as a function of

---

* Corresponding author.
E-mail address: kurt.kraeuchi@pukbasel.ch (K. Kräuchi).

0278-5919/05/$ – see front matter © 2005 Elsevier Inc. All rights reserved.
doi:10.1016/j.csm.2004.12.009   *sportsmed.theclinics.com*

warmer CBT, performance is also indirectly improved. Thermoregulation is a complex phenomenon and involves an intimate coupling between the central (core) and peripheral (shell) body compartments that exchange body heat. CBT and skin temperatures often change in parallel, depending on the location where they are measured. This aspect, which is the focus of this article, has not been sufficiently considered in studies dealing with the relationship between thermophysiology, sleepiness, and sleep.

Circadian regulation of the core and the shell

A circadian rhythm of CBT was described in the middle of the nineteenth century, when it was shown that oral temperature followed a daily rhythm that included a maximum temperature in the early evening and a minimum in the early morning hours, with a maximum–minimum range of 0.9°C [9]. For a long time, muscular activity (exercise) and digestive processes were considered the most important factors for the generation of the CBT rhythm [10]. However, Aschoff and his colleagues [11–13] systematically explored the underlying causes and showed that the circadian rhythm of CBT is determined by changes in heat production (measured by indirect calorimetry or indirectly by heart rate [14]) and heat loss. They concluded that heat production undergoes a circadian rhythm that is phase advanced with respect to the circadian rhythm of heat loss (ie, when heat production surpasses heat loss, CBT increases) and that the lag arises because of the body's inertia and because transport of heat takes time. That both heat production and heat loss are regulated results in a much finer tuning of the CBT rhythm than if only one of these components was regulated.

Therefore, changes in CBT can only be explained by knowing the relationship between heat production and heat loss. Under resting conditions, heat production depends mainly on the metabolic activity of inner organs, such as the liver, intestines, kidneys, the heart in the abdominal/thoracic cavity, and the brain, which together produce about 70% of the entire resting metabolic rate of the human body [13]. However, this heat is generated in only 8% of the body mass, which is surrounded by a small proximal skin surface whose shape is too flat for a good heat transfer to the environment. In other words, heat has to be transferred from the core to more peripheral parts of the body (ie, the extremities) with better heat transfer conditions [13]. These distal parts of the body have ideal (round) surface shapes, which are good properties for heat transfer to the environment. Under thermoneutral conditions, blood is the main medium for transporting heat from the core to distal skin regions (convectively), driven and distributed by the cardiovascular system. Therefore, in thermophysiologic terms, the human body consists of two compartments: the heat-producing core, and the heat-loss regulating shell [13].

The core (especially the brain) is homeostatically regulated around a set point of about 37°C, whereas the shell is not. Shell temperature depends largely on ambient temperature changes and can be considered poikilothermic, similar to the body of a lizard. From this point of view, humans have bodies that are homeothermic and poikilothermic. In a hot environment the shell is small; in a cold environment it is large, and thus acts as a buffer to protect the core from dangerous cooling [13]. This regulation occurs very rapidly before CBT has enough time to change. This so-called "feed-forward regulation" [15] with respect to CBT is an important property of the thermophysiologic "core/shell" principle. Another feed-forward regulation serves the counter-current heat exchange in the extremities (ie, legs and arms). In a cold environment, venous blood returns by way of inner blood vessels located near the arteries that prewarm the back-streaming blood, thereby efficiently protecting the core from cooling out [16]. In contrast, in a warm environment the venous blood streams back by way of outer veins near the skin surface, thereby enhancing additional heat loss by way of the lower extremities [16]. Furthermore, it is known that when shunts (ie, arteriovenous anastomoses [AVAs], exclusively found in distal skin regions) between arterioles and venules are open, the blood streams back also by way of these outer veins, thereby enhancing the heat-loss function of opened AVAs [17]. Blood flows more rapidly through AVAs (about 10,000 times more blood volume per second) than through capillary blood flow [17] directly from arterioles to the dermal venous plexus, which enables an efficient heat exchange. All these autonomically regulated mechanisms of shell size occur through constriction or dilatation of blood vessels (arterioles and AVAs) in distal skin regions [17]. There is now substantial evidence indicating that homeostatic control of CBT is mediated by a hierarchically organized set of neuronal mechanisms, with the anterior hypothalamic-preoptic areas at the top of the hierarchy [18]. In addition to the homeostatic principle, a rostral projection from the circadian pacemaker (localized in the suprachiasmatic nuclei [SCN]) to the preoptic areas serves the circadian modulation of CBT [19].

The mechanisms for changing shell size according to changing ambient temperature also take place over 24 hours when the underlying endogenous circadian CBT rhythm is regulated under constant ambient temperature. Distal skin temperature rises in the evening, whereas heat production [14], proximal skin temperature, and CBT decline; in the morning the inverse occurs [14], as is described later. A crucial role for the circadian regulation of heat loss is played by the nocturnally secreted pineal hormone melatonin. Melatonin selectively augments distal skin blood flow, most likely through opening AVAs, either by central or peripheral mechanisms (or both), while leaving proximal skin blood flow and cerebral blood flow unaffected [20]. Until now, no direct evidence exists for the existence of melatonin receptors (Mt1 or Mt2) in distal blood vessels in humans. Melatonin initiates not only distal vasodilatation but also sleepiness, acting therefore as the hormonal trigger between body heat loss and induction of sleep in the evening (opening of the sleep gate) [21–25].

The following sections will discuss the relationship between thermophysiology, sleepiness, and sleep, as elucidated in a series of studies performed under constant routine conditions. This protocol provided the necessary controlled environmental conditions to study the relationship between thermoregulation, sleepiness, and sleep [14,26] whereby external influences ("masking effects") are minimized (eg, constant room temperature, 22°C; humidity, 60%; light, less than 8 lux; constant bed rest in supine body position; no sleep allowed; food and fluid intake in small isocaloric portions at hourly intervals).

Sleepiness in relation to skin temperatures and core body temperature

Three major processes are involved in the daily time course of sleepiness (Fig. 1). First, there is a homeostatic increase of sleepiness (process H) dependent on time spent awake which dissipates during sleep [27,28]. Neither the central localization nor the neurobiologic mechanisms of the sleepiness/sleep homeostat have been discovered. Second, a circadian process (C), driven by the circadian pacemaker in the SCN, produces a maximal drive for sleepiness during the subjective night in all diurnal species [27,28] and an alerting signal during the subjective day. Third, a process of sleep inertia (I) describes the

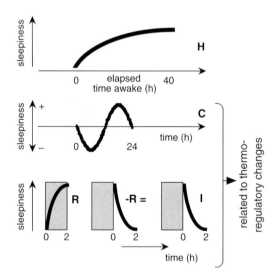

Fig. 1. Schematic illustration of the three-process model of sleepiness regulation. Process H represents the homeostatic component of sleepiness which increases with time elapsed awake, regulated by a sleep homeostat. H describes an exponential curve. The circadian component of sleepiness (C) is driven by the SCN producing a waking signal (-) during the subjective day and a sleepiness signal (+) during the subjective night. The sleep inertia process (I) describes a fast process that is active immediately after sleep and disappears in the following 1 to 2 hours in an exponential manner (gray area represents previous sleep duration). The exponential process R describes a relaxation-induced sleepiness, which starts immediately after lights-off or lying down (gray area). -R represents the inverse process of R occurring after lights-on or standing up (therefore, -R = I). Note: Processes C, R, and -R (I) are coupled with thermophysiologic changes (distal vasodilatation), whereas H is not coupled.

phenomenon of low vigilance on awakening even though sleepiness should be lowest at the end of a sleep episode [29,30]. The underlying neurobiologic and physiologic mechanisms for sleep inertia are unknown. All three processes have been mathematically described by the three-process model for sleepiness [29,31], which is a further development of the two-process model of sleep regulation [27,28].

The relationship between sleep and thermoregulation is tightly coupled to the question: "Why do we sleep?" From a thermophysiologic point of view, the proposed answer has been: "We sleep to conserve energy." This answer was derived from the observation that all living organisms, whether nocturnal or diurnal, sleep or rest when their metabolism (heat production) is low. However, this statement does not seem to be true, at least not for humans. In the past, one important observation had not been taken into account: not only did heat production decline in the evening, but also changes in heat loss occur via accelerated distal skin blood flow. Thus, the relationship between thermophysiology and sleep is rather the opposite: we sleep at times when distal skin blood flow starts to increase. The following summary of our studies concerning thermophysiology, sleepiness, and sleep deals with the question: "How are the three processes involved in sleep regulation related to thermophysiologic changes?"

Circadian and homeostatic aspects of sleepiness and its relation to changes in body temperatures

Numerous studies have indicated that the circadian profile of subjective and objective sleepiness is a mirror image of the endogenous CBT rhythm, with maximum sleepiness occurring around the CBT minimum [7]. From a homeostatic perspective, sleepiness should increase steadily with increased elapsed time awake; however, this is not the case. In the evening humans are often in a productive and alert state, especially evening chronotypes. From a homeostatic point of view this is a paradoxical phenomenon, explained by the fact that the circadian drive for alertness from the SCN is at its maximum right before humans usually fall asleep, thereby counteracting the homeostatic drive for sleep in the evening [32–34]. This so-called "wake maintenance zone" (or "forbidden zone to sleep") occurs at the circadian phase where the inner heat conductance is at its minimum: distal vasoconstriction is high in spite of the elevated CBT. Thus, the sleepiness/sleep homeostat interacts with the circadian clock in an additive or nonadditive way (which is still a matter of debate [35]), and determines the actual state of an individual's sleepiness. Usually humans choose their bedtimes shortly after the SCN-alerting signal has declined and the "sleep gate" has been opened [25], which occurs at the time of the maximum decline rate of CBT and the maximum increase rate of body heat loss [24].

Fig. 2 shows the results of a constant routine study illustrating circadian and homeostatic aspects of sleepiness together with the circadian patterns of CBT, distal, and proximal skin temperatures [14]. To illustrate the homeostatic component of sleepiness, an exponential curve (H) has been added to the

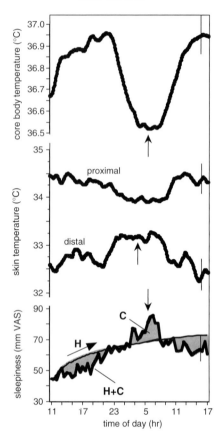

Fig. 2. Mean time course of CBT (rectal) and skin temperatures are shown in addition to subjective ratings of sleepiness (100 mm visual analog scale [VAS]). Seven men were studied in a constant routine protocol for 35 hours (sleep not allowed). Proximal indicates weighted mean of following skin regions: infraclavicular, stomach, forehead, and thigh, and distal indicates mean of hands and feet. The vertical bar at the right of the curves indicates plus and minus averaged SEM of all time points. To emphasize the homeostatic rise of sleepiness, an exponential curve (*thick line H*) has been added. The residuals (*gray areas*) indicate the circadian component C. Vertical arrows indicate circadian phase positions of the parameters derived from the mean of up- and downwards midrange crossing values. Note: The circadian rhythm of sleepiness is in phase with CBT; both are phase delayed compared with distal skin temperature. (*Data from* Kräuchi K, Wirz-Justice A. Circadian rhythm of heat production, heart rate, and skin and core body temperature under unmasking conditions in men. Am J Physiol 1994;267:R819–26.)

original subjective sleepiness rating (H + C). The residuals (C) describe the underlying circadian component of sleepiness (*gray areas*). The circadian regulation of sleepiness is in phase with CBT and phase delayed with respect to distal skin temperature, confirming other studies [36]. The fact that sleepiness is phase delayed relative to distal skin temperature explains the finding that increased distal skin temperature before nocturnal sleep is a better predictor for short sleep-onset latency than the decline in CBT [26,37]. Therefore, the circadian component of sleepiness is related to thermophysiologic changes most closely coupled to distal skin vasodilatation. Interestingly, beside their circadian time courses, CBT, distal, and proximal skin temperatures are not changed in the course of a 35-hour sleep deprivation, indicating no or very small influence of increased sleep pressure (process H) on the thermophysio-logic system during constant routine conditions. Thus, the thermostat seems to be sleep-pressure compensated or independent of the sleep homeostat. This phenomenon can be explained by two counteracting processes, resulting in no effect on the thermoregulatory system. That is, with increasing elapsed time awake, distal vasodilatation should also increase when sleepiness increases. However, to stay awake, distal vasoconstriction is induced, counteracting the former process and resulting in no changes.

Influence of sleep on the thermoregulatory system

Very early studies concluded that when subjects remained still and quiet in bed, neither sleep nor waking affected CBT [38]. However, more recent studies found a reduction of CBT during a nocturnal sleep episode [38]. This so-called "sleep evoked effect" on CBT has been replicated in several studies, also under constant routine conditions (CBT reduction of 0.3°C during an 8-hour night sleep episode) [39]. However, is this reduction of CBT really induced by sleep per se? To separate the true influence of sleep on the thermoregulatory system from behavioral changes related to sleep (eg, lying down, relaxation) we per-formed a constant routine for many hours before the start of a nocturnal sleep episode [26]. As described previously, proximal skin temperature and CBT decline before lights off, and the distal skin temperature increase was followed by an increase in sleepiness (Fig. 3a). After lights off, an additional phenome-non can be observed: distal and proximal skin temperatures increase rapidly to a similar level because of relaxation-induced withdrawal of the sympathetic vasoconstrictor tonus in precapillary muscles (see Fig. 3a).

When sleep is not allowed at this circadian phase, distal skin temperatures remain about 0.8°C lower than proximal skin temperatures (see Fig. 2). During sleep, however, the core-shell difference is lost completely, as indexed by very similar levels of proximal and distal skin temperatures. However, the increase in skin temperatures after lights-off does not lead to efficient heat loss, because cardiac output is decreased in parallel [40]; CBT declines very slowly under normal environmental conditions [13]. When the data were adjusted with respect to the timing of sleep stage 2 onset, no additional thermoregulatory changes occur thereafter (Fig. 3b) [41]. This analysis indicated that a long-lasting redistribution of heat from the core to the shell begins immediately after lights-off before the onset of sleep [41,42]. In contrast to a previously claimed hypothesis [43,44], slow-wave sleep, which dominantly occurs at the beginning of a sleep episode [27,28] has therefore minor, if any, thermoregulatory functions. Taken together, the process of relaxation (R) begins immediately after

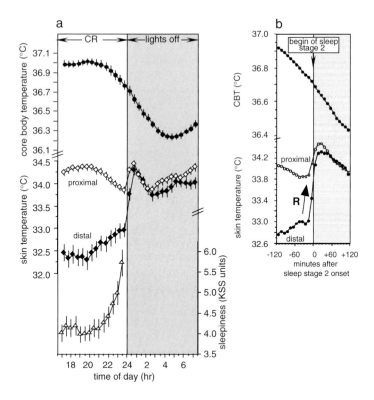

Fig. 3. (*a*) Mean curves (± SEM; N = 18 men) of CBT, skin temperatures, and subjective ratings of sleepiness before and during nocturnal sleep aligned to lights-off. Note: Distal and proximal skin temperatures show an inverse time course before lights-off, but increase in parallel to a similar level thereafter. (*Data from* Kräuchi K, Cajochen C, Werth E, Wirz-Justice A. Functional link between distal vasodilation and sleep-onset latency? Am J Physiol 2000;278:R741–8.) (*b*) Mean time courses of CBT and skin temperatures (N = 36 men), adjusted to onset of sleep stage 2. Note: skin temperatures have already increased before sleep stage 2 onset, indicating a relaxation-induced effect (R). KSS, Karolinska sleepiness scale. (*Data from* Kräuchi K, Cajochen C, Werth E, et al. Thermoregulatory changes begin after lights off and not after onset of sleep stages 2. Sleep 2001;24:165–6.)

lights-off before sleep starts; it is not sleep that induces thermoregulatory changes but rather the relaxation process per se. Because sleep is a very relaxed state, especially deep sleep, a complete loss of the core/shell principle occurs at this time. Therefore, a logical question is: "What happens to the core/shell principle after waking up from a sleep episode?"

Sleep inertia is related to thermoregulatory after-effects of relaxation

To answer that question we analyzed data of a controlled constant routine study 2 hours before, during, and 2 hours following an afternoon nap from 16 to18 hours (Fig. 4) [45]. This circadian phase around the CBT maximum was chosen to separate thermophysiologic changes induced during and after a

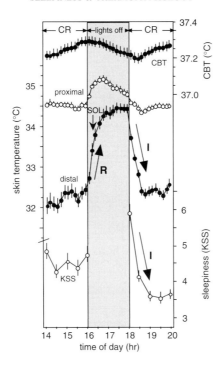

Fig. 4. Mean curves (± SEM; N = 8 men and 8 women) of CBT, skin, and subjective ratings of sleepiness 2 hours before, during, and after a nap between 4 PM and 6 PM. Note: Subjective ratings of sleepiness and distal skin temperatures showed a similar time course after lights on. -R equals I. KSS, Karolinska sleepiness scale; SOL, sleep stage 2 onset. (*Data from* Kräuchi K, Brunner DP, Cajochen C, et al. Time course or rectal temperature and heart rate during baseline and recovery sleep. J Sleep Res 1994;3(Suppl.1):132.)

sleep episode from the endogenous circadian thermoregulatory changes in the evening. However, very similar results were also found after a nocturnal 8-hour sleep episode (see Fig. 3) [26] with the confounding circadian changes in thermophysiology. In both experiments, immediately after lights-off, distal and proximal skin temperatures increased rapidly (before onset of sleep stage 2) to nearly a similar level at the end of the nap, whereas CBT declined marginally and slowly (see Fig. 4).

Proximal skin temperature peaked 50 minutes after lights-off, distal skin temperature later at the end of the nap, and CBT declined slowly to reach its lowest value ($-0.08°C$) 30 minutes after lights-on. Sleepiness ratings were highest in the first assessment right after lights-on and declined thereafter within about 1 hour, very similar to the time course of distal skin temperature. Proximal skin temperature declined after the maximum within the nap and reached its lowest value 40 minutes after lights-on. The distal skin temperature and sleepiness ratings declined after lights-on could be fitted to an exponential "cooling-out" function with a similar time constant. This indicates a close temporal association between subjective sleepiness ratings and distal vaso-dilatation after lights-on. Sleep inertia on waking showed a similar rate of dissipation to the cooling-out rate of the extremities, which had been warmed up by the redistribution of blood during the dark period. Thus, as the readiness to fall asleep is correlated with distal vasodilatation, so is the waking-up process (or disappearance of sleep inertia) correlated with distal vasoconstriction. Taken together, the symmetry between the thermoregulatory processes initiating sleepi-ness [26,37] and those dissipating it is striking and provide a physiologic rationale for a "power nap" being short: redistribution of blood to the extremi-ties is incomplete after less than 20 minutes of scheduled sleep or relaxation. This may lead to less distal vasodilatation on wake-up and less sleep inertia. A simple test of our hypothesis would be cold water applied directly to the extremities on waking, which should rapidly increase distal vasoconstriction and, in turn, alertness. In the following section the simple behavior of lying down to go to sleep will be revisited from a thermophysiologic point of view.

Lying down-induced sleepiness is related to relaxation-induced effects

A further relaxation effect can be induced by changes in body position (eg, from upright to a supine position). We have shown that distal and proximal skin temperatures increase rapidly after lying down, together with increased sleepiness ratings and decreased CBT (Fig. 5a) [46]. The opposite pattern was found in another study after a change from supine to upright body position (Fig. 5b) [46]. Here again, distal and proximal skin temperatures change in the same direction as during and after a sleep episode, indicating that relaxation-induced sleepiness may be differently regulated by the thermostat than by the circadian process of sleepiness, where distal and proximal skin temperatures show inverse patterns.

Changes in distal skin temperatures seem to be the crucial thermophysio-logic correlate for relaxation-induced sleepiness, and not the decrease in CBT or changes in proximal skin temperature. The same conclusion can be drawn from experiments involving eating ice (200 g), where CBT and distal skin tempera-ture decline and sleepiness decreases [47]. Thus, it is the increase in distal skin temperature that is associated with an increase in sleepiness, whereas the decrease in distal skin temperature is associated with a decrease in sleepiness (ie, alerting effect). This leads to the question: "Which mechanisms are involved in the coupling between distal vasodilatation and sleepiness induction?"

Putative mechanisms involved in coupling sleepiness and distal vasodilatation

Changes in acral skin blood flow are easily demonstrable by distal skin temperature, most prominently in fingertips, and are a commonly used indicator for sympathetic reflex responses to various stimuli. However, skin temperatures are a function of inner and outer heat transport and transfer conditions, leading

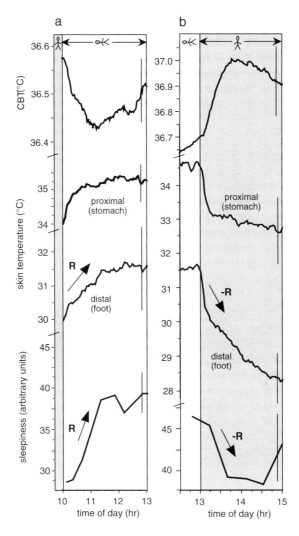

Fig. 5. (*a*) Mean curves (N = 8 men) of CBT, skin temperatures, and subjective ratings of sleepiness immediately after lying down from an upright position. The vertical bar at the right of the curves indicates plus and minus averaged SEM of all time points. Note: Distal and proximal skin temperatures increased together with subjective ratings of sleepiness. (*b*) Mean curves (N = 9 men) of CBT, skin temperatures, and subjective ratings of sleepiness after standing up from a supine position. The vertical bar at the right of the curves indicates plus and minus averaged SEM of all time points. Note: Distal and proximal skin temperatures decreased together with subjective ratings of sleepiness. (*Data from* Kräuchi K, Cajochen C, Wirz-Justice A. A relationship between heat loss and sleepiness: effects of postural change and melatonin administration. J Appl Physiol 1997;83:134–9; and Kräuchi K, Werth E, Wüst D, et al. Interaction of melatonin with core body cooling: sleepiness is primarily associated with heat loss and not with a decrease in core temperature. Sleep 1999; 22(Suppl 1):285–6.)

to a nonlinear relationship between skin blood flow and skin temperature; only a certain range of blood flow skin temperatures can be used as a good indicator for skin blood flow [13]. In many studies, the relationship between distal skin blood flow and sleepiness has been challenged by diverse interventions [48]. For example, distal skin temperature can be strongly affected during hypnosis, when images used for suggesting cold and warmth include experiences of physical temperature and physiologic stress or relaxation [49]. Furthermore, thermal biofeedback training in raising hand temperature increases not only finger-skin temperature [50] but also promotes a rapid sleep onset [51]. Therefore, sympathetic nerve activity seems to be the most important mechanism determining blood flow through arterioles by way of adrenergic constrictor nerves, and is also a good indicator for the arousal system. There is now emerging evidence from physiologic and neuroanatomic studies to indicate that changes in body temperatures may trigger somnogenic brain areas (eg, medial preoptic area [52], ventrolateral preoptic area [53]) to initiate sleep, either indirectly through nerve afferents activated by cold and warm receptors located in the dermis and in the core, or directly through changes in core blood temperature leading to changed spinal cord and brain temperatures [54]. However, the interrelationship between thermoregulatory and sleepiness/sleep regulatory mechanisms is rather complex. Recent studies have indicated that the medial preoptic area controls sleep and temperature through independent, but overlapping, neuronal circuits [53,55,56]. However, the disadvantage of these animal studies is that the behavior of an animal cannot be independently controlled for sleep, which is crucial to separate the influence of the three components of sleepiness regulation (C, H, and I). There is good reason to believe that future studies in humans using imaging techniques (eg, functional MRI) will shed more light on how thermoregulatory and sleepiness/sleep regulatory mechanisms are related in the human brain.

Acknowledgments

The studies reviewed here were supported by SNF Grants #32-4245.94 and #31-49254.96, and the Kneipp Stiftung Würzburg, Germany.

References

[1] Johns MW. A new method for measuring daytime sleepiness: the Epworth sleepiness scale. Sleep 1991;14(6):540–5.
[2] Åkerstedt T, Gillberg M. Subjective and objective sleepiness in the active individual. Intern J Neurosci 1990;52:29–37.
[3] Folkard S, Åkerstedt T. Trends in the risk of accidents and injuries and their implications for models of fatigue and performance. Aviat Space Environ Med 2004;75(3 Suppl):A161–7.
[4] Kleitman N. Sleep and Wakefulness. Chicago: The University of Chicago Press; 1987.

[5] Coleshaw SR, van Someren RN, Wolff AH, et al. Impaired memory registration and speed of reasoning caused by low body temperature. J Appl Physiol 1983;55:27–31.

[6] Giesbrecht GG, Arnett JL, Vela E, et al. Effect of task complexity on mental performance during immersion hypothermia. Aviat Space Environ Med 1993;64:206–11.

[7] Johnson MP, Duffy JF, Dijk DJ, et al. Short-term memory, alertness and performance: a reappraisal of their relationship to body temperature. J Sleep Res 1992;1:24–9.

[8] Wright Jr KP, Hull JT, Czeisler CA. Relationship between alertness, performance, and body temperature in humans. Am J Physiol Regul Integr Comp Physiol 2002;283:R1370–7.

[9] Gierse A. Quaeniam sit ratio caloris organici [MD Thesis] [What is the cause of organic heat?]. Halle; 1842 [in German].

[10] Hardy JD. Physiology of temperature regulation. Physiol Rev 1961;41:521–606.

[11] Aschoff J. The circadian rhythm of body temperature as a function of body size. In: Taylor R, Johanson K, Bolis L, editors. A Comparison to animal physiology. Cambridge, England: Cambridge Univ Press; 1982. p. 173–89.

[12] Aschoff J, Heise A. Thermal conductance in man: its dependence on time of day and of ambient temperature. In: Itoh S, Ogata K, Yoshimura H, editors. Advances in climatic physiology. Tokyo: Igako Shoin; 1972. p. 334–48.

[13] Aschoff J. Temperaturregulation. In: Gauer OH, Kramer K, Jung R, editors. Energiehaushalt und Temperaturregulation [Energy budget and temperature regulation]. Physiologie des Menschen. München: Urban & Schwarzenberg; 1971. p. 43–112 [in German].

[14] Kräuchi K, Wirz-Justice A. Circadian rhythm of heat production, heart rate, and skin and core body temperature under unmasking conditions in men. Am J Physiol 1994;267:R819–26.

[15] Mrosovsky N. Rheostasis. The physiology of change. New York: Oxford University Press; 1990.

[16] Aschoff J, Wever R. Kern und Schale im Wärmehaushalt des Menschen [Core and shell in human energy budget]. Naturwissenschaften 1958;45:477–85 [in German].

[17] Hales JRS. Skin arteriovenous anastomoses, their control and role in thermoregulation. In: Johansen K, Burggren WW, editors. Cardiovascular shunts. Alfred Benzon Symposium 21. Copenhagen, Denmark: Munksgaard; 1985. p. 433–51.

[18] Satinoff E. Neural organization and evolution of thermal regulation in mammals. Science 1978;201:16–22.

[19] Moore RY, Danchenko RL. Paraventricular-subparaventricular hypothalamic lesions selectively affect circadian function. Chronobiol Int 2002;19:345–60.

[20] van der Helm - Van Mil AH, van Someren EJ, van den Boom R, et al. No influence of melatonin on cerebral blood flow in humans. J Clin Endocrinol Metabol 2003;88:5989–94.

[21] Cajochen C, Kräuchi K, von Arx MA, et al. Daytime melatonin administration enhances sleepiness and theta/alpha activity in the waking EEG. Neurosci Lett 1996;207:209–13.

[22] Cagnacci A, Kräuchi K, Wirz-Justice A, et al. Homeostatic versus circadian effects of melatonin on core body temperature in humans. J Biol Rhythms 1997;12:509–17.

[23] Cajochen C, Kräuchi K, Wirz-Justice A. Role of melatonin in the regulation of human circadian rhythms and sleep. J Neuroendocrinol 2003;15:432–7.

[24] Campbell SS, Broughton RJ. Rapid decline in body temperature before sleep: fluffing the physiological pillow? Chronobiol Int 1994;11:126–31.

[25] Lavie P. Melatonin: role in gating nocturnal rise in sleep propensity. J Biol Rhythms 1997; 12(6):657–65.

[26] Kräuchi K, Cajochen C, Werth E, et al. Functional link between distal vasodilation and sleep-onset latency? Am J Physiol Regul Integr Comp Physiol 2000;278:R741–8.

[27] Daan S, Beersma DG, Borbély AA. Timing of human sleep: recovery process gated by a circadian pacemaker. Am J Physiol 1984;246:R161–83.

[28] Borbély AA. A two-process model of sleep regulation. Hum Neurobiol 1982;1:195–204.

[29] Åkerstedt T, Folkard S. A model of human sleepiness. In: Horne J, editor. Sleep '90. Bochum, Germany: Pontenagel Press; 1990. p. 310–3.

[30] Dinges DF. Are you awake? Cognitive performance and reverie during the hypnotic state. In: Bootzin R, Kihlstrom J, Schachter D, editors. Are you awake? Washington, DC: American Psychological Association; 1990. p. 159–75.

[31] Folkard S, Åkerstedt T. A three-process model of the regulation of alertness-sleepiness. In: Broughton RJ, Ogilvie RD, editors. Sleep, arousal, and performance. Boston: Birkhäuser; 1992. p. 11–26.

[32] Dijk DJ, Duffy JF, Czeisler CA. Circadian and sleep/wake dependent aspects of subjective alertness and cognitive performance. J Sleep Res 1992;1:112–7.

[33] Ebbecke U. Schüttelfrost in Kälte, Fieber und Affekt. Klin Wochenschr 1948;39/40(15.Okt.):609–13.

[34] Edgar DM, Dement WC, Fuller CA. Effect of SCN lesions on sleep in squirrel monkeys: evidence for opponent processes in sleep-wake regulation. J Neurosci 1993;13(3):1065–79.

[35] Achermann P, Borbely AA. Mathematical models of sleep regulation. Front Biosci 2003;8:s683–93.

[36] Gradisar M, Lack L. Relationships between the circadian rhythms of finger temperature, core temperature, sleep latency, and subjective sleepiness. J Biol Rhythms 2004;19(2):157–63.

[37] Kräuchi K, Cajochen C, Werth E, et al. Warm feet promote the rapid onset of sleep. Nature 1999;401:36–7.

[38] Aschoff J. Circadian control of body temperature. J Therm Biol 1983;8:143–7.

[39] Barrett J, Lack L, Morris M. The sleep-evoked decrease of body temperature. Sleep 1993;16:93–9.

[40] Somers VK, Dyken ME, Mark AL, et al. Sympathetic-nerve activity during sleep in normal subjects. N Engl J Med 1993;328(5):303–7.

[41] Kräuchi K, Cajochen C, Werth E, et al. Thermoregulatory changes begin after lights off and not after onset of sleep stage 2. Sleep 2001;24(Abstr Suppl):165–6.

[42] Lack L, Gradisar M. Acute finger temperature changes preceding sleep onsets over a 45-h period. J Sleep Res 2002;11(4):275–82.

[43] Sewitch DE. Slow wave sleep deficiency insomnia: a problem in thermo-downregulation at sleep onset. Psychophysiol 1987;24(2):200–15.

[44] McGinty D, Szymusiak R. Keeping cool: a hypothesis about the mechanisms and functions of slow-wave sleep. Trends Neurosci 1990;13(12):480–7.

[45] Kräuchi K, Cajochen C, Wirz-Justice A. Waking up properly: is there a role of thermoregulation in sleep inertia? J Sleep Res 2004;13:121–7.

[46] Kräuchi K, Cajochen C, Wirz-Justice A. A relationship between heat loss and sleepiness: effects of postural change and melatonin administration. J Appl Physiol 1997;83:134–9.

[47] Kräuchi K, Werth E, Wüst D, et al. Interaction of melatonin with core body cooling: sleepiness is primarily associated with heat loss and not with a decrease in core temperature. Sleep 1999;22(Suppl 1):285–6.

[48] van Someren EJW. Sleep propensity is modulated by circadian and behavior-induced changes in cutaneous temperature. J Therm Biol 2004;29:437–44.

[49] Kistler A, Mariauzouls C, Wyler F, et al. Autonomic responses to suggestions for cold and warmth in hypnosis. Forsch Komplementärmed 1999;6:10–4.

[50] Freedman RR, Morris M, Norton DA, et al. Physiological mechanism of digital vasoconstriction training. Biofeedback Self Regul 1988;13(4):299–305.

[51] Lushington K, Greeneklee H, Veltmeyer M, et al. Biofeedback training in hand temperature raising promotes sleep onset in young normals. J Sleep Res 2004;13(Suppl 1):460.

[52] Szymusiak R, Steininger T, Alam N, et al. Preoptic area sleep-regulating mechanisms. Arch Ital Biol 2001;139(1–2):77–92.

[53] Saper CB. The central autonomic nervous system: conscious visceral perception and autonomic pattern generation. Annu Rev Neurosci 2002;25:433–69.

[54] van Someren EJ. More than a marker: interaction between circadian regulation of temperature and sleep, age-related changes, and treatment possibilities. Chronobiol Int 2000;17:313–54.

[55] van Someren EJ, Raymann RJ, Scherder EJ, et al. Circadian and age-related modulation of thermoreception and temperature regulation: mechanisms and functional implications. Ageing Res Rev 2002;1:721–78.

[56] Kumar VM. Body temperature and sleep: Are they controlled by the same mechanism? Sleep Biol Rhythms 2004;2:103–24.

CLINICS
IN SPORTS
MEDICINE

Clin Sports Med 24 (2005) 301–317

It's Practice, with Sleep, that Makes Perfect: Implications of Sleep-Dependent Learning and Plasticity for Skill Performance

Matthew P. Walker, PhD[a],*, Robert Stickgold, PhD[b]

[a]Sleep and Neuroimaging, Center for Sleep and Cognition, Department of Psychiatry,
Beth Israel Deaconess Medical Center, Harvard Medical School,
330 Brookline Avenue, Boston, MA 02215, USA
[b]Center for Sleep and Cognition, Department of Psychiatry, Harvard Medical School,
Beth Israel Deaconess Medical Center, 330 Brookline Avenue, Boston, MA 02215, USA

When contemplating the learning of new skilled actions and behaviors, particularly those involved in athletic endeavors, practice is often believed to be the only determinate of improvement. Although repeatedly performing a new task often results in learning benefits, leading to the adage "practice makes perfect," a collection of studies over the past decade has begun to change this concept. Instead, these reports suggest that after initial training, the human brain continues to learn in the absence of further practice, and that this delayed improvement develops during sleep. This article reviews these studies of what is now becoming known as sleep-dependent memory processing and focuses on the effects of sleep in the development of procedural skills.

Definitions

Before interactions between sleep and memory can be discussed, what these terms represent and encompass must first be understood. The process of sleep, with its varied stages and equally diverse physiology and biology, has already

This work was supported by grants from the National Institutes of Health (MH 48,832, MH 65,292, MH 69,935, and MH 67,754) and the National Science Foundation (BCS-0121953).
* Corresponding author.
E-mail address: mwalker@hms.harvard.edu (M.P. Walker).

been described elsewhere in this issue. Just as sleep cannot be considered homogeneous, the spectrum of memory categories that are believed to exist in the human brain and the unique stages that create and sustain memory appear equally diverse.

Memory categories

Although it is often used as a unitary term, *memory* is not a single entity. Human memory has been subject to several different classification schemes. The most popular is based on the distinction between declarative and nondeclarative memory (Fig. 1A) [1,2]. Declarative memory refers to consciously accessible memories of fact-based information (ie, knowing "what"). Several subcategories of the declarative system exist, including episodic memory (ie, memory for events of one's past) and semantic memory (ie, memory for general knowledge, not tied to a specific event) [1]. In contrast, nondeclarative memory can be regarded as nonconscious. The nondeclarative category includes procedural memory (ie, knowing "how"), such as the learning of actions and complex skills, and nonconscious implicit learning. However, although these

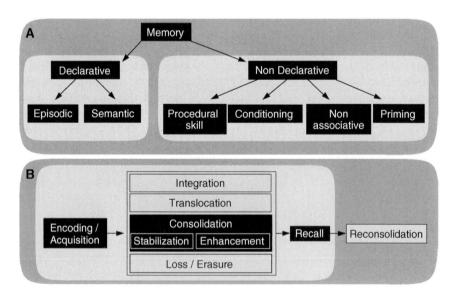

Fig. 1. Memory systems and memory stages. (*A*) Memory systems. Human memory is most commonly divided into declarative forms, subdivided into episodic and semantic, and nondeclarative forms, subdivided into an array of different types, including procedural memory required for learning skilled actions and movements. (*B*) Developing stages of memory. Following initial encoding/ acquisition of a memory, several ensuing stages are proposed, beginning with consolidation, and including integration of the memory representation, translocation of the representation, or erasure of the memory. Following later recall, the memory representation is believed to become unstable again, requiring periods of reconsolidation.

categories offer convenient and distinct divisions, they rarely operate in complete isolation and commonly work together to achieve cognitive goals.

Memory stages

Because memory is not monolithic, there is not one individual event that creates or develops it. Instead, memory appears to evolve in several unique stages over time (Fig. 1B). Memories are initially formed or acquired by engaging with an object or performing an action, leading to the rapid formation (within seconds to minutes) of a memory representation within the brain. The most efficient time for actively encoding or acquiring memory representations occurs not in sleep, but while we are awake, during a state of focused perceptual attention to external stimuli and the conscious performance of motor output.

Following acquisition, the most commonly recognized next-stage of memory formation is consolidation. Classically, consolidation refers to a stabilizing process whereby a memory becomes increasingly resistant to interference from competing or disrupting factors over time (within hours to days) [3]. However, recent findings suggest that memory consolidation is more specifically determined by time spent in unique brain states, such as sleep and the different stages of sleep. Furthermore, these studies have begun to indicate that consolidation can result not only in stabilizing memories, but actually enhancing them across sleep [4]. Although this article focuses on consolidation and the enhancing effects that develop across sleep periods, several additional memory stages beyond consolidation are also proposed, although they are currently not as well understood (Fig. 1B).

To summarize, human memory can be classified into a variety of forms, including procedural skill memory. Furthermore, the development of efficient and improved memory representations does not occur in a single step, but instead progresses through a number of distinct stages that appear to depend on the passage of time in specific brain states, such as sleep and its different stages.

Behavioral studies of sleep and memory

Sleep-dependent memory consolidation has been found in numerous species and across a range of memory systems. This article focuses on nondeclarative procedural skill memory in humans, spanning motor and sensory perceptual systems (eg, visual, auditory).

Motor learning and overnight sleep

Motor skills have been broadly classified into two forms: motor adaptation (eg, learning to use a computer mouse) and motor sequence learning (eg, learning a piano scale) [5]. However, real-life skilled procedures often involve combined use of these systems. An excellent illustration would be a pommel horse gymnastic routine. Not only is there a critical need to execute a series of hand and leg movements in a temporally correct sequential order (motor sequence learning) but these movements must adapt to each limb's speed and rotation at any given moment in time, compensating for the weight, velocity, and gravitational forces with which they are moving (motor adaptation learning). Clearly, these different forms of motor skill ability are equally essential in athletic performance, and therefore evidence describing sleep-dependent memory enhancement across these different motor skill forms should be considered.

Beginning with motor sequence learning, the authors have demonstrated that a night of sleep can trigger significant performance improvements in speed and accuracy of a sequential finger-tapping task [6]. In the first of a series of studies, subjects trained on the motor sequence task either at 10 AM or 10 PM and then retested at subsequent intervals across 24 hours. Initial practice on the motor skill task significantly improved performance within the training session for all groups equally, regardless of time of day. However, subjects then demonstrated remarkably different time courses of subsequent motor skill improvement, specifically dependent on sleep. Subjects who were trained at 10 AM in the morning showed no significant improvement when retested later that same day after 12 hours of wake time (Fig. 2A). However, when retested a second time the next morning following a night of sleep, they averaged a 20% improvement in speed and a 39% improvement in accuracy. In contrast, subjects trained at 10 PM in the evening immediately demonstrated equally large improvements the next morning following sleep, yet showed no significant additional improvement after another 12 hours of wake time later that day (Fig. 2B). Thus,

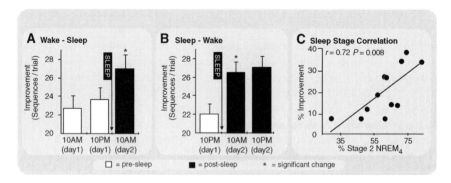

Fig. 2. Sleep-dependent motor skill learning in the human brain. (*A*) Wake–sleep. After morning training (10 AM, *clear bar*) subjects showed no significant change in performance when tested after 12 hours of wake time (10 PM, *clear bar*). However, when tested again following a night of sleep (10 AM, *filled bar*), performance had improved significantly. (*B*) Sleep–wake. After evening training (10 PM, *clear bar*), subjects displayed significant performance improvements just 12 hours after training following a night of sleep (10 AM, *filled bar*), yet expressed no further significant change in performance following an additional 12 hours of wake time (10 PM, *filled bar*). (*C*) The amount of overnight improvement on the motor skill task correlated with the percentage of stage-2 NREM sleep in the last (fourth) quarter of the night (stage-2 NREM₄). Asterisks indicate significant improvement relative to training and error bars indicate SEM.

significant delayed learning without further practice was only seen across a night of sleep and not over an equivalent period of time awake, regardless of whether the time awake or time asleep came first.

An alternative explanation of these results, however, is that motor activity during the daytime interfered with memory consolidation, and thus sleep is simply a passive time of hand rest that allows for memory enhancement. To eliminate this possibility, an additional group of subjects were trained at 10 AM, and then wore mittens for the duration of the waking interval to prevent skilled finger movements and the potential for interference before being retesting at 10 PM. Once again, the waking episode, even with total hand rest, conferred no significant improvement in performance, and actually led to a decrease in accuracy. However, when subjects returned following a night of sleep, large improvements in speed and accuracy were expressed again at retesting. Finally, when the degree of overnight learning was correlated with sleep-stage recordings, a significant positive correlation with the percentage of stage-2 non–rapid eye movement (NREM) sleep was evident, particularly in the last quarter of the night (eg, the last 2 hours of an 8-hour night of sleep) (Fig. 2C). This window corresponds to a time when sleep spindles, which are a defining electrophysiologic characteristic of stage-2 NREM, reach peak density late in the night [7]. Spindles may trigger key intracellular mechanisms required for synaptic plasticity [8], and are known to increase following training on a motor skill task [9]. As such, this late-night sleep, laden with spindles, may offer an ideal environment for triggering events that result in plastic brain changes leading to improved skill performance. Furthermore, this late-night correlation is of particular interest when considering optimal skill learning in athletes, suggesting that early morning awakenings may prevent maximization of learning potential by cutting short a critical sleep-consolidation time window.

Fischer et al [10] confirmed these findings of sleep-dependent motor-sequence learning using a similar task, although they reported a correlation with rapid eye movement (REM) sleep. They also demonstrated that if subjects were deprived of sleep the first night after training, and then allowed a night of recovery sleep before being retested, normal overnight consolidation improvements were blocked. This finding indicates that sleep on the first night following training is critical for the development of consolidation and delayed learning. From the perspective of motor-memory consolidation, it appears that one cannot accumulate a sleep debt and hope to repay it at a later time. Instead, the sleep-dependent consolidation process critically depends on sleep within the first 24 hours after training.

In another study, the authors investigated the temporal evolution of motor learning before and after sleep, the effects of different training regimens, and the long-term development of motor learning across multiple nights of sleep [11]. These data demonstrate that doubling the duration of initial training does not alter or inhibit the amount of subsequent sleep-dependent learning. Furthermore, the data show that the amount of practice-dependent learning during initial training does not correlate with the amount of subsequent sleep-dependent learning overnight, suggesting that these two stages (initial acquisition of the skill and the later sleep-dependent skill enhancement) are functionally distinct and regulated by different brain mechanisms. Finally, while the majority of sleep-dependent motor skill learning appears to occur during the first night of sleep, two additional nights of sleep trigger continued consolidation enhancement, with speed improving by 26% overall, and accuracy improving by nearly 50%.

Because most of the skills acquired throughout life are of a multi-limb and multi-digit nature, the authors studied the effects of increasing task complexity on sleep-dependent motor learning [12]. In this study, subjects trained on a variety of task configurations involving either a short or long motor sequence, coordinated between either one or two hands. The more complex the task became (depending on the combinations of these factors), the greater the overnight, sleep-dependent memory enhancement. This indicates that as task difficulty increases, the overnight sleep-dependent process responds with even greater performance improvements, further emphasizing the importance of sleep in learning many real-life motor skill routines.

These findings alone, however, do not reveal how the sleep-dependent process triggered significant improvements in motor performance speed and accuracy. Therefore, a more detailed analysis focused on performance changes within these motor sequences [12]. Before sleep, individual key-press transitions within the sequence were uneven (Fig. 3A, *clear circles*), with some transitions seemingly easy (fast) and others problematic (slow), as if the entire sequence was being parsed into smaller subsequences during initial learning (a phenomenon

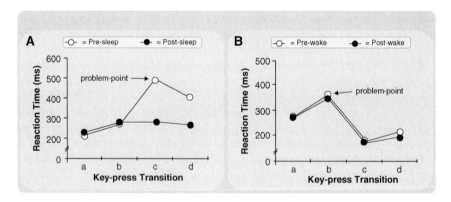

Fig. 3. Single-subject examples of changes in transition speeds. Within a five element motor sequence (eg, "4-1-3-2-4"), there are four unique key press transitions: (1) from 4 to 1, (2) from 1 to 3, (3) from 3 to 2, and (4) from 2 to 4. (*A*) The transition profile at the end of training before sleep (○) demonstrated considerable variability, with certain transitions being particularly slow (most difficult; "problem points"), whereas other transitions appear to be relatively rapid (easy). Following a night of sleep (●), there was a specific reduction (improvement) in the time required for the slowest problem point transition. (*B*) Similarly, at the end of training before a waking interval, transition profiles were uneven (○); with some particularly slow transitions ("problem points"), and other relatively fast transitions (easy). However, in contrast to postsleep changes, no change in transition profile was observed following 8 hours of wake (●).

termed *chunking* [13]).After a night of sleep, the problematic slow transitions improved, whereas transitions that had already been effectively mastered before sleep did not change (see Fig. 3A, *filled circles*). In contrast, if subjects were retested after an 8-hour waking interval across the day, the authors observed no improvement in the profile of key-press transitions at any location within the sequence (Fig. 3B). These changes suggest that the sleep-dependent consolidation process may involve the unification of smaller motor memory units into one single memory element by selectively improving problem regions of the sequence. This overnight process would therefore offer a greater degree of performance automation and effectively optimize skill speed throughout the entire motor program.

A recent study by Robertson et al [14] indicates that awareness of what is being learned can modify the sleep-dependent nature of delayed learning on a visuomotor sequence task. If subjects learn a motor sequence implicitly, that is, without conscious awareness because the sequence length exceeds the limits of explicit knowledge (eg, a particularly long 12-element motor sequence), then delayed learning improvements can develop across time awake in addition to during sleep. However, if subjects are explicitly aware of the sequence being learning, usually during shorter motor sequences, then delayed improvements again only develop across sleep, and this overnight learning correlates positively with NREM sleep. This suggests that an individual's level of awareness of what is being learned can modify the influence of wake and sleep. However, it remains unknown whether the improvements that develop implicitly across wake and sleep are achieved by similar or different underlying brain mechanisms.

Moving from motor sequence learning to motor adaptation learning, Smith and MacNeill [15] have shown that selective sleep deprivation impairs retention of a visuomotor adaptation task. All subjects trained on the task and were retested 1 week later. Some subjects were either completely or selectively deprived of different sleep stages across the first night following memory acquisition. Not all subjects retained the skill memory at the later retest session. Those subjects who were deprived of stage-2 NREM sleep expressed the most pronounced deficits in motor performance, again suggesting that stage-2 NREM is crucial to successful motor memory enhancement.

Huber et al [16] similarly demonstrated that following initial memory acquisition of a motor-reaching adaptation task, delayed learning is observed exclusively across a night of sleep, and not across equivalent periods awake. Furthermore, using high-density electroencephalography (EEG), they were able to show that daytime motor skill practice was accompanied by a discrete increase in the subsequent amount of NREM slow-wave EEG activity over the parietal cortex. They also demonstrated that this increase in slow-wave activity was proportional to the amount of delayed learning that developed overnight, and that the subjects who showed the greatest increase in slow-wave activity in the parietal cortex demonstrated the largest motor skill enhancements the next day.

In summary, these reports build a convincing argument in support of sleep-dependent learning across several forms of motor skill memory. All of these studies indicate that a night of sleep triggers delayed learning, without the need for further training. In addition, overnight improvements consistently display a strong relationship to NREM sleep, and, in some cases, to specific NREM sleep-stage windows at different times in the night.

Perceptual learning and overnight sleep

Often skilled performance is believed to involve only movement actions such as those described earlier. However, almost all of these motor actions are guided by other sensory perceptual systems, such as vision, hearing, and touch. Therefore, these systems also represent memory domains that play a significant role in skill perfection. Similar to motor skill studies, investigations of perceptual skill learning in the visual and auditory systems have offered support for the critical role of sleep in memory consolidation and associated learning enhancement.

In the visual system, Karni and colleagues [17] demonstrated that learning of a visual texture discrimination task (identifying different oriented line bars) improves significantly following a night of sleep. Furthermore, they established that selective disruption of REM, but not NREM, sleep results in a loss of these performance gains. Gais et al [18] selectively deprived subjects of early sleep, which is normally dominated by NREM slow-wave sleep (SWS), or late-night sleep, which is normally dominated by REM and stage-2 NREM, and concluded that consolidation enhancements on this task were initiated by NREM SWS-related processes, whereas REM sleep promotes additional enhancement.

Using the same task, the authors have shown that these enhancements are specifically sleep- and not time-dependent, similar to the characteristics of motor skill learning [19]. Furthermore, overnight learning correlated positively with the amount of early-night SWS and late-night REM sleep, proposing a two-step process requiring the sequential contribution of these different sleep stages. In addition, it was established that obtaining less than 6 hours of sleep the night following training results in no significant overnight learning, and that total first-night sleep deprivation, even when followed by two subsequent recovery nights of sleep, blocks normal sleep-dependent improvement [20]. Again these data not only highlight the importance of sleep in the evolution of delayed learning but also indicate that adequate sleep within the first 24 hours following memory acquisition is a requirement for subsequent sleep-dependent learning enhancement.

More recent studies have begun to explore sleep-dependent auditory skill learning. Gaab et al [21] used a pitch memory task to show that regardless of whether subjects train in the morning or evening, delayed performance improvements develop only across a subsequent night of sleep and not across similar waking time periods, regardless of whether the sleep episode comes first. Atienza and colleagues [22,23] have also described evidence of time- and sleep-dependent auditory memory consolidation, together with sleep-dependent changes in brain-evoked response potentials. Although posttraining sleep deprivation did not prevent continued improvements in behavioral performance, changes in evoked responses that are normally associated with the automatic shift of attention to relevant stimuli failed to develop following a night of posttraining sleep deprivation. Finally, Fenn et al [24] have shown that periods of wake following training on a synthetic speech recognition task actually result in deterioration of task performance across the day; an impairment that was not simply a consequence of circadian test time. However, if subjects were retested following a subsequent night of sleep, performance was restored to posttraining levels, reflecting a process of sleep-dependent consolidation capable of rescuing and reestablishing previously learned auditory skills.

In summary, learning of perceptual skills, like motor skills, appears to depend on sleep for the development of delayed learning, with evidence that several different sleep stages may be involved in triggering this form of overnight consolidation.

Daytime naps and skill learning

Although the majority of sleep-dependent studies have investigated learning across a night of sleep, several reports have examined the benefits of daytime naps on perceptual and motor skill tasks.

Based on evidence that motor learning continues to develop overnight, the authors explored the influence of daytime naps using the sequential finger-tapping task [25]. Two groups of subjects trained on the task in the morning. One group then obtained a 60- to 90-minute midday nap while the other group remained awake. When retested later that same day, subjects who experienced a 60- to 90-minute nap displayed a significant learning enhancement of nearly 16%, whereas subjects who did not nap failed to show any significant improvement in performance speed across the day (Fig. 4). However, when subjects were retested a second time following a subsequent full night of sleep, those subjects in the nap group showed only an additional 7% overnight increase in speed, whereas subjects in the control group, who had not napped the previous day, displayed speed enhancements of nearly 24% following the night of sleep (see Fig. 4).

These results demonstrate that as little as 60 to 90 minutes of midday sleep is sufficient to produce significant improvements in motor skill performance, whereas equivalent periods of wake time produce no enhancement. These data also suggest that there may be a limit to how much sleep-dependent motor skill improvement can occur over 24 hours, and that napping changes the time course of when learning occurs but not how much total delayed learning ultimately accrues. Thus, although both groups improved by approximately the same total amount 24 hours later (see Fig. 4), the temporal evolution of this enhancement was modified by a daytime nap. These findings offer the exciting possibility that naps may protect motor skill memories against the detrimental effects of subsequent sleep deprivation [10], suggesting a prophylactic strategy against learning deficits if overnight sleep loss can be predicted in advance.

As with motor skill learning, daytime naps also appear to benefit visual skill learning, although the characteristics of these effects are subtly different. Med-

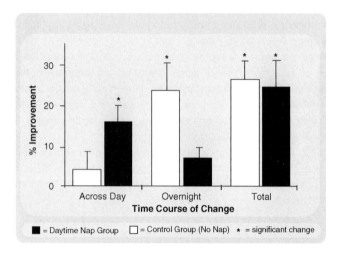

Fig. 4. Daytime naps and motor skill learning. Subjects practiced the motor skill task in the morning, and either obtained a 60- to 90-minute midday nap, or remained awake across the first day. When retested later that same day, subjects who experienced a 60- to 90-minute nap (*filled bar*; "Across Day") displayed significant performance speed improvements of 16%, whereas subjects who did not nap showed no significant enhancements (*clear bars*; "Across Day"). When retested a second time after a full night of sleep the next day, subjects in the nap group showed only an additional 7% increase in speed overnight (*filled bar*; "Overnight"), whereas subjects in the control group expressed a significant 24% overnight improvement following sleep (*clear bar*; "Overnight"). Therefore, 24 hours later, both groups averaged the same total amount of delayed learning (*filled & clear bars*; "Total"). Asterisks indicate significant improvement and error bars indicate SEM.

nick and colleagues [26] have shown that if a visual skill task is repeatedly administered across the day, performance does not improve or remain stable, but deteriorates. This may reflect a selective fatigue of brain regions recruited during task performance, a characteristic not observed in the motor system. However, if a short 30 to 60 minute daytime nap is introduced during these repeat administrations of the visual skill task, the performance deterioration is ameliorated. If a longer nap period is introduced that ranges from 60 to 90 minutes and contains REM sleep and NREM SWS, performance not only returns to baseline, but is enhanced [27]. Furthermore, these benefits did not prevent additional significant improvements across the following night of sleep, in contrast to findings reported earlier for a motor skill task.

These studies build a cohesive argument that daytime naps confer a robust learning benefit to visual and motor skills, and in the case of visual skill learning, are capable of restoring performance deterioration caused by repeated practice across the day. From the standpoint of athletic training regimens, it will be important to determine the optimal nap duration to generate maximal learning improvements and identify whether naps at different circadian times across the day (resulting in different sleep-stage compositions and electrophysiologic characteristics) are more or less effective at enhancing different forms of procedural skills. For example, delayed motor learning that develops across just a

60 to 90 minute nap (almost equivalent to a night of sleep) may be related to the distribution and incidence of sleep spindles at this time of day. Moreover, the efficacy of shorter naps (10–20 minutes) in triggering delayed skill learning, such as those often used when one cannot pay the price of sleep inertia (discussed by Lack et al elsewhere in this issue), have not yet been evaluated. Determining optimal nap duration represents an important future research goal, considering that immediate performance after awakening from longer sleep bouts (>60 minutes) can result in short-term performance impairments caused by transient sleep inertia, potentially masking sleep-dependent improvements.

Intermediate summary

Studies in humans demonstrate that sleep is necessary for consolidation and delayed-learning enhancement across a range of human procedural skills; is able to restore previously deteriorated task performance; and can trigger additional learning improvements without the need for added practice. Furthermore, different memory systems appear to require subtly different sleep stages, or even sleep-stage time windows, for consolidation and overnight improvement.

Sleep-dependent brain plasticity

Memory formation depends on a process termed *brain plasticity*, which is a lasting structural or functional change in the neural response to a stimulus, such as an experience. Evidence of sleep-dependent plasticity would greatly strengthen the claim that sleep is a critical mediator of memory consolidation. In the following section, the authors consider data describing sleep-dependent brain plasticity in humans, complementing the effects of sleep on behavioral performance.

Modification of post-training sleep and brain activation

Several studies have investigated whether initial daytime training is capable of modifying functional brain activation during later sleep episodes. Based on earlier studies involving animals, neuroimaging experiments have explored whether the signature pattern of brain activity elicited while practicing a memory task actually reemerges or is replayed during sleep.

Using brain imaging, Maquet and colleagues [28] have shown that patterns of brain activity expressed during motor skill training reappear during subsequent REM sleep, whereas no change in REM sleep brain activity occurred in subjects who received no daytime training (Fig. 5). Furthermore, these researchers demonstrated that the extent of learning during daytime practice exhibits a positive relationship to the amount of reactivation during REM sleep [29]. These find-

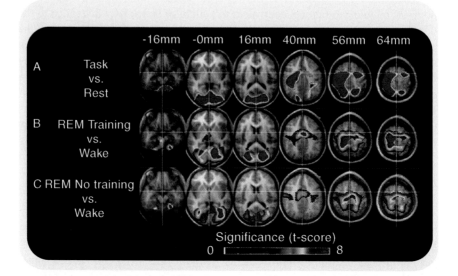

Fig. 5. Task-dependent reactivation of human brain activity during REM sleep. Statistical activation maps of different experimental contrasts. Maps are displayed at six different brain levels (from 16 mm below to 64 mm above the bicommissural plane), superimposed on the average MRI image of subjects. All maps are thresholded at $P < .001$ (uncorrected), except for (A), which is thresholded at voxel-level-corrected $P < .05$. (A) Brain regions activated during daytime performance of the motor skill task (Task versus Rest). (B) Brain regions activated during subsequent REM sleep in subjects that received daytime training (REM Sleep Training versus Wake). Note considerable overlap with daytime task-dependent activity patterns. (C) Brain regions activated during REM sleep in subjects who did not receive any daytime training (REM Sleep No Training versus Wake). (From Maquet P, Laureys S, Peigneux P, et al. Experience-dependent changes in cerebral activation during human REM sleep. Nat Neurosci 2000;3(8):831–6; with permission.)

ings suggest that simply experiencing the task is not what modifies subsequent sleep physiology, it is the process of learning itself. The function of sleep-dependent replay may be to modify the strength of synaptic connections between neurons within specific brain networks, strengthening some synaptic connections while weakening others in the endeavor of refining skill memory.

Overnight reorganization of memory representations

An alternative approach to investigating sleep-dependent plasticity is to compare patterns of brain activation before and after a night of sleep. In contrast to measuring changes in functional activity during sleep, this approach aims to find evidence that the neural representation of a memory has been reorganized following a night of sleep.

Although the behavioral characteristics of sleep-dependent motor-sequence learning are now well established, the neural basis of this overnight learning is still unknown. Using a motor-sequence task, the authors recently explored differences between patterns of brain activation before and after sleep using functional magnetic resonance imaging (fMRI) [30]. Following a night of sleep, relative to an equivalent intervening period awake, the authors identified increased postsleep activation in motor control structures of the right primary motor cortex (Fig. 6A) and left cerebellum (Fig. 6B)—changes that likely allow faster motor output and more precise mapping of key-press movements. There were also regions of increased activation in the medial prefrontal lobe and hippocampus (Figs. 6C and 6D), structures that support improved sequencing of motor movements in the correct order. In contrast, the authors identified decreased activity postsleep bilaterally in the parietal cortices (Fig. 6E), possibly reflecting a reduced need for conscious spatial monitoring, and regions of signal decrease throughout the limbic system (Figs. 6F and 6G), indicating a decreased emotional task burden. These results suggest that sleep-dependent motor learning is associated with a large-scale plastic reorganization of memory throughout several brain regions, allowing skilled motor movements to be executed more quickly, accurately, and automatically following sleep. Furthermore, these findings hold important implications for understanding the brain-basis for perfecting real-life skills, and may also signify a potential role for sleep in clinical rehabilitation following brain damage.

Maquet et al [31] also demonstrated sleep-dependent plasticity using a combined visuomotor adaptation task. Subjects trained on the task and then were retested 3 days later, with half the subjects deprived of sleep the first night following training. The remaining half, who slept all 3 nights, showed enhanced behavioral performance at retest and a selective increase in activation in the superior temporal sulcus, a region involved in the evaluation of complex motion patterns. In contrast, subjects deprived of sleep the first night showed no such enhancement of either performance or brain activity, indicating that sleep deprivation had interfered with a latent process of neural plasticity and consolidation.

Using the sleep-dependent visual texture discrimination task described previously, Schwartz et al [32] compared performance-related fMRI patterns of brain activity 24 hours after training, relative to a naïve, untrained condition. They observed significantly greater activation in the 24-hour posttraining condition in the primary visual cortex, suggesting that this functional area representing the visual memory had expended. However, these findings did not distinguish between changes that occurred during training, across posttraining wake time, or across a subsequent night of sleep.

Extending these findings, the authors examined regional brain activity patterns before and after sleep, following equivalent amounts of initial practice on this visual skill task [33]. Postsleep retesting was not only associated with significantly increased activity in the primary visual cortex but in several other visual processing regions following sleep, including at the occipital-temporal junction and in the medial temporal and inferior parietal lobes (regions involved in object detection and identification). In addition, decreased activity postsleep occurred in the right temporal pole, a region involved in emotional visual processing. These findings strengthen the claim that a night of sleep reorganizes

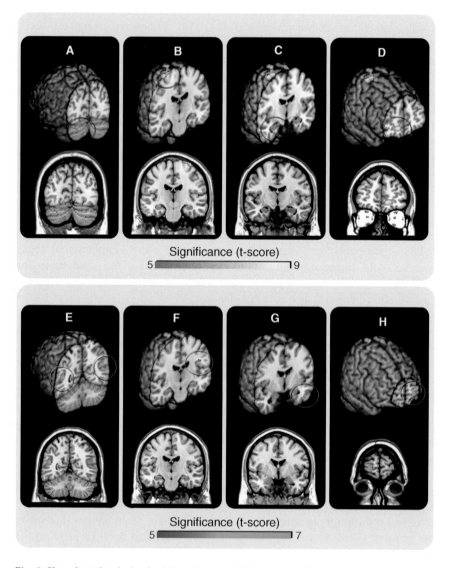

Fig. 6. Sleep-dependent brain plasticity and motor skill learning. Subjects were trained on a sleep-dependent motor sequence task and retested 12 hours later, either following a night of sleep or following intervening wake, during an fMRI brain scanning session. (*A–D*) Increased fMRI activity (*red/yellow*) and (*E–H*) decreased signal activity (*blue*) postsleep, relative to postwake. Activation patterns are displayed on three-dimensional rendered brains (top panel of each graphic), together with corresponding coronal sections (bottom panel of each graphic). Following sleep, regions of increased activation were identified in the right primary motor cortex (*A*), the left cerebellum (*B*), the right hippocampus (*C*), and the right medial prefrontal cortex (*D*). Regions of decreased activity post-sleep were expressed bilaterally in the parietal lobes (*E*), together with the left insula cortex (*F*), left temporal pole (*G*), and left fronto-polar area (*H*), all regions of the extended limbic system. All data are displayed at a corrected threshold of $P < .05$.

the representation of a visual skill memory, with greater activation throughout the visual system following sleep perhaps offering improved identification of the visual stimulus form and its location in space.

Intermediate summary

Learning and memory are dependent on processes of brain plasticity, and sleep-dependent learning and memory consolidation must be mediated by such processes. Using brain-imaging techniques, several studies have now identified changes in the functional patterns of brain activity during posttraining sleep periods, and the reorganization of newly formed skill memories following a night of sleep. These plastic brain changes likely contribute to the refinement of the memory representation, resulting in improved next-day behavioral performance.

Summary and implications

Although the functions of the sleeping brain remain uncertain, rapidly increasing literature now supports the role of sleep in modifying and improving memory. These reports provide an abundance of converging evidence indicating that sleep-dependent mechanisms of neural plasticity lead to skill memory consolidation and consequently to delayed performance improvements. Different forms of simple and complex skill memory appear to require subtly different types of sleep for overnight memory enhancement, and several studies indicate that sleep within the first 24 hours following initial practice is essential for consolidation to develop. Furthermore, growing evidence indicates that naps can also confer a beneficial effect on skill memory, offering protection from performance deterioration and triggering memory enhancements similar to those observed across a normal night of sleep. Most recently, these findings of sleep-dependent learning have been complimented by evidence of sleep-dependent plasticity within the human brain, offering a brain-based explanation for these overnight performance enhancements.

Key future research goals will be to (1) further characterize the range of sensory and motor skills that are dependent on sleep for delayed learning, (2) elucidate whether leaning concurrent skill sets involved in a single complex action (eg, learning motor adaptation and motor sequence programs simultaneously, such as in a common real-life sports scenario) either facilitates or modifies the characteristics of sleep-dependent learning, (3) determine optimal daytime nap and nighttime sleep durations for facilitating skill perfection, and how these may vary for different skill tasks, and (4) identify how much initial daytime practice should occur before an intervening sleep period is inserted, thereby developing the most optimal training routine to allow the fastest learning curve possible.

The implications for learning skilled movements and actions are considerable, and nowhere is this more important than in the learning of procedural memory required for athletic sports. It is not uncommon to train athletes consistently across the day, only to rouse them early the next morning for the purpose of further practice. Based on current evidence, however, such a regime would appear detrimental, and by curtailing sleep durations, one runs the risk of short-changing the brain of sleep-dependent consolidation and plasticity. Instead, building sufficient sleep periods, or even daytime sleep epochs, into training programs may offer the biologically necessary periods of sleep required to maximize skill potential, advancing learning beyond that achieved during initial practice without the need for further task engagement. If efficient skill learning is the goal, long-held beliefs may need to be modified, and the realization made that it is practice, with sleep, that ultimately leads to perfection.

Acknowledgments

We wish to thank Mysha Mason, who conducted the motor napping study reported in this manuscript.

References

[1] Tulving E. How many memory systems are there? Am Psychol 1985;40:385–98.
[2] Squire LR, Zola SM. Structure and function of declarative and nondeclarative memory systems. Proc Natl Acad Sci USA 1996;93(24):13515–22.
[3] McGaugh JL. Memory–a century of consolidation. Science 2000;287(5451):248–51.
[4] Walker MP. A refined model of sleep and the time course of memory formation. Behav Brain Sci 2005;28(1).
[5] Doyon J, Penhune V, Ungerleider LG. Distinct contribution of the cortico-striatal and cortico-cerebellar systems to motor skill learning. Neuropsychologia 2003;41(3):252–62.
[6] Walker MP, Brakefield T, Morgan A, et al. Practice with sleep makes perfect: sleep dependent motor skill learning. Neuron 2002;35(1):205–11.
[7] De Gennaro L, Ferrara M, Bertini M. Topographical distribution of spindles: variations between and within NREM sleep cycles. Sleep Res Online 2000;3(4):155–60.
[8] Sejnowski TJ, Destexhe A. Why do we sleep? Brain Res 2000;886(1–2):208–23.
[9] Fogel S, Jacob J, Smith C. Increased sleep spindle activity following simple motor procedural learning in humans. Paper presented at: Congress Physiological Basis for Sleep Medicine. Uruguay, October 21–26, 2001.
[10] Fischer S, Hallschmid M, Elsner AL, et al. Sleep forms memory for finger skills. Proc Natl Acad Sci USA 2002;99(18):11987–91.
[11] Walker MP, Brakefield T, Seidman J, et al. Sleep and the time course of motor skill learning. Learn Mem 2003;10(4):275–84.
[12] Kuriyama K, Stickgold R, Walker MP. Sleep-dependent learning and motor skill complexity. Learn Mem 2004;11:705–13.
[13] Sakai K, Kitaguchi K, Hikosaka O. Chunking during human visuomotor sequence learning. Exp Brain Res 2003;152(2):229–42.
[14] Robertson EM, Pascual-Leone A, Press DZ. Awareness modifies the skill-learning benefits of sleep. Curr Biol 2004;14(3):208–12.

[15] Smith C, MacNeill C. Impaired motor memory for a pursuit rotor task following Stage 2 sleep loss in college students. J Sleep Res 1994;3(4):206–13.

[16] Huber R, Ghilardi MF, Massimini M, et al. Local sleep and learning. Nature 2004;430(6995): 78–81.

[17] Karni A, Tanne D, Rubenstein BS, et al. Dependence on REM sleep of overnight improvement of a perceptual skill. Science 1994;265(5172):679–82.

[18] Gais S, Plihal W, Wagner U, et al. Early sleep triggers memory for early visual discrimination skills. Nat Neurosci 2000;3(12):1335–9.

[19] Stickgold R, Whidbee D, Schirmer B, et al. Visual discrimination task improvement: a multi-step process occurring during sleep. J Cogn Neurosci 2000;12(2):246–54.

[20] Stickgold R, James L, Hobson JA. Visual discrimination learning requires sleep after training. Nat Neurosci 2000;3(12):1237–8.

[21] Gaab N, Paetzold M, Becker M, et al. The influence of sleep on auditory learning: a behavioral study. Neuroreport 2004;15(4):731–4.

[22] Atienza M, Cantero JL, Dominguez-Marin E. The time course of neural changes underlying auditory perceptual learning. Learn Mem 2002;9(3):138–50.

[23] Atienza M, Cantero JL, Stickgold R. Posttraining sleep enhances automaticity in perceptual discrimination. J Cogn Neurosci 2004;16(1):53–64.

[24] Fenn KM, Nusbaum HC, Margoliash D. Consolidation during sleep of perceptual learning of spoken language. Nature 2003;425(6958):614–6.

[25] Mason M. The effects of naps and interference training on a sleep-dependent procedural motor skill learning task [Honor's Thesis]. Cambridge, Massachusetts: Harvard University; 2004.

[26] Mednick SC, Nakayama K, Cantero JL, et al. The restorative effect of naps on perceptual deterioration. Nat Neurosci 2002;5(7):677–81.

[27] Mednick S, Nakayama K, Stickgold R. Sleep-dependent learning: a nap is as good as a night. Nat Neurosci 2003;6(7):697–8.

[28] Maquet P, Laureys S, Peigneux P, et al. Experience-dependent changes in cerebral activation during human REM sleep. Nat Neurosci 2000;3(8):831–6.

[29] Peigneux P, Laureys S, Fuchs S, et al. Learned material content and acquisition level modulate cerebral reactivation during posttraining rapid-eye-movements sleep. Neuroimage 2003; 20(1):125–34.

[30] Walker MP, Stickgold R, Alsop D, et al. Sleep-dependent plasticity and motor skill learning in the human brain. Sleep 2004;27(Abstract Suppl):A405.

[31] Maquet P, Schwartz S, Passingham R, et al. Sleep-related consolidation of a visuomotor skill: brain mechanisms as assessed by functional magnetic resonance imaging. J Neurosci 2003; 23(4):1432–40.

[32] Schwartz S, Maquet P, Frith C. Neural correlates of perceptual learning: a functional MRI study of visual texture discrimination. Proc Natl Acad Sci USA 2002;99(26):17137–42.

[33] Walker MP, Yoo SS, Stickgold R. The functional anatomy of sleep-dependent visual skill learning. Sleep 2004;27(Abstract Suppl):A406.

ELSEVIER
SAUNDERS

CLINICS
IN SPORTS
MEDICINE

Clin Sports Med 24 (2005) 319–328

Sleep and Circadian Rhythms in Children and Adolescents: Relevance for Athletic Performance of Young People

Mary A. Carskadon, PhD

Sleep and Chronobiology Research Laboratory, E.P. Bradley Hospital,
1011 Veterans Memorial Parkway, East Providence, RI 02915, USA

As described in the article by Van Dongen and Dinges elsewhere in this issue, sleep is regulated by two intrinsic systems: the basic sleep–wake homeostatic system and the circadian timing system. The basic sleep–wake homeostatic system essentially tracks the accumulation of pressure for sleep while we are awake and the dissipation of this pressure while we sleep. This system is also able to track the build up of sleep pressure, or "sleep debt," if an insufficient amount of sleep is obtained over days. The circadian timing system, by contrast, regulates the timing of sleep and waking across each daily cycle. Both systems undergo a developmental progression in humans during the first two decades. Of equal importance to the development of sleep–wake patterns are changes that occur in the psychosocial milieu as youngsters mature.

The intrinsic regulatory systems appear functional in humans at or near birth, but manifest significant maturation in early life. In human newborns, for example, Jenni et al [1] has shown an overnight electroencephalography (EEG) pattern that appears to reflect sleep homeostasis, though occurring in an EEG frequency band different from the proposed homeostatic marker in adults [2], in whom activity in the slowest EEG frequencies (≤ 4 Hz) during sleep is thought to mark the homeostatic process. Confirmation of the findings of Jenni et al with experimental interventions may be necessary; however, we can be sure that

This work was supported by Grants MH52415, AA013252, and NR08381 from the National Institutes of Health.

E-mail address: mary_carskadon@brown.edu

by school age, children have a robust sleep–wake homeostatic process and a copious amount of EEG slow-wave activity (SWA) during sleep.

Where the circadian timing mechanism is concerned, the neural components are extant and viable prenatally in primates [3] and appear to be functionally engaged in regulating sleeping and waking, as marked by activity/inactivity rhythms in the first few months after birth [4,5]. This vigorous regulatory process plays a major role in young children and can even "rule the roost" if parents fail to provide the infant with appropriate time cues to give the internal clock a 24-hour synchronizing stimulus. In these instances, the child's internal day length, typically different from 24 hours, leads to a "free-running" pattern that makes the timing of sleeping and waking incomprehensible for parents [6].

In terms of understanding the sleep–wake and circadian systems in the context of athletic performance, the focus of this article targets older children and the transition to adolescence. Many recent advances in developmental and experimental research underlie a reasonably comprehensive understanding of sleep needs and abilities in young people.

Sleep and psychosocial factors

The roles of parents and lifestyle in the sleep–wake patterns of children and adolescents cannot be overstated. When parents are attentive to setting clear and firm bedtimes in school children (eg, of age 10), most will sleep about 10 hours and wake spontaneously whether on school days or weekends [7]. As parents stop setting bedtimes at the cusp of adolescence, children stay up later and parents' attention focuses more on wake-up time because spontaneous arousals are less likely. This pattern worsens as children pass into adolescence, when many important psychosocial factors attain greater salience. As children get older, school work becomes more demanding and time consuming; youngsters have greater autonomy and more activities available in the evenings, including dating; and many youngsters begin to devote more time to extracurricular events, clubs, and community service. In the last two decades, more and more children and adolescents have "arousing" activities available at all hours and often in their bedrooms, such as television, play stations, Internet connections, cellular phones, and instant messaging. Part-time employment is common among adolescents, with working hours increasing with age; consumption of caffeinated beverages and alcoholic beverages increases, which is also associated with poor sleep patterns; and finally, activities related to athletics, such as lengthy practices and away games, eat into youngsters' time budgets. With all of these competing activities and often early school starting times, young people live in a nearly constant state of chronic insufficient sleep.

Coping with this state of affairs for many young people often involves coming to school late or missing school altogether because the child is over-tired [8]. The student athlete may "bunk" school in the morning to be awake for an after-school practice. Oftentimes, neither the school schedule nor the practice and events schedules are friendly to a young person's sleep needs, and young people are set up to do poorly. The preponderance of evidence indicates that students with short nights and irregular sleep patterns perform poorly in school and in other aspects of their lives, including a tendency for depressed mood [9,10]. These behavioral and psychosocial features of a young person's lifestyle affect sleep in important ways, and the maturational changes in the intrinsic sleep–wake regulatory processes are interwoven with the more external processes.

Maturation of bioregulatory factors

Sleep need in children and adolescents

Older school children, such as those in fourth and fifth grades, appear to require roughly 10 hours of sleep each night. This sleep requirement is not true of every child; just as with many biological factors, the normal requirement is a range around this mean value. A good rule of thumb for determining sleep need is that a child's sleep need is met when he or she wakes spontaneously in the morning and does not sleep more on weekends than weekdays. A landmark longitudinal study by the Stanford group demonstrated that from ages 10, 11, and 12 to approximately ages 15, 16, and 17, children will sleep over 90% of a 10-hour opportunity, roughly 9.2 hours a night. The children were often awake at the end of the 10-hour sleep period when they were preteens; however, they always required a wake-up call after achieving midpuberty [11]. Furthermore, at midpuberty, the children manifested a midday increase in physiologically measured sleepiness, even though they slept the same amount at night. Early on, this finding was taken to mean that teenagers not only require as much sleep as their younger counterparts, but required more. Subsequent research has explained the sleep–wake pattern in terms of ways in which the homeostatic and circadian regulatory processes change across the transition to adolescence [12]. Of critical importance, however, is that a teenager's need for sleep appears just about identical to when he or she was a preteen, even though nearly every teen succumbs to the adolescent lifestyle (and the constraints of school schedules) by getting less sleep than required on most school nights and partially compensating by oversleeping on weekend days.

Maturation of sleep-wake homeostasis in school children

Longitudinal and cross-sectional studies of sleep in children and adolescents usually measure sleep in the laboratory using the child's typical sleep schedule [13–16]. Even so, other than a reduction in sleep quantity with age (and a concomitant reduction of rapid eye movement [REM] sleep), few consistent changes are found. The one exception is that these studies consistently demonstrate a significant reduction in the amount of deep slow-wave sleep (SWS), the type of sleep most closely tied to the homeostatic sleep–wake system. Even with a well-controlled longitudinal study in which sleep was kept at 10 hours nightly rather than changing with typical patterns, the chief change was a 40% decline in the amount of SWS across the early years of the second decade [17].

One interpretation of this finding is that the homeostatic sleep–wake process that dissipates sleep pressure early in the night changes across this developmental phase, the decline indicating an overall reduction in sleep need. More recent research using spectral analysis of sleep EEG to examine the homeostatic parameters of nocturnal SWA shows rather that the process itself is not altered by pubertal development [18]. Overall EEG spectral power declines in most frequency ranges and in REM and nonrapid eye movement (NREM) sleep, indicating that a non–state-specific process is responsible. The most likely explanatory hypothesis is that cortical EEG amplitude declines in association with cortical synaptic pruning [19,20] and is therefore more phenomenological than functional.

Although the sleep-pressure–dissipating aspect of the sleep–wake homeostatic process does not demonstrate a functional difference across adolescent development, the accumulation of sleep pressure across a waking day does. We have converging evidence of this developmental shift from sleep propensity and sleep recovery data in response to sleep deprivation in pre- and late pubertal children. In the first place, the speed of falling asleep after about 14 hours is significantly faster in prepubertal children aged approximately 11 and 12 years as compared with pubertal 13- and 14-year-old children [21]. Furthermore, simulations including sleep recordings before and after sleep deprivation in these groups of children indicate that the accumulation of "process S," the sleep pressure that builds during wakefulness, is faster in the prepubertal than pubertal youngsters [22]. One interpretation of this set of findings is that it becomes easier for young people to stay awake longer as they mature, even though other evidence indicates that they do not need less sleep. When this "permissive" brain pattern is combined with the maturational changes of the circadian timing system described below, the teenager faces a very tough challenge to obtaining adequate sleep.

Maturation of the circadian timing system in school children

Measurement of the circadian timing system in human children and adolescents requires examining behavioral estimates of circadian-phase preference or biological signals generated by the circadian clock, often taking such measures under challenging laboratory protocols. A prominent feature of sleep patterns in the transition from childhood to adolescence is that the schedule becomes later for bedtime and waking (except, of course, when wake-up time is forced to an early hour by school schedules) [10]. A small study provided one of the first indications that this adolescent delay in the timing of sleep emanated in part from circadian timing rather than simply as a result of adolescent lifestyle choices. The study showed that phase preference favored eveningness over morningness in parallel with self-reported progression of pubertal development [23]. This finding was subsequently confirmed using the phase of melatonin secretion to mark the circadian timing system and physician ratings of pubertal development [24].

The precise nature of the maturational changes in the circadian timing system across adolescence is not yet known, although several features have been examined. One of the mechanisms by which circadian timing can delay is through lengthening the period of the circadian clock; that is, a longer internal day length [25]. Under normal day-to-day circumstances, features of the environment that have a 24-hour period, particularly the light–dark cycle, entrain the internal clock to 24 hours. The phase angle with which the internal clock time aligns with the external day, however, is determined in part by the intrinsic circadian period: the phase angle of entrainment is delayed in parallel with the extent to which the internal day length exceeds 24 hours. Thus, a major question has been whether the internal day lengthens during the adolescent transition.

Although the hypothesis is simple, testing it is difficult because the method for measuring period involves prolonged (2- to 3-week) laboratory stays under carefully controlled conditions. Fig. 1 illustrates an experimental protocol used to assess period in adolescents by collecting serial measures of salivary mela-

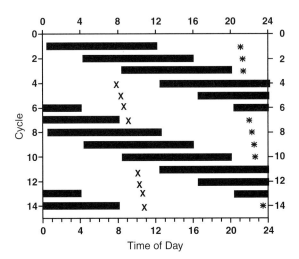

Fig. 1. Schematic diagram of the forced desynchrony protocol used to determine intrinsic period of the circadian timing system. Scheduled sleep episodes (black bars) are shown for a 28-hour day length on 14 consecutive cycles. Participants live in the laboratory under dim light conditions (approximately 15 lux) so that dim-light melatonin onset and offset phases can be determined from serial saliva samples. A hypothetical pattern of the melatonin onset (*) and offset (x) phase determinations is shown, indicating that the circadian timing system is running free of the 28-hour day length at a period of about 24.2 hours.

tonin onset and offset across 12 cycles on a 28-hour day, or forced desynchrony [26]. Our initial analysis of intrinsic period in adolescents showed that
the circadian period appeared longer than reported by others in young adults;
however the number of adolescent subjects was insufficient to test the pubertal
hypothesis [27]. A subsequent analysis compared the distribution of values for
intrinsic period in the adolescent sample with samples of adults in whom period
was also derived from melatonin phase markers in a 28-hour forced desynchrony
paradigm [28,29]. The results demonstrate that mean period of the circadian
clock in the combined adolescent sample is significantly longer than in the adult
sample [30]. These findings suggest that longer internal day lengths may
emerge in adolescence and contribute to the delay of sleep and to a reorganization
of sleep timing to the circadian day.

In conclusion, the circadian and lifestyle changes conspire to place sleep of
adolescents in a markedly delayed time relative to younger children and to adults.
In fact, a recent analysis of self-reported sleep data and chronotype in a sample
of thousands of Europeans defined a marker for "the end of adolescence,"
designated as the age when the pattern of sleep delay begins to reverse [31].

*Sleep–wake homeostasis and the circadian timing system: consequences for
timing of sleep, wake, and alertness*

One consequence of the maturational changes in sleep homeostasis, circadian
rhythms, and lifestyle choices is an alteration in the alignment of sleep to the
underlying timing system. Thus, the timing of sleep delays with respect to the
external clock time, but actually is earlier in its alignment to the internal clock
[12]. As a consequence, if sleep is optimal—that is, when the young person
obtains adequate sleep routinely—then the prepubertal youngster is alert and
wide awake throughout the day, and the pubertal adolescent manifests a
midafternoon decline in alertness and performance occurring approximately
8 hours after waking. This decline reverses spontaneously, as alertness is
buffered in a clock-dependent manner due to the circadian timing system.
If, by contrast, sleep is not adequate and a sleep deficit (such as it described
by Dement elsewhere in this issue) has accumulated, then children are most tired
in the afternoon and into the evening, whereas pubertal adolescents are extremely
impaired in the morning because they wake close to the circadian trough of
alertness without the buffering effect of restorative sleep. Nevertheless, the older
adolescent, even when under conditions of chronic insufficient sleep, experiences
a lifting of energy late in the day, benefiting from clock-dependent alerting in
the evening [12].

The role of napping has not been well studied with respect to athletic performance. As noted by Van Dongen and Dinges in this issue, sleep termination
is accompanied by obtunded performance called *sleep inertia*, which may last
for 30 to 60 minutes. Under conditions of insufficient sleep (5 hours a night for
1 week), a 45-minute midday nap occurring approximately 6 hours after waking

was found to support alertness and mood for approximately 8 hours [32]. On the other hand, participants showed no benefit the next morning from an afternoon nap. In other words, sleepiness in the prenap morning hours worsened with each day on the schedule [32].

How and when is athletic performance affected by sleep and circadian systems?

Little work has been done to assess the issues of athletic performance, sleep, and circadian rhythms in children and adolescents. Yet, as Van Dongen and Dinges note, Walter and Stickgold describe, and Dement portrays elsewhere in this issue, reaction time, vigilance, learning, and alertness are impaired by insufficient sleep. Mood and motivation also suffer negative effects from poor sleep. Based on data from studies of children and adolescents and findings of adult studies, we can derive the following presumptions regarding likely outcomes for athletic performance:

- Prepubertal children and adolescents generally function better early in the day than in late afternoon and evening;
- Pubescent and postpubescent adolescents manifest worst performance in the morning;
- Performance in children and adolescents benefits from adequate sleep obtained routinely on a regular schedule;
- Adolescent travel teams heading westward across time zones have an advantage over home teams early in the day;
- High-school or collegiate travel athletic teams taking extended training trips (eg, spring break) of a week or more may experience schedule difficulties on the return home. This scenario is most problematic for teams on the east coast that travel west, as student athletes may return home with a significant sleep-phase delay that is difficult to correct.

Role of melatonin and gonadotropins

Melatonin is a pineal hormone secreted in the brain during nighttime, and suppressed by light through suppression of an enzyme (hydroxyindole-o-methyltransferase) in the metabolic pathway. Melatonin has been alluded to as the "hands on the circadian clock," identifying the boundaries of the biological night. On another level, however, melatonin may also be involved in the timing of puberty. Melatonin is thought by some to inhibit gonadotropin releasing hormone (GnRH) secretion, thus delaying the GnRH initiation of nocturnal pulsatile release of luteinizing hormone and follicle stimulating hormone. According to one hypothesis, nocturnal pineal melatonin release remains constant, but the effective level declines as physical growth increases the volume of distribution; when melatonin falls below a threshold, GnRH is freed of its inhibitory influence and begins the pubertal cascade [33]. The augmentation of nocturnal gonadotropin release occurs before the physical signs of puberty are apparent. Typically, girls achieve these milestones at younger ages than boys by a year or two, and a secular trend for earlier age of pubertal onset over the last century and in westernized societies is tied to improved nutrition and growth.

The interactions among exercise, heavy training, melatonin, and puberty are not known. One might speculate that in young female athletes whose training regimen restricts weight gain (eg, gymnasts), the onset of puberty and associated physical changes may be delayed because small stature may prevent melatonin levels from falling below the critical threshold to disinhibit GnRH. Exercise may also affect melatonin secretion. Although data are not consistent, one study showed that melatonin levels were increased in association with exercise in adolescent girls [34,35], which would be consistent with the theory that melatonin will delay pubertal onset. Whether melatonin plays a role in the amenorrhea experienced by adolescent and young adult females undergoing rigorous physical training has not been clearly defined.

Most male athletes are not required to maintain small stature and low weight. In contrast, with the possible exception of wrestling and some gymnastic events, male athletes are often encouraged to increase physical size and strength. The onset of puberty is associated with an augmentation of these efforts. The effects of steroid supplements on melatonin, sleep, and circadian rhythms of young athletes are not well described.

In terms of administering melatonin to alter circadian timing—whether to assist with advancing sleep timing in a phase-delayed adolescent, to assist in adjusting to a time-zone change, or to modify pubertal timing—several concerns are relevant:

- Exogenous melatonin may affect reproductive maturation [36];
- The timing of melatonin administration is crucial to its effects on the circadian timing system and if mistimed can have an effect opposite of the intended direction of change [35];
- Natural daylight or artificial light, when appropriately timed, is more effective at phase resetting than is melatonin [35];
- Melatonin, through its potential soporific effect, may impair performance;
- Though some have speculated that the hypothermic effect of melatonin may be beneficial for extending temperature-dependent physical exertion endurance, current evidence is unconvincing [35].

References

[1] Jenni OG, Borbely AA, Achermann P. Development of the nocturnal sleep electroencephalogram in human infants. Am J Physiol Regul Integr Comp Physiol 2004;286(3):R528–38.
[2] Borbely AA. A two process model of sleep regulation. Hum Neurobiol 1982;1(3):195–204.

[3] Hao H, Rivkees SA. The biological clock of very premature primate infants is responsive to light. Proc Natl Acad Sci USA 1999;96(5):2426 – 9.

[4] Rivkees SA. Emergence and influences of circadian rhythmicity in infants. Clin Perinatol 2004;31(2):217 – 28 [v–vi.].

[5] Rivkees SA, Mayes L, Jacobs H, et al. Rest-activity patterns of premature infants are regulated by cycled lighting. Pediatrics 2004;113(4):833 – 9.

[6] Ferber R. Solve your child's sleep problems. New York: Simon and Schuster; 1985.

[7] Anders TF, Carskadon MA, Dement WC, et al. Sleep habits of children and the identification of pathologically sleepy children. Child Psychiatry Hum Dev 1978;9(1):56 – 63.

[8] Wahlstrom K. Changing times: findings from the first longitudinal study of later school start times. National Association of Secondary School Principals Bulletin 2002;86:3 – 21.

[9] Wolfson AR, Carskadon MA. Understanding adolescents' sleep patterns and school performance: a critical appraisal. Sleep Med Rev 2003;7(6):491 – 506.

[10] Wolfson AR, Carskadon MA. Sleep schedules and daytime functioning in adolescents. Child Dev 1998;69(4):875 – 87.

[11] Carskadon MA, Harvey K, Duke P, et al. Pubertal changes in daytime sleepiness. Sleep 1980; 2(4):453 – 60.

[12] Carskadon MA, Acebo C. Regulation of sleepiness in adolescents: update, insights, and speculation. Sleep 2002;25(6):606 – 14.

[13] Coble PA, Kupfer DJ, Taska LS, et al. EEG Sleep of normal healthy children. Part 1: Findings using standard measurement methods. Sleep 1984;7:289 – 303.

[14] Feinberg I, Koresko R, Heller N. EEG sleep patterns as a function of normal and pathological aging in man. J Psychiatr Res 1967;1:107 – 44.

[15] Karacan I, Anch M, Thornby JI, et al. Longitudinal sleep patterns during pubertal growth: four-year follow-up. Pediatr Res 1975;9:842 – 6.

[16] Williams RL, Karacan I, Hursch CJ. Electroencephalography (EEG) of human sleep: clinical applications. New York: John Wiley and Sons; 1974.

[17] Carskadon MA. The second decade. In: Guilleminault C, editor. Sleeping and waking disorders: indications and techniques. Menlo Park, CA: Addison Wesley; 1982. p. 99 – 125.

[18] Jenni OG, Carskadon MA. Spectral analysis of the sleep electroencephalogram during adolescence. Sleep 2004;27(4):774 – 83.

[19] Feinberg I. Schizophrenia: caused by a fault in programmed synaptic elimination during adolescence? J Psychiatr Res 1982;17(4):319 – 34.

[20] Sowell ER, Thompson PM, Tessner KD, et al. Mapping continued brain growth and gray matter density reduction in dorsal frontal cortex: inverse relationships during postadolescent brain maturation. J Neurosci 2001;21(22):8819 – 29.

[21] Taylor DJ, Carskadon MA, Acebo C, et al. Changes in levels of daytime sleepiness across puberty. Sleep 2003;26(Suppl):A189.

[22] Jenni O, Achermann P, Carskadon MA. Maturational changes of sleep homeostasis across puberty. J Sleep Res 2004;12:361.

[23] Carskadon MA, Vieira C, Acebo C. Association between puberty and delayed phase preference. Sleep 1993;16(3):258 – 62.

[24] Carskadon MA, Acebo C, Richardson GS, et al. An approach to studying circadian rhythms of adolescent humans. J Biol Rhythms 1997;12(3):278 – 89.

[25] Aschoff J. Free-running and entrained rhythms. In: Aschoff J, editor. Handbook of behavioral neurology: biological rhythms. New York: Plenum Press; 1981. p. 81 – 93.

[26] Czeisler CA, Allan JS, Kronauer RE. A method for assaying the effects of therapeutic agents on the period of the endogenous circadian pacemaker in man. In: Godbout R, editor. Sleep and biological rhythms: basic mechanisms and applications to psychiatry. New York: Oxford University Press; 1990. p. 87 – 98.

[27] Carskadon MA, Labyak SE, Acebo C, et al. Intrinsic circadian period of adolescent humans measured in conditions of forced desynchrony. Neurosci Lett 1999;260(2):129 – 32.

[28] Czeisler CA, Duffy JF, Shanahan TL, et al. Stability, precision, and near-24-hour period of the human circadian pacemaker. Science 1999;284(5423):2177 – 81.

[29] Wright KP, Hughes RJ, Kronauer RE, et al. Intrinsic near-24-h pacemaker period determines limits of circadian entrainment to a weak synchronizer in humans. Proc Natl Acad Sci USA 2001;98(24):14027–32.

[30] Carskadon MA, Acebo C, Jenni OG. Regulation of adolescent sleep: implications for behavior. Ann N Y Acad Sci 2004;1021:276–91.

[31] Roenneberg T, Kuehnle T, Pramstaller PP, et al. A marker for the end of adolescence. Curr Biol 2004;14(24).

[32] Carskadon MA, Dement WC. Effects of a daytime nap on sleepiness during sleep restriction. Sleep Res 1986;15:69.

[33] Silman R. Melatonin and the human gonadotrophin-releasing hormone pulse generator. J Endocrinol 1991;128(1):7–11.

[34] Barriga C, Marchena JM, Ortega E. Melatonin levels and exercise in adolescent boys and girls. Biog Amines 2000;15:643–65.

[35] Atkinson G, Drust B, Reilly T, et al. The relevance of melatonin to sports medicine and science. Sports Med 2003;33(11):809–31.

[36] Silman RE. Melatonin: a contraceptive for the nineties. Eur J Obstet Gynecol Reprod Biol 1993;49(1–2):3–9.

CLINICS
IN SPORTS
MEDICINE

ELSEVIER
SAUNDERS

Clin Sports Med 24 (2005) 329–341

Sleep Apnea and Sports Performance

Helene A. Emsellem, MD[a,b,*], Karen E. Murtagh, CRNP[a]

[a]The Center for Sleep & Wake Disorders, 5454 Wisconsin Avenue, Suite 1725, Chevy Chase,
MD 20815, USA
[b]The George Washington School of Medicine, 2300 Street, NW, Washington, DC 20037, USA

The image of the elite athlete in our society is one of an individual who is in excellent condition and physically fit for the demands of the chosen sport. Elite athletes are not thought of as being at risk for medical conditions that are generally associated with middle age, obesity, and deconditioned status. Nonetheless, physical characteristics associated with optimal performance in certain sports may predispose athletes to obstructive sleep apnea-hypopnea syndrome (OSA).

OSA is a significant and often under-recognized health issue in our society. It is characterized by repeated episodes of partial or complete pharyngeal airflow obstruction during sleep, despite continued respiratory effort. These obstructive events result in oxygen desaturations, increased sympathetic tone, and arousals, fragmenting sleep continuity and resulting in nonrestorative sleep and daytime sleepiness. Snoring is a common feature of OSA. In some patients, there may be a progression over time from mild snoring, to loud disruptive snoring with arousals (termed *upper airway resistance syndrome*), to actual episodes of airflow obstruction and OSA. OSA has been linked with the development of hypertension, cardiovascular disease, stroke, cognitive impairment, mood disorder, and sexual dysfunction [1]. Not only are the effects on sleep quality, quantity, and continuity believed to play a role in the etiology of these related health issues but also the metabolic consequences and oxidative stress associated with the disorder [2–4].

* Corresponding author. The Center for Sleep & Wake Disorders, 5454 Wisconsin Avenue, Suite 1725, Chevy Chase, MD 20815.
    E-mail address: sleepdoc@sleepdoc.com (H.A. Emsellem).

0278-5919/05/$ – see front matter © 2005 Elsevier Inc. All rights reserved.
doi:10.1016/j.csm.2005.01.002   *sportsmed.theclinics.com*

OSA must be distinguished from central sleep apnea, which is a rare, independent condition associated with central nervous system disorders and a failure of the central respiratory drive mechanisms.

Prevalence and risk factors

OSA affects 2% to 4% of the middle-aged population [5] and is more common in men than women. In addition, there is an increased prevalence among Blacks, Hispanics, and Pacific Islanders. Certain anatomic features can be risk factors for OSA at any age. A body mass index (BMI) more than 28 kg/m^2 or a heavy neck, particularly with a circumference greater than 40 cm, are correlated with the diagnosis. Retrognathia, tonsillar or adenoidal hypertrophy, macroglossia, a large uvula, and a low soft palate all predispose to OSA. Medical conditions associated with apnea include Marfan's syndrome, acromegaly, polycystic ovary syndrome, and hypothyroidism [1].

Symptomatology

Snoring is the most common symptom associated with apnea. Age of over 40 years, obesity, witnessed episodes of gasping or stoppage of airflow during sleep, and daytime sleepiness increase the predictive value of snoring for OSA [6]. Other nighttime symptoms include reflux (resulting from elevated gastric and abdominal pressures related to breathing effort), nocturia, a choking sensation, and frequent awakenings. Sleep is often reported as nonrestorative despite the number of hours slept. Daytime symptoms can include morning headache, depression, irritability, anxiety, concentration and attentional difficulties, memory impairment, diminished dexterity, decreased libido, fatigue, and sleepiness [1].

Pathophysiology

OSA arises as a result of airway closure at a pharyngeal level (Fig. 1). Given the relationship of the pharynx to the esophagus and the role pharyngeal structures play in phonation, it is necessary for segments of the pharynx to be compliant. Active neuromuscular innervation of the pharynx is required for patency to be maintained. With inspiration, negative pressure generated by diaphragmatic contraction results in a drop in pharyngeal intraluminal pressure. This action pulls the pharyngeal structures inward. The net pharyngeal lumen size during inspiration is therefore determined by the dynamic balance between the forces that would serve to collapse the airway (negative inspiratory pressure) versus

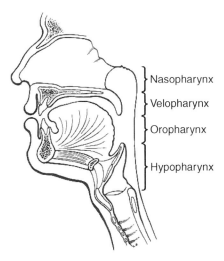

Fig. 1. Anatomy of the upper airway. (*From* Van Lunteren E, Strohl KP. Striated muscles of the upper airways. In: Matthew OP, Sant' Ambrogio G, editors. Respiratory function of the upper airway. New York: Marcel Dekker; 1988. p. 87–123; with permission.)

those that would keep it open (muscle tonus) (Fig. 2). There is potential for obstruction at any level of the pharynx, and in 75% of patients who have OSA there is more than one site of partial or full obstruction [7].

At sleep onset, muscle tone in the pharynx decreases, narrowing the lumen. This narrowing results in greater resistance to airflow, thereby predisposing to snoring and obstruction. Continued efforts to ventilate against an obstructed or partially obstructed airway cause an increase in sympathetic activity and blood pressure. Oxygen saturation decreases and PCO_2 rises. Ultimately, the apnea terminates, typically with a gasp, snort, or loud snore and an arousal or even an awakening [8]. The severity of apnea is related to how frequently the events

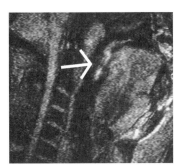
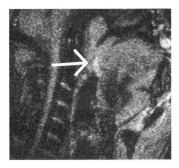

Fig. 2. CT on left illustrates patent pharyngeal airway. Figure on right documents pharyngeal collapse during inspiration in patient with obstructive sleep apnea.

occur on an hourly basis, the duration of each event, the degree of associated hypoxemia, and the intensity of arousals with the restitution of airflow.

Health consequences of obstructive sleep apnea

Cardiovascular

OSA is associated with the metabolic syndrome, arrhythmias, hypertension, dyslipidemia, cardiovascular disease, and stroke, although the exact mechanisms are not yet fully elucidated [9–13]. OSA may also be associated with pulmonary hypertension and right ventricular hypertrophy [13]. Oxidative stress resulting from repeated episodes of hypoxia is believed to result in the expression of a number of redox-sensitive genes, such as the inflammatory cytokines tumor necrosis factor α (TNF-α) and interleukin-6. The downstream effects of endothelial cell damage/dysfunction and the promotion of atherosclerosis can occur as a consequence of the expression of a number of these redox-sensitive genes [2,3]. Low-density lipoprotein is more susceptible to oxidation in OSA and can also promote further endothelial damage and atherosclerosis [14]. Endothelial dysfunction is thought to exist in OSA, even in the absence of overt cardiovascular disease [15,16].

Metabolic/endocrinologic

OSA has been associated with obesity, impaired glucose tolerance, insulin resistance, and hyperleptinemia. The insulin resistance and hyperleptinemia have been shown to be independent of BMI in OSA patients [17]. TNF-α, which is elevated in OSA and obesity, is associated with insulin resistance and also stimulates leptin secretion [18]. In addition to its effects on appetite and energy expenditure, leptin is a respiratory stimulant [19], though the degree to which this plays a role in untreated OSA is not clear. Insulin resistance, in addition to hyperandrogenism, is also seen in women who have polycystic ovary syndrome and have an increased incidence of OSA [20]. The above metabolic abnormalities, particularly with regard to leptin and glucose regulation, can further promote cardiovascular disease and weight gain. This effect serves to worsen the OSA, and it is not uncommon for an increase to occur in daytime eating in an effort to feel better or more alert, thereby further worsening what is a vicious pathologic cycle.

Sexual dysfunction in men is a potential consequence of OSA. There is dysfunction of the pituitary-gonadal axis in men, resulting in decreased testosterone levels. This effect is reversible with treatment for the OSA [21,22]. Virtually no information on sexual dysfunction in women with OSA is reported in the literature.

Growth hormone (GH) stimulates growth of skin, muscle, cartilage, bone, and visceral tissues. It also induces lipolysis and insulin resistance. GH is regulated by way of a feedback loop, though other factors can also affect its secretion. Exercise, fasting, hypoglycemia, and stress can increase GH levels, whereas obesity and hyperglycemia reduce them [23]. GH, which is secreted in a circadian pulsatile fashion and peaks with the first cycle of slow-wave sleep, is lower in patients who have untreated OSA. Treatment of apnea and restoration of slow-wave sleep has been shown to improve GH levels from baseline pretreatment levels [24]. Although GH excess and deficiency have been linked with cardiovascular morbidity [23,25], the role of altered GH levels in OSA, with regard to cardiovascular risk, is unclear at this time.

Neurocognitive

Alertness issues and neurocognitive deficits associated with OSA are well-recognized. It is not clear what the relative contribution is of the repetitive episodes of hypoxia versus the fragmentation of sleep associated with apneic events, but both are thought to play a role in the etiology of fatigue and cognitive impairment in OSA [3,4]. Daytime sleepiness is a significant societal issue, not just in terms of productivity and quality of life but also in terms of safety while engaged in potentially dangerous activities, such as driving. More than 800,000 drivers were involved in OSA-related collisions in 2000, and it has been estimated that treating all drivers who have OSA would save 980 lives per year and billions of dollars in collision costs [26].

Diagnosis of obstructive sleep apnea

Index of suspicion

There should be a high index of suspicion for OSA in those individuals who report loud disruptive snoring and daytime sleepiness, particularly if obesity, hypertension, and witnessed episodes of apnea are observed. Reflux, morning headache, dry mouth, nasal congestion, and evidence of anatomic narrowing of the pharyngeal airway on examination increase the suspicion further, as does an increased neck circumference. Retrognathia, tonsillar or adenoidal hypertrophy, macroglossia, a large uvula, and a low soft palate all predispose to OSA [1,6] and may represent significant risk factors in nonobese patients who have normal neck circumference. Daytime sleepiness and fatigue are common complaints associated with OSA and must be taken seriously, given their negative impact on performance and quality of life. In the setting of a regulated sleep–wake cycle with adequate allocation of time for sleep (minimum 6.5 to 7 hours per night), the Epworth Sleepiness Scale (ESS) [27] can be easily administered to quickly assess sleepiness. The ESS is a subjective rating scale that has been validated in controlled studies against the Multiple Sleep Latency Test, an objec-

---

THE EPWORTH SLEEPINESS SCALE

Name: _____

Today's date: _____ Your age (years): _____

Your sex (male = M; female = F): _____

How likely are you to doze off or fall asleep in the following situations, in contrast to feeling just tired? This refers to your usual way of life in recent times. Even if you have not done some of these things recently try to work out how they would have affected you. Use the following scale to choose the *most appropriate number* for each situation:

0 = would *never* doze
1 = *slight* chance of dozing
2 = *moderate* chance of dozing
3 = *high* chance of dozing

Situation	Chance of dozing
Sitting and reading	_____
Watching TV	_____
Sitting inactive in a public place (eg, a theater or a meeting)	_____
As a passenger in a car for an hour without a break	_____
Lying down to rest in the afternoon when circumstances permit	_____
Sitting and talking to someone	_____
Sitting quietly after a lunch without alcohol	_____
In a car, while stopped for a few minutes in traffic	_____

Thank you for your cooperation

Fig. 3. The Epworth Sleepiness Scale.

tive sleep laboratory-based test for sleepiness. The ESS asks patients to reflect on their sleepiness and report their chance of dozing in key life situations (Fig. 3).

Polysomnography

The diagnosis of OSA is made by polysomnography, an overnight monitoring of physiologic parameters including electroencephalogram, nasal and oral airflow, EKG, chest and abdominal movements, oxygen saturations, eye movements, chin electromyogram, and limb movements. This provides a detailed assessment of the cycling through the stages of sleep (sleep architecture), the degree of disordered breathing, desaturations, arousals, and limb movements. Disordered breathing events are categorized and tallied. An apnea is defined as a cessation of airflow lasting 10 seconds or longer. An hypopnea is an abnormal respiratory event also lasting 10 seconds or longer with at least a 30% reduction in airflow and at least a 4% drop in oxygen saturations [28]. These events are totaled and an apnea-hypopnea index (AHI) of disordered breathing per hour of sleep is calculated allowing for standardization of results. In some individuals airway resistance may cause more subtle airflow changes with less than 4% desaturation, yet still cause arousal. These respiratory effort–related arousals may be included with apneas and hypopneas to calculate a more sensitive measure of airflow resistance, the respiratory disturbance index (RDI). An AHI of 5 to 15 per hour is considered mildly abnormal in adults and an AHI over 30 per hour is severe. In addition to the AHI, severity of OSA is also related to the extent to which arousals following disordered breathing events fragment sleep continuity and the degree of oxygen desaturation. Treatment decisions are based on the these parameters and the patient's clinical presentation, and must be individualized.

Although the most accurate means of evaluating for OSA is in a sleep laboratory, there is a variety of portable monitoring devices available, each having varying efficacy, for use as home screening devices for sleep apnea.

Treatment modalities

Continuous positive airway pressure

Continuous nasal positive airway pressure (CPAP) is the gold standard for the treatment of OSA and is the treatment of choice for patients who have moderate to severe obstructive sleep apnea. The concept of treatment is to splint the airway open with air above ambient room air pressure, delivered to the patient by a mask worn over the nose during sleep [29,30]. With a CPAP device the patient is exposed to equal inspiratory and expiratory air pressure. Some patients have difficulty exhaling against the pressure and may benefit from using a bilevel positive airway pressure (BiPAP) device that allows for independent adjustment of the inspiratory and expiratory pressures. Sophisticated equipment is also currently available that senses airflow resistance and adjusts the pressure as required according to a preprogrammed algorithm (autotitrating CPAP). Patient usage may be tracked by some CPAP equipment with memory chips that record dates and hours of use. Although some patients are resistant to the idea of CPAP at the outset, the great benefit derived from the treatment usually outweighs the initial reservations. Compliance may be enhanced by patient education and support [31].

Surgical and medical interventions

The American Sleep Disorders Association Practice Parameters [44] for the treatment of OSA advise that surgery may be indicated in patients who have a specific, underlying, surgically correctable abnormality that is causing the sleep apnea, and may also be indicated in patients for whom other noninvasive treatments have been unsuccessful or rejected. There are several surgical interventions aimed at maintaining patency of the upper airway. These procedures are all plagued with success rates as low as 50% and difficulty selecting candidates who may benefit. The procedures can include tonsillectomy/adenoidectomy, septoplasty, turbinectomy, and uvulopalatopharyngoplasty. Laser-assisted uvulopalatoplasty, somnoplasty, and injection snoreplasty are less invasive procedures performed in the outpatient setting to reduce snoring with very limited efficacy for the management of OSA. Other more extensive surgeries involving jaw advancement are available and may be effective on selected patients, though are not generally recommended as a first-line treatment [30,32]. Treatment of allergies and chronic sinus disease may not only facilitate treatment but may improve apnea. See the article by Komarow and Postolache elsewhere in this issue for further discussion of seasonal allergies.

Oral appliances

Oral appliances designed to reposition the mandible and base of the tongue forward during sleep may be useful in the management of mild OSA, snoring, and upper airway resistance syndrome, or when CPAP is not tolerated. These devices are generally not a first-line treatment for the patient who has moderate to severe OSA [33]. The efficacy of oral appliances is limited by the range of motion of the temporomandibular joints and tolerability.

Behavioral changes

Weight loss and exercise should be encouraged in the obese patient who has OSA. The poor success rate of most diet programs limits the efficacy of dieting as a primary intervention. Alcohol should be avoided before bedtime, as it can disrupt sleep architecture and because its muscle relaxant properties contribute to an increase in upper airway resistance, thus worsening apnea. When apnea is predominantly positional (supine), management can include avoidance of this position during sleep.

Treatment efficacy

Treatment efficacy may be assessed subjectively by the resolution of symptoms such as snoring, observed apneic episodes, and daytime sleepiness. Serial administration of the ESS may help to quantify residual daytime sleepiness. Repeat polysomnographic monitoring is reserved for use in the setting of persistent, unexplained symptoms.

Obstructive sleep apnea in athletes

Hypoxic training

There is little data available on the incidence of OSA in athletes. For athletes training at altitude, an increase in sleep-disordered breathing has been observed [34]. The concept of training at altitude is based on increasing performance by exposure to hypoxia, thereby stimulating erythropoietin production and increasing exercise performance [35]. The stress associated with intermittent hypoxia is also thought to be cross-protective for other stressors. With altitude training, there is an induction of stress-related proteins and antioxidant enzymes, and protection of the myocardium has been observed [36].

Not all athletes benefit from intermittent hypoxic training, however [37]. In the review of the effects of intermittent hypoxia by Neubauer [3], she cites data showing an increase in right ventricular mass associated with chronic intermittent hypoxia in animal models, thought to be related to pulmonary hypertension and vascular remodeling. She also cites support for the intermittent hypoxia alone as being causative for the hypertension seen in OSA. The chronicity of intermittent hypoxia may determine whether a response is protective or pathologic. This raises the question of what amount, if any, of intermittent hypoxic training is beneficial for the athlete and what level then becomes deleterious either to short-term or long-term health, or both. More research is needed to determine if prior exposure to intermittent hypoxemia caused by sleep apnea puts effected athletes at greater risk for complications of sleep apnea, such as fatigue, when they are subjected to further hypoxemia at altitude.

Effects of physical activity

Ari et al [38] evaluated the effects of exercise in physically active elderly men who did not have OSA compared with sedentary controls. There were significant positive differences in maximal oxygen uptake, testosterone levels, GH levels, reaction time, and insulin-like growth factor seen in the active group.

Giebelhaus et al [39] evaluated exercise as a potential treatment for OSA using a small sample. After 6 weeks of physical exercise twice weekly, they found an improvement in the RDI on repeat polysomnography in the absence of a change in BMI. The results were postulated to be associated with a stabilization of airway muscle tone or an increased respiratory drive. However, most of the improvement was seen in two out of only eleven individuals.

Shifflett et al [40] studied exercise tolerability at pretreatment and 4 weeks posttreatment for moderate to severe OSA in a small sample of patients. They found an improvement in perceived exertion posttreatment for OSA, with more improvement seen in the more severely affected patients. However, a wide range of treatment compliance existed in this small group of only nine patients.

Vanuxem et al [41] evaluated the effect of exercise tolerance and muscle metabolism in patients who had OSA versus a matched control group. They found that the OSA patients had a lower maximum load and lower peak oxygen uptake, in addition to lower maximal lactate concentration and elimination. They postulated that OSA patients have impaired glycolytic metabolism and oxidative metabolism. Sauleda et al [42] documented an increase in type II muscle fiber diameter in patients who had OSA compared with controls. There was also an increase in phosphofructokinase and cytochrome oxidase activity, demonstrating structural and bioenergetic changes in the skeletal muscle of apnea patients.

All of these studies were performed using small samples, making generalizations for the larger population of patients who have OSA questionable. They are interesting to consider with regard to the athlete, however. One question for further exploration would be whether the increase in GH and testosterone levels in the physically active adult offset the decreases seen in OSA. Does superior conditioning protect against apnea by improving airway muscle tonus and ventilatory response? What is the role of skeletal muscle change in terms of endurance and strength and are the changes comparable in the athlete and nonathlete?

Obstructive sleep apnea in professional athletes

Football players are the only professional athletes in whom OSA has been studied [43]. The large neck circumference, relatively high BMI, and male gender indicate a possibility of sleep apnea in this group. More than 20% of questionnaire respondents scored abnormally on the ESS and 92% had large neck circumferences, which are two of the risk factors for OSA. ESS scores were higher in habitual snorers. Of the players stratified into a high-risk group for apnea, 34% had an abnormal AHI of greater than ten, compared with 7% in the low-risk group. The rate of OSA in these professional football players greatly exceeded the population prevalence estimates with nearly a five times higher risk of OSA in the entire group and an eleven-fold increased risk in the questionnaire-identified high-risk group. Excessive daytime sleepiness was present in a high percentage of players, but not all occurrences were accounted for by the sleep disordered breathing. Further study is required to determine the extent to which sleep apnea may negatively impact performance in this group.

Because of the high BMI and large neck circumferences of the players, one might have expected even more instances of OSA in this group overall. The low occurrence raises the question of whether the risk factors of snoring, BMI, and large neck circumference are perhaps offset by an improved chemoreceptor sensitivity, hypoxic ventilatory response, and pharyngeal tone caused by physical activity with or without the effects of intermittent hypoxia.

Implications for sports performance

Obstructive sleep apnea is increasingly recognized as a significant medical diagnosis with wide-ranging consequences on general physical and mental health. The extent to which the nonrestorative and fragmented sleep, intermittent hypoxia, and daytime sleepiness of OSA can negatively impact athletic performance and the degree to which performance may be enhanced by treatment of apnea have not been completely defined and are areas for future research. Preliminary studies indicate a higher prevalence of sleep apnea in professional football players. Other potentially high-risk groups of athletes who have abnormal BMI and large neck circumference and who may have OSA include wrestlers, boxers, and weight lifters. However, it is not only athletes such as these who may be at risk for OSA; retrognathia may be a risk factor for apnea in thin male or female athletes. Screening designed to identify risk factors for OSA, including loud, disruptive snoring; BMI; neck circumference; jaw structure; daytime sleepiness; and fatigue (ESS over 10), is recommended for high-risk athletes. Further workup and referral to a sleep center should be considered in any athlete who is identified as being at risk.

A high index of suspicion for OSA will facilitate prompt diagnosis and minimize the potential negative cardiovascular, metabolic, endocrinologic, and neurocognitive sequelae, allowing for improved overall health and optimal athletic performance. Polysomnography should be considered in any athlete who has risk factors predictive of OSA, and treatment implemented for those found to have the disorder. Reversible, noninvasive treatment interventions such as CPAP or oral appliances are recommended. Response to treatment should be assessed on an individual basis.

References

[1] Bassiri AG, Guilleminault C. Clinical features and evaluation of obstructive sleep apnea-hypopnea syndrome. In: Kryger MH, Roth T, Dement WC, editors. Principles and practice of sleep medicine. 3rd edition. Philadelphia: WB Saunders Co; 2000. p. 869–78.

[2] Lavie L. Obstructive sleep apnoea syndrome—an oxidative stress disorder. Sleep Med Rev 2003;7(1):35–51.

[3] Neubauer JA. Physiological and genomic consequences of intermittent hypoxia. Invited review: physiological and pathophysiological responses to intermittent hypoxia. J Appl Physiol 2001; 90(4):1593–9.

[4] Veasey SC, Davis CW, Fenik P, et al. Long-term intermittent hypoxia in mice: protracted hypersomnolence with oxidative injury to sleep-wake brain regions. Sleep 2004;27(2):194–201.

[5] Young T, Palta M, Dempsey J, et al. The occurrence of sleep-disordered breathing among middle-aged adults. N Engl J Med 1993;328:1230–5.

[6] Hoffstein V. Snoring. In: Kryger MH, Roth T, Dement WC, editors. Principles and practice of sleep medicine. 3rd edition. Philadelphia: WB Saunders Co; 2000. p. 813–26.

[7] Kuna S, Remmers JE. Anatomy and physiology of upper airway obstruction. In: Kryger MH, Roth T, Dement WC, editors. Principles and practice of sleep medicine. 3rd edition. Philadelphia: WB Saunders Co; 2000. p. 840–58.

[8] Weiss JW, Launois SH, Anand A. Cardiorespiratory changes in sleep-disordered breathing. In: Kryger MH, Roth T, Dement WC, editors. Principles and practice of sleep medicine. 3rd edition. Philadelphia: WB Saunders Co; 2000. p. 859–68.

[9] Coughlin SR, Mawdsley L, Mugarza JA, et al. Obstructive sleep apnoea is independently associated with an increased prevalence of metabolic syndrome. Eur Heart J 2004;25(9):735–41.

[10] Peppard PE, Young T, Palta M, et al. Prospective study of the association between sleep-disordered breathing and hypertension. N Engl J Med 2000;342:1378–84.

[11] Dyken ME, Somers VK, Yamada T, et al. Investigating the relationship between stroke and obstructive sleep apnea. Stroke 1996;27:401–7.

[12] Bassetti C, Aldrich MS. Sleep apnea in acute cerebrovascular diseases: final report on 128 patients. Sleep 1999;22(2):217–33.

[13] Wolk R, Somers VK. Cardiovascular consequences of obstructive sleep apnea. Clin Chest Med 2003;24:195–201.

[14] Barcelo A, Miralles C, Barbe F, et al. Abnormal lipid peroxidation in patients with sleep apnoea. Eur Respir J 2000;16:644–7.

[15] Kato M, Roberts-Thomson P, Phillips BG, et al. Impairment of endothelium-dependent vasodilation of resistance vessels in patients with obstructive sleep apnea. Circulation 2000; 102:2607–10.

[16] Carlson JT, Rangemark C, Hedner JA. Attenuated endothelium-dependent vascular relaxation in patients with sleep apnoea. J Hypertens 1996;14(5):577–84.

[17] Vgontzas AN, Papanicolaou DA, Bixler EO, et al. Sleep apnea and daytime sleepiness and fatigue: relation to visceral obesity, insulin resistance, and hypercytokinemia. J Clin Endocrinol Metab 2000;85(3):1151–8.

[18] Mantzoros CS, Moschos S, Avramopoulos I, et al. Leptin concentrations in relation to body mass index and the tumor necrosis factor-alpha system in humans. J Clin Endocrinol Metab 1997;82(10):3408–13.

[19] Tankersley CG, O'Donnell C, Daood MJ, et al. Leptin attenuates respiratory complications associated with the obese phenotype. J Appl Physiol 1998;85:2261–9.

[20] Vgontzas AN, Legro RS, Bixler EO, et al. Polycystic ovary syndrome is associated with obstructive sleep apnea and daytime sleepiness: role of insulin resistance. J Clin Endocrinol Metab 2001;86(2):517–20.

[21] Luboshitzky R, Aviv A, Hefetz A, et al. Decreased pituitary-gonadal secretion in men with obstructive sleep apnea. J Clin Endocrinol Metab 2002;87(7):3394–8.

[22] Meston N, Davies RJ, Mullins R, et al. Endocrine effects of nasal continuous positive airway pressure in male patients with obstructive sleep apnoea. J Intern Med 2003;254(5):447–54.

[23] Burr RE. Neuroendocrinology. Disorders of the hypothalamus and pituitary gland. In: Noble J, Greene HL, Levinson W, et al, editors. Textbook of primary care medicine. 2nd edition. St. Louis, MO: Mosby; 1996. p. 532–44.

[24] Saini J, Krieger J, Brandenberger G, et al. Continuous positive airway pressure treatment. Effects on growth hormone, insulin and glucose profiles in obstructive sleep apnea patients. Horm Metab Res 1993;25(7):374–81.

[25] Rosen T, Bengtsson BA. Premature mortality due to cardiovascular disease in hypopituitarism. Lancet 1990;336(8710):285–8.

[26] Sassani A, Findley LJ, Kryger M, et al. Reducing motor-vehicle collisions, costs, and fatalities by treating obstructive sleep apnea syndrome. Sleep 2004;27(3):453–8.

[27] Johns MW. A new method for measuring daytime sleepiness: the Epworth sleepiness scale. Sleep 1991;14(6):540–5.

[28] Department of Health & Human Services Centers for Medicare & Medicaid Services Medicare coverage issues manual [Transmittal 150]. December 26, 2001.

[29] Grunstein R, Sullivan C. Continuous positive airway pressure for sleep breathing disorders. In: Kryger MH, Roth T, Dement WC, editors. Principles and practice of sleep medicine. 3rd edition. Philadelphia: WB Saunders Co; 2000. p. 894–912.

[30] Thorpy M, Chesson A, Derderian S, et al. Practice parameters for the treatment of obstructive sleep apnea in adults: the effect of surgical modifications of the upper airway. Sleep 1996;19: 152–5.

[31] Hoy CJ, Vennelle M, Kingshott RN, et al. Can intensive support improve continuous positive airway pressure use in patients with the sleep apnea/hypopnea syndrome? Am J Respir Crit Care Med 1999;159(4 pt 1):1096–100.

[32] Riley RW, Powell NB, Li KK, et al. Surgical therapy for obstructive sleep apnea-hypopnea syndrome. In: Kryger MH, Roth T, Dement WC, editors. Principles and practice of sleep medicine. 3rd edition. Philadelphia: WB Saunders Co; 2000. p. 913–28.

[33] American Sleep Disorders Association. Practice parameters for the treatment of snoring and obstructive sleep apnea with oral appliances. Sleep 1995;18(6):511–3.

[34] Kinsman TA, Hahn AG, Gore CJ, et al. Respiratory events and periodic breathing in cyclists sleeping at 2,650-m simulated altitude. J Appl Physiol 2002;92:2114–8.

[35] Fulco CS, Rock PB, Cymerman A. Improving athletic performance: is altitude residence or altitude training helpful? Aviat Space Environ Med 2000;71(2):162–71.

[36] Zhuang JG, Zhou ZN. Protective effects of intermittent hypoxic adaptation on myocardium and its mechanisms. Biol Signals Recept 1999;8:316–22.

[37] Chapman RF, Stray-Gundersen J, Levine BD. Individual variation in response to altitude training. J Appl Physiol 1998;85:1448–56.
[38] Ari Z, Kutlu N, Uyanik BS, et al. Serum testosterone, growth hormone, and insulin-like growth factor-1 levels, mental reaction time, and maximal aerobic exercise in sedentary and long-term physically trained elderly males. Int J Neurosci 2004;114(5):623–37.
[39] Giebelhaus V, Strohl KP, Lormes W, et al. Physical exercise as an adjunct therapy in sleep apnea—an open trial. Sleep Breath 2000;4(4):173–6.
[40] Shifflett DE, Walker EW, Gregg JM, et al. Effects of short-term PAP treatment on endurance exercise performance in obstructive sleep apnea patients. Sleep Med 2001;2:145–51.
[41] Vanuxem D, Badier M, Guillot C, et al. Impairment of muscle energy metabolism in patients with sleep apnoea syndrome. Respir Med 1997;91:551–7.
[42] Sauleda J, Garcia-Palmer FJ, Tarraga S, et al. Skeletal muscle changes in patients with obstructive sleep apnoea syndrome. Respir Med 2003;97:804–10.
[43] George CF, Kab V, Kab P, et al. Sleep and breathing in professional football players. Sleep Med 2003;4:317–25.
[44] Thorpy M, Chesson A, Derderian S, et al. Practice parameters for the treatment of obstructive sleep apnea in adults: the efficacy of surgical modifications of the upper airway. Report of the American Sleep Disorders Association. Sleep 1996;19:152–5.

ELSEVIER
SAUNDERS

Clin Sports Med 24 (2005) 343–353

CLINICS
IN SPORTS
MEDICINE

Nonpharmacologic Techniques for Promoting Sleep

Roger J. Cole, PhD

Synchrony Applied Health Sciences, 12759 Via Felino Del Mar, CA 92014, USA

Good sleep improves psychomotor performance, so it is crucial for competitive athletes to sleep well (see Van Dongen and Dinges report elsewhere in this issue). A specialist who understands how the interaction of circadian rhythms, homeostatic drive, and sleep inertia regulate human sleep and performance can design a customized sleep/nap schedule to help a particular athlete be optimally well rested and ready to perform on a particular day at a particular hour. Discussions on homeostatic drive and sleep inertia can be found elsewhere in this issue in articles by Van Dongen and Dinges, and Kräuchi et al, respectively. Such a schedule might recommend specific times to fall asleep at night or to nap during the day. To benefit from such a program, however, athletes must be able to actually fall asleep when the schedule dictates. If athletes have difficulty initiating sleep, they may choose to use a hypnotic medication, but they must choose carefully because some hypnotics can produce negative hangover effects on performance [1]. To avoid this problem, some athletes might prefer to use nonpharmacologic methods for promoting sleep onset.

This article discusses the possible physiologic basis and the potential utility of several of these nonpharmacologic methods. It focuses on simple, practical, drug-free techniques that athletes might self-administer acutely while attempting to fall asleep, or just before the attempt. It should be borne in mind, however, that there exist other, nonacute, nonpharmacologic sleep-promotion techniques

E-mail address: rcole5@san.rr.com

doi:10.1016/j.csm.2004.12.010　　　　　　　　　　　*sportsmed.theclinics.com*

not discussed here, but which have been proven effective for promoting sleep. Examples include cognitive behavior therapy/stimulus control/sleep restriction for nocturnal insomnia [2,3] and bright light treatment to correct circadian phase misalignment [4]. Postolache and Oren provide further discussion of bright light treatment elsewhere in this issue. It seems likely that the acute techniques this article describes could complement these non-acute techniques.

Physiologic foundation

Healthy people typically fall asleep rather quickly (but not too quickly), remain asleep for many hours, wake up quickly, then remain awake for many hours. They do not dwell long in the transitional states of falling asleep or waking up. This reflects the organization of the neural systems that control sleep. In many of these systems, neurons that keep the brain awake tend to activate other wake-inducing neurons and inhibit sleep-inducing neurons, and vice versa. Therefore, in transitional periods when both systems are partially active at the same time, whichever is more active soon becomes fully engaged and shuts off the opposing system, establishing a clear state of sleep or wakefulness. Once a state is established, it tends to be self-sustaining and to resist transition to the opposing state. In engineering terms, sleep/wake control circuits function like a "flip-flop" switch that is stable in either of its extreme positions (asleep or awake), but unstable in between [5–8].

In order for any intervention to help a person fall asleep, it must make it easier to flip the switch. This means it must directly or indirectly inhibit wake-promoting neurons or stimulate sleep-promoting neurons.

Fig. 1 illustrates part of the neural circuitry that controls sleep and wakefulness. Early sleep researchers discovered that cortical electroencephalogram (EEG) arousal and behavioral wakefulness are maintained by the activity of neurons in the brainstem, especially the midbrain reticular formation (MRF) [9]. They also found that sleep-active neurons in the anterior hypothalamus [10] and in the solitary tract nucleus (STN) in the medulla oblongata [11–13] promote cortical EEG synchronization and behavioral sleep.

More recent research has confirmed this general picture and added to it (for example, see Stiller and Postolache article elsewhere in this issue). This new research has identified specific wake-promoting nuclei; for example, the dorsal raphe nucleus (DRN) and the locus coeruleus (LC) in the brainstem and the tuberomammillary nucleus (TMN) in the hypothalamus [6,7]. It has also identified the key sleep-promoting centers in the anterior hypothalamus: the ventrolateral preoptic area (VLPO) [5–8] and the median preoptic nucleus (MnPN) [14]. Many other important sleep-related neural systems exist in the brain, but for the sake of simplicity this discussion is limited to those mentioned previously. The key point is that either electrical or pharmacologic stimulation

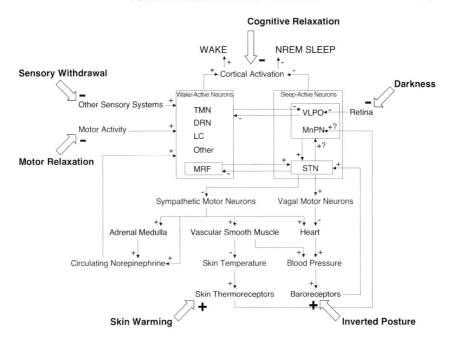

Fig. 1. Possible physiological pathways for nonpharmacologic sleep promotion. Plus symbol indicates stimulation and minus symbol indicates inhibition. TMN, tuberomammillary nucleus; DRN, dorsal raphe nucleus; LC, locus coeruleus; MRF, midbrain reticular formation; VLPO, ventrolateral preoptic area; MnPN, median preoptic nucleus; STN, solitary tract nucleus.

of the STN or preoptic hypothalamus often induces EEG slowing and sleep, whereas stimulation of the MRF and other wake-active areas induces arousal. This suggests that behavioral interventions that stimulate the STN, VLPO, or MnPN while withdrawing stimulation from the MRF and other activating centers should promote sleep onset.

Compared with wakefulness, non–rapid eye movement (NREM) sleep is characterized by a clear reduction in sympathetic nervous system activity and a shift of the sympathovagal balance toward parasympathetic (vagal) dominance [15], as reported elsewhere in this issue by Stiller and Postolache. These characteristics suggest, at the very least, that behaviors or stimuli that intensify sympathetic activity will antagonize sleep onset. As discussed later, this turns out to be the case, and the inverse is also true: interventions that inhibit sympathetic activity can promote sleep onset. The main mediator of these effects may be the STN. STN activity does more than just slow the EEG, it also inhibits sympathetic motor neurons and excites vagal motor neurons in the brainstem [16]. Thus, the natural shift to parasympathetic dominance that accompanies spontaneous sleep onset, and the evoked shift to parasympathetic dominance that accompanies some of the sleep-promoting stimuli described here, may be caused, in part or in full, by increased STN activity.

Overview of potential nonpharmacologic interventions

To predict what sorts of acute nonpharmacologic interventions might help flip the "sleep switch" from wakefulness to sleep, it is useful to consider what conditions can prevent such a switch. Many studies have investigated non-pharmacologic ways to help sleepy people stay awake. Reviewing the evidence, Bonnet [17] listed the following as conditions that may antagonize sleep: (1) upright posture, (2) excessively hot or cold temperature, (3) motor activity, (4) bright light, (5) noise, and (6) stress. This list naturally suggests a corresponding list of opposite conditions that might be expected to promote sleep: (1) inverted posture, (2) appropriately warm or cool temperature, (3) motor relaxation, (4) sensory withdrawal, and (5) cognitive relaxation. In addition, the scientific literature suggests that certain breathing techniques might create conditions conducive to sleep. Box 1 lists putative sleep-promoting conditions, along with practical interventions one might apply to create those conditions.

Inverted posture

Upside-down postures increase blood pressure locally at the baroreceptors located in the carotid sinus and aortic arch. Postures that invert the trunk lift the heart higher than the baroreceptors, so arterial blood flows "downhill" to them, increasing hydrostatic pressure there [18]. This distends the receptors, causing them to increase the rate at which they send afferent impulses, by way of the glossopharyngeal nerve (from the carotid sinus) or the vagus nerve (from the aortic arch), to the STN [19]. The STN, in turn, stimulates vagal motor neurons, slowing the heart. At the same time, it inhibits sympathetic outflow to the heart, vascular smooth muscle, and adrenal medulla (see Fig. 1) [16,20]. This further slows the heart, promotes peripheral vasodilatation, and reduces circulating norepinephrine levels. Thus, the general effect of inverted posture is to shift sympathovagal balance toward parasympathetic dominance, that is, toward a more NREM–sleep-like state.

It has been recognized since ancient times that baroreceptor stimulation can promote sleep. According to the American Heritage Dictionary, "[The word] 'carotid' [derives from the] Greek... *karoun* to stupefy (it was once thought that pressure on the carotids causes a stupor)" [21]. Balinese indigenous medicine traditionally used carotid massage as a soporific [22]. For millennia, Indian yoga has used inverted postures to induce mental calm. Referring to inverted postures, one modern yoga text states, "With the trunk and legs taken over the head, the brain relaxes" [23].

The soporific influence of baroreceptor activity has also been recognized by sleep scientists for decades. From the 1930s to the 1970s, dozens of studies showed that either mechanical or electrical stimulation of the carotid sinus, aortic arch, or their afferent nerves can produce EEG and behavioral signs of sleep in dogs, cats, or monkeys [13]. Some of these studies determined

Box 1. Putative acute nonpharmacologic methods for promoting sleep onset

Inverted posture

  Neck/chest below heart
  Legs above heart

Skin warming/core cooling

  Prior hot bath
  Hot footbath
  Warm blankets, socks, and so forth
  Thermal biofeedback
  Ice consumption

Motor relaxation

  Prior stretching
  Prior inactivity
  Completely supported posture
  Voluntary muscular relaxation

Sensory withdrawal, or masking and habituation

  Visual: darkness (sleep mask, dark room)
  Auditory: quiet, rhythmic sound, or white noise
  Tactile, proprioceptive, vestibular: comfort, stillness

Breathing techniques

  Prolonged exhalation
  Carbon dioxide elevation

Cognitive relaxation

  Relaxation training
  Biofeedback

that the STN mediates these effects. Mechanical stimulation of the carotid sinus has also been observed to produce EEG slowing in humans [24,25].

Despite the enormous amount of anecdotal and empirical evidence suggesting that inverted postures could help promote sleep, no published clinical trials address this issue to date. The existing literature does, however, suggest some hypotheses about how inversions might best be applied. Several studies found that the soporific effect of baroreceptor stimulation does not appear immediately, but requires up to several minutes to evolve [13]. This suggests that inverted postures may have to be held for some minimum period to be effective. Some investigators noted that baroreceptors exert their soporific effect most reliably against a slow, drowsy EEG background, and that excessive EEG activation at the time of stimulus can block the effect altogether [13]. This observation suggests that it might be most efficient to precede or combine inverted postures with other sleep-promoting methods that set up favorable conditions. Furthermore, this investigator has observed (unpublished) in humans that steep inversion can sometimes cause EEG activation (ie, reduced theta activity), whereas mild inversion can reliably elicit EEG slowing (ie, dramatically increased theta). The steep inversion was a 60° head-down tilt; the mild one was reclining supine with the legs, pelvis, and lower trunk supported horizontally on a long bolster and the head and shoulders resting on the floor about 15 to 25 cm below.

Skin warming/core cooling

Kräuchi et al explain elsewhere in this issue that in humans, "the readiness to fall asleep is correlated with distal vasodilatation." That is, shortly before people fall asleep, blood flow to their skin increases, especially in the fingers and toes. This causes the skin to become warmer and the core cooler. Kräuchi et al note that key neural centers that control body temperature lie in the preoptic hypothalamus, where they overlap those that control sleep. They suggest that hot or cold receptors in the skin, body core, or central nervous system might somehow help trigger sleep onset by activating sleep-promoting neurons in the VLPO or medial preoptic area. Therefore, it is possible that sleep onset may be promoted by manipulating skin or core body temperature.

There is substantial empirical evidence to support this hypothesis. First, Kräuchi et al point out that thermal biofeedback, in which participants learn to voluntarily raise hand temperature, helps them fall asleep quickly [26]. Second, several studies have shown that taking a warm bath before bed, which warms the skin and the body core, promotes sleepiness or shortens sleep latency [27–30]. Third, Sung [30] found that warming only the feet in a warm footbath before bedtime also shortens sleep latency, although it does not raise core temperature. Finally, Van Someren et al [31] found that artificially warming the proximal skin of the body with a water-heated suit hastens sleep onset. Van Someren et al also found that drinking an iced beverage, which mildly cools the body core, promotes sleep better than drinking a warm beverage, which mildly heats the core. Drinking an iced beverage and wearing a heated suit at the same time shortened sleep onset latency more than any other combination of a warm or cold beverage with a warm or cold suit. Thus, simultaneously cooling the core and warming the skin was the most effective way to induce sleep.

The increase in skin temperature during natural sleep onset, sleep promotion by artificial temperature manipulation, and sleep promotion by head-down posture may all be related through the STN. Blood flow (and therefore temperature) in the skin of the extremities is controlled primarily by sympathetic innervation of smooth muscle that surrounds arterioles. Sympathetic activity constricts the arterioles, reducing blood flow, lowering temperature, and raising blood pressure [32]. The STN inhibits these sympathetic nerves, promoting vasodilatation [16]. Stimulating the baroreceptors can trigger this effect by activating the STN. Neurons in the preoptic area of the hypothalamus potentiate the baroreflex [33].

The important role of the STN circulatory regulation suggests a possible chain of events that might occur during spontaneous sleep onset. Increased preoptic activity might directly or indirectly depolarize neurons in the STN, making them more sensitive to the prevailing level of baroreceptor input. As a result, the neurons' firing rate would increase in the absence of an increase in blood pressure. The increased firing would inhibit arteriolar sympathetic nerves, producing the peripheral vasodilatation and skin warming that is characteristic of sleep onset.

But what might cause the initial increase in activity of the preoptic area? If thermoreceptors in the skin can trigger it, then the chain of sleep onset could be started by artificially warming the skin. A warm bath might be an efficient way to do this, but if this is unavailable one might simply cover the skin with a blanket. However, the heat that accumulates under a blanket comes from the skin itself. If the skin is cold to begin with, its arterioles will be constricted, and there may not be enough blood flow near the surface to rapidly warm the air trapped underneath the blanket. Here is where inverted posture might be useful. It would stimulate the baroreceptors, causing reflex vasodilatation. This could bring enough blood to the surface to speed the process of warming the skin under the blanket. Incidentally, it is not necessary to invert the trunk to obtain reflex vasodilatation; postures in which the trunk remains horizontal but the legs are elevated also produce reflex peripheral vasodilatation [34]. This leg-elevation effect is probably not mediated by the high-pressure sino-aortic baroreceptors but rather by low-pressure volume receptors in the right atrium [34].

Motor relaxation

Motor activity inhibits sleep-active neurons in the STN [12] and is tightly coupled with strong activation of arousal-related neurons in the TMN [35], which may help explain why walking, even for 5 minutes, immediately before lying down for a nap produces an activating effect that significantly delays sleep onset [36]. On the other hand, systematically relaxing skeletal muscles helps people fall asleep faster [3], suggesting that a person who wishes to fall asleep quickly should remain as inactive as possible before the sleep attempt, or perhaps should perform gentle stretching exercises to reduce muscle tone. During the sleep attempt itself, one's posture should be supported to allow complete muscle relaxation and physical stillness.

Sensory withdrawal, or masking and habituation

Common sense tells us that various types of sensory stimuli, such as noise, touch, and body discomfort, make it difficult to fall asleep. When such stimuli cannot be avoided, it might sometimes be useful to mask them with monotonous stimuli to which sensory receptors might habituate. For example, white noise can help induce sleep [37]. One study found that presenting auditory stimuli rhythmically in synchrony with beat-to-beat baroreceptor afferent activity substantially shortened sleep-onset latency [38].

Blocking light from the eyes has special importance for sleep promotion. The VLPO receives direct input from light-sensitive retinal ganglion cells [39]. This input is apparently inhibitory, because even dim light immediately slows the activity of preoptic hypnogenic neurons [40], and therefore just a small amount of light reaching the eyes can make it harder to fall asleep. Furthermore, at night, if the light is bright enough, it will suppress melatonin secretion, further inhibiting sleep [41]. Therefore, it is advisable to block as much light from the eyes as possible when attempting sleep, day or night.

Breathing techniques

Sleep profoundly affects breathing, so it is reasonable to hypothesize that breathing exercises could greatly affect sleep. However, few treatment studies have systematically addressed this question.

Spontaneous exhalation reduces cardiac sympathetic activity and increases parasympathetic activity [42]. This phenomenon is consistent with the claim made by yoga practitioners that voluntarily prolonging exhalation produces a feeling of calm [43]. Therefore, it might be worthwhile to test whether a breathing practice that emphasizes long exhalations might promote sleep.

Carbon dioxide tension (pCO_2) spontaneously rises during sleep [44]. Two independent studies found that voluntarily breathing in ways that elevate pCO_2 can rapidly promote drowsiness [45,46]. However, elevated pCO_2 can also cause anxiety, so this sort of breathing exercise may be difficult to apply reliably [45].

Cognitive relaxation

Cognitive relaxation methods presumably work by using mentation to directly reduce cortical arousal. Some semicognitive methods, such as skin temperature biofeedback, also target specific physiologic systems that affect sleep [26]. Many types of relaxation and biofeedback training have been shown to improve sleep in various ways, so this approach can be recommended in general. However, no specific technique has been clearly demonstrated to be the best [3].

References

[1] Grobler LA, Schwellnus MP, Trichard C, et al. Comparative effects of zopiclone and loprazolam on psychomotor and physical performance in active individuals. Clin J Sport Med 2000;10(2):123–8.

[2] Edinger JD, Wohlgemuth WK, Radtke RA, et al. Cognitive behavioral therapy for treatment of chronic primary insomnia: a randomized controlled trial. JAMA 2001;285(14):1856–64.

[3] Morin CM, Hauri PJ, Espie CA, et al. Nonpharmacologic treatment of chronic insomnia. An American Academy of Sleep Medicine review. Sleep 1999;22(8):1134–56.

[4] Terman M, Terman JS. Light therapy. In: Kryger MH, Roth T, Dement WC, editors. Principles and practice of sleep medicine. 3rd edition. Philadelphia: WB Saunders; 2000. p. 1258–74.

[5] Lu J, Greco MA, Shiromani P, et al. Effect of lesions of the ventrolateral preoptic nucleus on NREM and REM sleep. J Neurosci 2000;20(10):3830–42.

[6] Chou TC, Bjorkum AA, Gaus SE, et al. Afferents to the ventrolateral preoptic nucleus. J Neurosci 2002;22(3):977–90.

[7] Sherin JE, Elmquist JK, Torrealba F, et al. Innervation of histaminergic tuberomammillary neurons by GABAergic and galaninergic neurons in the ventrolateral preoptic nucleus of the rat. J Neurosci 1998;18(12):4705–21.

[8] Szymusiak R, Steininger T, Alam N, et al. Preoptic area sleep-regulating mechanisms. Arch Ital Biol 2001;139(1–2):77–92.

[9] Moruzzi G, Magoun HW. Brain stem reticular formation and activation of the EEG. Electroencephalogr Clin Neurophysiol 1949;1:455–73.

[10] Sterman MB, Clemente CD. Forebrain inhibitory mechanisms: sleep patterns induced by basal forebrain stimulation in the behaving cat. Exp Neurol 1962;6:103–17.

[11] Magnes J, Moruzzi G, Pompeiano O. Synchronization of the EEG produced by low-frequency electrical stimulation of the region of the solitary tract. Arch Ital Biol 1961;99:33–67.

[12] Eguchi K, Satoh T. Convergence of sleep-wakefulness subsystems onto single neurons in the region of cat's solitary tract nucleus. Arch Ital Biol 1980;118(4):331–45.

[13] Gottesmann C. The neurophysiology of sleep and waking: intracerebral connections, functioning and ascending influences of the medulla oblongata. Prog Neurobiol 1999;59(1):1–54.

[14] McGinty D, Gong H, Suntsova N, et al. Sleep-promoting functions of the hypothalamic median preoptic nucleus: inhibition of arousal systems. Arch Ital Biol 2004;142(4):501–9.

[15] Burgess HJ, Trinder J, Kim Y. Cardiac autonomic nervous system activity during presleep wakefulness and stage 2 NREM sleep. J Sleep Res 1999;8(2):113–22.

[16] Ganong WF. Review of medical physiology. Los Altos, CA: Lange; 1983. p. 483.

[17] Bonnet MH. Sleep deprivation. In: Kryger MH, Roth T, Dement WC, editors. Principles and practice of sleep medicine. 3rd edition. Philadelphia: WB Saunders; 2000. p. 53–71.

[18] Gauer OH, Thron HL. Postural changes in the circulation. In: Hamilton WF, Dow P, editors. Handbook of Physiology: Sec 2. Circulation: Vol 3. Washington: Am Physiol Soc; 1965. p. 2409–39.

[19] Barr ML. The human nervous system: an anatomical viewpoint. 2nd edition. Hagerstown, MD: Harper & Row; 1974. p. 133–5.

[20] Aviado DM, Schmidt CF. Reflexes from stretch receptors in blood vessels, heart and lungs. Physiol Reviews 1955;35(2):247–300.

[21] Morris W, editor. The American Heritage Dictionary of the English Language. Boston: Houghton Mifflin; 1976. p. 205.

[22] Schlager E, Meier T. A strange Balinese method of inducing sleep (with some notes about Balyans). Acta Trop 1947;4:127–34.

[23] Mehta S, Mehta M, Mehta S. Yoga the Iyengar Way. New York: Knopf; 1990. p. 110.

[24] Bridgers SL, Spencer SS, Spencer DD, et al. A cerebral effect of carotid sinus stimulation: observation during intraoperative electroencephalographic monitoring. Arch Neurol 1985;42: 574–7.

[25] Sinha S, Westmoreland BF, Sharbrough FW. EEG changes with carotid sinus baroreflex during carotid endarterectomy. Am J Electroneurodiagnostic Technol 2004;44(2):95–7.

[26] Lushington K, Greeneklee H, Veltmeyer M, et al. Biofeedback training in hand temperature raising promotes sleep onset in young normals. J Sleep Res 2004;13(Suppl 1):460.

[27] Kanda K, Tochihara Y, Ohnaka T. Bathing before sleep in the young and in the elderly. Eur J Appl Physiol Occup Physiol 1999;80(2):71–5.

[28] Horne JA, Reid AJ. Night-time sleep EEG changes following body heating in a warm bath. Electroencephalogr Clin Neurophysiol 1985;60(2):154–7.

[29] Horne JA, Shackell BS. Slow wave sleep elevations after body heating: proximity to sleep and effects of aspirin. Sleep 1987;10(4):383–92.

[30] Sung EJ, Tochihara Y. Effects of bathing and hot footbath on sleep in winter. J Physiol Anthropol Appl Human Sci 2000;19(1):21–7.

[31] Van Someren EJ, Drosopoulos RR, Collins S, et al. Effect of body temperature manipulation on pulse wave amplitude and sleep onset latency. Sleep 2002;25(Abstract Suppl):A128.

[32] Hales JRS. Skin arteriovenous anastomoses, their control and role in thermoregulation. In: Johansen K, Burggren WW, editors. Cardiovascular shunts. Alfred Benzon Symposium 21. Copenhagen: Munksgaard; 1985. p. 433–51.

[33] Inui K, Nomura J, Murase S, et al. Facilitation of the arterial baroreflex by the preoptic area in anaesthetized rats. J Physiol 1995;488(Pt 2):521–31.

[34] Roddie IC, Shepherd JT, Whelan RF. Reflex changes in vasoconstrictor tone in human skeletal muscle in response to stimulation of receptors in a low-pressure area of the intrathoracic vascular bed. J Physiol 1957;139(3):369–76.

[35] Inzunza O, Seron-Ferre MJ, Bravo H, et al. Tuberomammillary nucleus activation anticipates feeding under a restricted schedule in rats. Neurosci Lett 2000;293(2):139–42.

[36] Bonnet MH, Arand DL. Sleepiness as measured by modified multiple sleep latency testing varies as a function of preceding activity. Sleep 1998;21(5):477–83.

[37] Lopez HH, Bracha AS, Bracha HS. Evidence based complementary intervention for insomnia. Hawaii Med J 2002;61(9):192, 213.

[38] Velden M, Wolk C. Baroreceptor activity and the induction of sleep. Percept Mot Skills 1996;82(1):178.

[39] Lu J, Shiromani P, Saper CB. Retinal input to the sleep-active ventrolateral preoptic nucleus in the rat. Neuroscience 1999;93(1):209–14.

[40] Bremer F. Existence of a mutual tonic inhibitory interaction between the preoptic hypnogenic structure and the midbrain reticular formation. Brain Res 1975;96:71–5.

[41] Myers BL, Badia P. Immediate effects of different light intensities on body temperature and alertness. Physiol Behav 1993;54(1):199–202.

[42] Berntson GG, Cacioppo JT, Quigley KS. Respiratory sinus arrhythmia: autonomic origins, physiological mechanisms, and psychophysiological implications. Psychophysiology 1993; 30(2):183–96.

[43] Iyengar BKS. Light on pranayama: the yogic art of breathing. New York: Crossroad; 1981. p. 100.

[44] Naifeh KH, Kamiya J. The nature of respiratory changes associated with sleep onset. Sleep 1981;4(1):49–59.

[45] Naifeh KH, Kamiya J, Sweet DM. Biofeedback of alveolar carbon dioxide tension and levels of arousal. Biofeedback Self Regul 1982;7(3):283–99.

[46] Choliz M. A breathing-retraining procedure in treatment of sleep-onset insomnia: theoretical basis and experimental findings. Percept Mot Skills 1995;80(2):507–13.

ELSEVIER
SAUNDERS

Clin Sports Med 24 (2005) 355–365

CLINICS
IN SPORTS
MEDICINE

Effects of Exercise on Sleep

Shawn D. Youngstedt, PhD

Department of Exercise Science, Norman J. Arnold School of Public Health,
University of South Carolina, 1300 Wheat Street, Columbia, SC 29208, USA

Historically, perhaps no daytime behavior has been more closely associated with better sleep than exercise. The notion that exercise promotes sleep has been traced back to Biblical times [1], and persists today. For example, in a classic survey in Finland in which randomly selected respondents (N = 1190) were asked an open-ended question about what behaviors best promoted their sleep [2], exercise was listed as the most important behavior. Sleep experts have also endorsed the viewpoint that exercise promotes sleep, as noted in recent books [3–5]. On the National Sleep Foundation's Web site, regular exercise is listed as one of the ten "Healthy Tips for Better Sleep" (www.sleepfoundation.org).

The assumption that exercise promotes sleep has also been central to various hypotheses about the functions of sleep. Hypotheses that sleep serves an energy conservation function [6], a body tissue restitution function [7], or a temperature down-regulation function [8] have all predicted a uniquely potent effect of exercise on sleep because no other stimulus elicits greater depletion of energy stores, tissue breakdown, or elevation of body temperature, respectively.

Exercise offers a potentially attractive alternative or adjuvant treatment for insomnia. Sleeping pills have a number of adverse effects [9] and are not recommended for long-term use, partly on the basis of a significant epidemiologic association of chronic hypnotic use with mortality [10]. Other behavioral/cognitive treatments are more effective than hypnotics for chronic insomnia treatment [11], but difficult and costly to deliver. By contrast, exercise could be a healthy, safe, inexpensive, and simple means of improving sleep.

This work was supported by Grant No. HL71560 from the National Institutes of Health.
E-mail address: syoungstedt@sc.edu

Evidence that exercise promotes sleep

The evidence that exercise promotes sleep has been derived from epidemiologic studies and experimental studies of the sleep-promoting effects of acute or chronic exercise.

Epidemiologic studies

Most epidemiologic studies have indicated a significant positive association of self-reported exercise with better self-reported sleep [12–16]. However, there are a number of limitations in these studies and several alternative explanations for the epidemiologic association of exercise and sleep.

First, there is evidence that better sleep is associated with a greater willingness and ability to exercise [17]. Second, better health and less stress are associated with better sleep and greater ability or willingness to exercise. Third, people who exercise tend to practice many other healthy behaviors that could be conducive to sleep, such as avoidance of tobacco and avoidance of excessive caffeine and alcohol intake [18]. Fourth, outdoor exercise could be associated with a significant increase in daily bright-light exposure, which is associated with better sleep [19]. Epidemiologic studies have not generally controlled for these possibilities.

Surveys reflecting a perception that exercise promotes sleep might also reflect incorrect assumptions and attributions regarding benefits of exercise for sleep. For example, expectation that exercise promotes sleep is based partly on the incorrect assumption that sleepiness is synonymous with physical fatigue [20]. The feelings of greater energy that people report after becoming more physically fit [21] could be assumed to reflect better sleep, but these feelings might reflect physiologic adaptations to exercise, such as having lower resting heart rate and respiration.

Acute exercise studies

Most experimental studies of the influence of exercise on sleep have examined acute exercise in comparison with sedentary control treatments [22]. With few exceptions, these studies have focused on objective laboratory sleep measures, primarily using standard polysomnographic recordings and scoring procedures. A meta-analysis of the extant literature concluded that acute exercise had virtually no effect on sleep latency or the amount of wake time after sleep onset (WASO); a statistically significant but modest increase in total sleep time (TST) (median duration 10 minutes); a statistically significant but small increase in slow-wave sleep (SWS) (1.6 minutes); and a significant increase in rapid eye movement (REM) sleep latency (11.6 minutes) and decrease in REM sleep amount (6 minutes) [22].

In general, the fitness level of the subjects had little influence on the results. The moderating influence of various features of the exercise stimulus was also assessed.

The influence of exercise on sleep latency and WASO varied significantly with regard to the time in which exercise was completed relative to bedtime. The most positive effects occurred following exercise that took place 4 to 8 hours before bedtime, as opposed to more than 8 or less than 4 hours before bedtime. However, the data provided little support for the common assumption that late-night exercise disrupts sleep. Across the literature, exercise completed within 4 hours of sleep increased TST, decreased WASO, and only slightly delayed sleep onset latency (SOL). Furthermore, recent studies have failed to show a significant impairment in sleep following vigorous late-night exercise, neither in fit nor sedentary subjects [23,24]. This could be an important issue in adherence to exercise programs. For much of the population, the evening might be a practical time to exercise, perhaps especially true for endurance athletes who train twice daily.

The effects of exercise on sleep duration were significantly moderated by exercise duration, with negligible effects on sleep for durations of less than 1 hour (approximately 2 minutes), and progressively greater effects following exercise of 1 to 2 hours (approximately 11 min), and more than 2 hours (approximately 15 minutes) [22]. This finding suggests that endurance athletes might enjoy the most benefit, as many segments of the sedentary population might be unwilling to exercise for 1 hour or more.

On the other hand, the evidence indicates that exercise need not be intense to elicit a positive effect on sleep [22], which is good news for the general population. Similar effects on sleep were noted following light, moderate, and vigorous exercise. A significant linear trend for WASO has been observed. Light-intensity exercise has been associated with reductions in WASO (approximately 16 minutes), whereas high-intensity exercise has been associated with increases (approximately 4 minutes).

Another approach to examining the influence of acute exercise on sleep has been to examine whether day-to-day fluctuations in exercise are associated with differences in sleep in one's usual home environment. Studies that have used this approach have not found significant within-subjects associations of exercise with objective or subjective sleep [25].

In summary, the effects of acute exercise on sleep have been modest, even considering contrasts not only of general popular opinion but also of many sleep experts' viewpoints. The small increase in slow-wave sleep (SWS) following acute exercise is particularly noteworthy because it is generally assumed that exercise elicits a substantial increase in SWS and that SWS is particularly indicative of good sleep quality. Modest increases in SWS found in some exercise studies have typically occurred concomitantly with equivalent decreases in REM [26,27], and there is little compelling evidence to suggest that SWS is better than REM sleep [28]. Furthermore, it has never been shown that SWS changes after exercise are associated with reports of better subjective sleep or better daytime functioning. In fact, the only examination of this issue, of which we are aware, found a significant negative association of SWS with subjective sleep quality [29].

Although the effects of acute exercise on sleep have been modest, the literature on this topic has focused exclusively on good sleepers who are unlikely to demonstrate large improvements in sleep because of ceiling effects. It cannot be expected that any of the current sleep treatments would elicit much improvement in good sleepers. In extensive statistical comparisons, little differences in sleep were found following acute exercise and hypnotics when the literature was restricted to normal sleepers [30]. Of course, a prediction that exercise would have similar efficacy as hypnotics in treating insomnia cannot be extrapolated from these findings, but this is an important empirical question worthy of study.

Chronic exercise studies

Unfortunately, many of the chronic exercise studies have also been limited to normal sleepers [31–33]. Comparisons of chronic exercise versus a priori-selected control treatments (eg, waiting list, stretching treatments) have not demonstrated significantly greater improvements following exercise in normal sleepers [33–35].

Several studies have addressed whether exercise might promote sleep in older adults [33–36]. However, a recent Cochrane review [37], using a priori selected criteria, identified only one study of chronic exercise in a sample of predominantly older adults (at least 80% of sample ≥ 60 years of age) who had been screened for diagnoses of primary insomnia and absence of depression or dementia. In that study [36], 43 older adults who had moderate sleep complaints were randomized to a 16-week exercise training treatment or a waiting list control treatment. The exercise regimen involved aerobic exercise (60%–75% maximal capacity) three to four times per week (twice in a YMCA class, twice at home). Significantly greater improvements in self-reported sleep quality, sleep latency (net decrease versus control of 11.5 minutes), and total sleep time (net increase of 42 minutes) were found following exercise versus the waiting list control treatment.

Other studies of symptomatic older and middle-aged adults have also yielded promising results. Singh et al [38] randomly assigned older, depressed adults (N = 32, ages 60–84 years) to either a 10-week weight-training treatment (three times per week) or a health education control treatment. Significantly greater improvement in sleep and decreases in depression were found following weight training vs control, and these effects were significantly correlated. Guilleminault et al [39] randomly assigned 30 middle-aged (mean age 44 years) insomniacs to 4-week treatments involving sleep hygiene education (the control), sleep hygiene plus exercise (brisk walking for 45 minutes per day), and bright light treatment (30 minutes per day). Sleep was assessed through actigraphy and sleep logs. Whereas actigraphy revealed a mean increase in SOL (1 minute) and decrease in TST (3 minutes) in the control group, the exercise group had improvements in SOL and TST of 7 minutes and 17 minutes, respectively. Interestingly, the bright light group had even greater decreases in SOL (8 minutes) and increases in TST (44 minutes). Subjective sleep showed a similar pattern.

Although these changes were not statistically different between treatments, partly as a result of the small number subjects and high variability of the data, the data reinforce the notion that light exposure might be an important component in exercise studies.

In summary, chronic exercise studies have not provided much compelling evidence that exercise promotes sleep. However, much of this literature has also been limited to good sleepers. Controlled studies of individuals with insomnia or depression have shown significant sleep-promoting effects of exercise, but these effects have been limited to self-report measures. Given the unique expectancy that people have about the sleep benefits of exercise, further verification of these findings using objective sleep variables is needed.

Sleep apnea and restless legs syndrome

Loss of body weight is clearly a mechanism through which exercise could help prevent or alleviate sleep apnea. However, it has also been hypothesized that engagement of the pharyngeal and glossal muscles during exercise could strengthen these muscles, making them less susceptible to collapse associated with upper airway obstruction [40]. An epidemiologic study (N = 1104) found that number of hours of exercise per week was inversely associated with apnea-hypopnea severity, and this effect was independent of body mass index [41]. Furthermore, in uncontrolled trials, exercise training alone or in combination with caloric restriction has been associated with significant decreases in disturbed breathing that were not correlated with weight reduction.

Patients who have restless legs syndrome (RLS) report that exercise helps prevent and relieve their symptoms, and epidemiologic evidence indicates that lack of exercise is a significant risk factor for RLS [42]. In light of the adverse effects associated with pharmacologic treatment of RLS, which usually involves dopaminergic drugs, it is surprising that there has been such little experimental investigation of exercise as a treatment of RLS. Research by de Mello and colleagues [43] has shown that vigorous acute exercise and chronic exercise training [44] can significantly reduce RLS and periodic limb movements during sleep, and that these effects were not different from that of L-dopa, the primary pharmacologic treatment for RLS. Further study of these exciting results is needed.

Mechanisms by which exercise could promote sleep

Anxiety reduction

Perhaps the most plausible mechanism through which exercise could promote sleep is anxiety reduction. Disturbed sleep is a hallmark of anxiety [45], and chronic insomnia has been associated with increased physiological arousal [46]. Therefore, stimuli that reduce anxiety may promote sleep. It is well-established that acute exercise reduces state anxiety and that chronic exercise results in stable reductions in trait anxiety [47].

Antidepressant effects

There is compelling evidence that disturbed sleep is a risk factor for the development of depression and a common consequence of depression [48]. Thus, chronic exercise could promote sleep through its well-established antidepressant effects [49], as demonstrated by the study discussed previously that found significant improvement in sleep and reduction in depression with exercise [38].

An intriguing hypothesis is that antidepressant effects of exercise could be mediated by nightly decreases in REM sleep, which is one of the best-documented effects of acute exercise [22]. REM sleep reduction has been found in some antidepressant treatments [50]. Recent research found that nightly experimental attenuation of REM by merely 25% elicited significant antidepressant effects after a few weeks [51]. Thus, it is conceivable that daily exercise could have an analogous effect.

Thermogenic effect

Probably the most influential studies regarding exercise and sleep were elegantly designed by Horne and colleagues [26,52]. These studies suggested that increases in SWS following exercise were mediated by temperature elevation. The studies were particularly influential because their results were consistent with those showing increases in SWS following passive heating [53], and because the findings coincided with an emerging hypothesis that sleep might serve a down-regulation function [8]. This hypothesis, advanced largely by McGinty and colleagues [8], was based partly on evidence linking the anterior hypothalamus/preoptic area with sleep regulation (particularly SWS) and temperature down-regulation. This hypothesis has undergone several revisions, but remains one of the most vigorously-tested hypotheses of sleep function [54,55].

The impact of the studies by Horne and colleagues is based largely on the assumption that SWS is necessarily the best and deepest form of sleep. However, as reviewed by Rechtschaffen et al [28], this assumption is dubious. For example, REM can be considered the deepest of sleep by some arousal criteria [28], and there is also little compelling evidence indicating that SWS is associated with better outcomes (eg, in terms of daytime sleepiness) than REM sleep. The increases in SWS in the Horne et al studies were essentially matched by decreases in REM sleep, with no significant changes in total sleep time, or in sleepiness assessed at bedtime or wake time following any of the exercise versus control treatments. Other research has found a significant negative association of SWS with self-reported sleep quality after exercise [29]. Nonetheless, given the prominence of the temperature regulation hypothesis and the high quality of the Horne et al studies, the hypothesis as it applies to exercise is still tenable.

Chronic exercise could conceivably promote the sleep onset process by promoting more efficient temperature down-regulation, which typically precipitates sleep [56]. People with disturbed sleep, including insomniacs [57] and depressed individuals [58], have shown indications of attenuated temperature decline at night, which might be reversed following successful treatment [59]. It is plausible that the decrease of approximately 0.5 °C to 1°C in body temperature at night could more readily occur following heat acclimation associated with exercise.

Circadian phase-shifting effect

Exercise could also impact sleep through its influence on the circadian system. Circadian effects of exercise are particularly well-established in rodents (especially hamsters) [60].

In humans, exercise can shift the circadian system in normally entrained conditions [61] and constant-routine conditions [62–64], and can accelerate re-entrainment to a shifted light–dark cycle [65,66] or to a shortened sleep–wake period [67].

Preliminary analysis of a comprehensive exercise phase response curve (PRC) with over 200 subjects suggests that the exercise PRC is similar in shape to that of bright light [68]. Exercise delays the circadian system when performed in the nighttime, with maximal phase-delaying effects occurring at approximately the time of the body temperature minimum. Maximal phase-advancing effects occur soon after the body temperature minimum, with diminishing phase-advancing effects from approximately 1 to 5 hours after the body temperature minimum. This pattern was observed in the acrophases (24-hour fitted peaks) of urinary 6-sulphatoxymelatonin, urinary cortisol, and oral temperature. These data are consistent with recent research indicating that, under normally entrained conditions, exercise elicited phase delays and phase advances when administered just before and shortly after the body temperature minimum [61].

Buxton et al [63] described a different phase response curve for exercise, with phase advances following early evening exercise and phase delays at other times of day. However, there were few data points in this PRC (N = 29). Moreover, whereas the mean phase of melatonin onset advanced by 30 minutes from day 1 to 2 of the experiment, it delayed by 66 minutes from days 1 to 3. Thus, the initial shift was likely a transient pattern or a masking effect of acute exercise that was administered shortly before melatonin onset.

The magnitude of exercise-induced phase shifts have been similar to that observed for bright light of similar duration in comparable protocols. For example, Van Reeth et al [62] found that 2.5 hours of very modest exercise (mean intensity 50% of maximal capacity) elicited equivalent phase-shifting effects as 3 hours of bright light (5000 lux) under constant routine conditions. Furthermore, our research indicated that 1 hour of vigorous exercise (maximum of 65%–75%) elicited phase shifts that were 40% of those following 3 hours of bright light (3000 lux) [68], which is approximately the discrepancy observed between 1 hour and 3 hours of bright light [69].

Studies involving hamsters have shown that appropriately timed exercise and bright light can have dramatic synergistic and antagonistic effects [70]. Tantalizing preliminary evidence suggests that exercise and bright light might have similar phase-shifting interactions in humans [71].

These effects could be quite helpful in treating circadian sleep disorders because not everyone is responsive or tolerant to bright light. For example, advanced sleep-phase syndrome and delayed sleep-phase syndrome could be treated with nighttime and morning exercise (or bright light), respectively.

Summary

It is commonly assumed that exercise is one of the most important behavioral factors promoting sleep. Epidemiologic studies have generally shown positive associations of exercise with sleep. On the other hand, experimental studies have failed to demonstrate substantial sleep-promoting effects of either acute or chronic exercise. However, many experimental studies have been limited to good sleepers with little room for improvement because of ceiling/floor effects. The limited research on people with insomnia has yielded more promising results. Better-controlled research with objective sleep measures is needed to verify these findings. There are strong theoretical rationales for examining the efficacy of exercise sleep problems secondary to anxiety, depression, or circadian malsynchronization. Evidence of exercise as an effective treatment for RLS should also be expanded.

References

[1] Ancoli-Israel S. "Sleep is not tangible" or what the Hebrew tradition has to say about sleep. Psychosom Med 2001;63:778–87.
[2] Urponen H, Vuori I, Hasan J, et al. Self-evaluations of factors promoting and disturbing sleep: an epidemiological survey in Finland. Soc Sci Med 1988;26:443–50.
[3] Dement WC, Vaughan C. The promise of sleep. New York: Delacorte Press; 1999.
[4] Ancoli-Israel S. All I want is a good night's sleep. Chicago: Mosby-Year Book Inc; 1996.
[5] Lavie P. The enchanted world of sleep. New Haven, CT: Yale University Press; 1996.
[6] Berger RJ, Phillips NH. Comparative aspects of energy metabolism, body temperature and sleep. Acta Physiol Scand 1988;133(Suppl 574):S21–7.
[7] Adam K. Sleep as a restorative process and a theory to explain why. Prog Brain Res 1980; 53:289–305.
[8] McGinty D, Szymusiak R. Keeping cool: a hypothesis about the mechanisms and functions of slow-wave sleep. Trends Neurosci 1990;13:480–7.
[9] Kripke DF. Chronic hypnotic use: deadly risks, doubtful benefit. Sleep Med Rev 2000;4:5–20.
[10] Kripke DF, Klauber MR, Wingard DL, et al. Mortality hazard associated with prescription hypnotics. Biol Psychiat 1998;43:687–93.
[11] Morin CM, Colecchi C, Stone J, et al. Behavioral and pharmacological therapies for late-life insomnia: a randomized controlled trial. JAMA 1999;281:991–9.
[12] Sherrill DL, Kotchou K, Quan SF. Association of physical activity and human sleep disorders. Arch Intern Med 1998;158:1894–8.

[13] Kim K, Uchiyama M, Okawa M, et al. An epidemiological study of insomnia among the Japanese general population. Sleep 2000;23:41–7.

[14] Liu X, Uchiyama M, Kim K, et al. Sleep loss and daytime sleepiness in the general adult population of Japan. Psychiatry Res 2000;93:1–11.

[15] Ohida T, Kamal AM, Uchiyama M, et al. The influence of lifestyle and health status factors on sleep loss among the Japanese general population. Sleep 2001;24:333–8.

[16] Morgan K. Daytime activity and risk factors for late-life insomnia. J Sleep Res 2003;12:231–8.

[17] Weaver TE, Laizner AM, Evans LK, et al. An instrument to measure functional status outcomes for disorders of excessive sleepiness. Sleep 1997;20:835–43.

[18] Sun YH, Yu TS, Tong SL, et al. A cross-sectional study of health-related behaviors in rural eastern China. Biomed Environ Sci 2002;15:347–54.

[19] Youngstedt SD, Kripke DF, Elliott JA, et al. Light exposure, sleep quality, and depression in older adults. In: Holick MF, Jung EG, editors. Biologic effects of light 1998. Boston: Kluwer Academic Publishers; 1999. p. 427–35.

[20] Dawson D, Fletcher A. A quantitative model of work-related fatigue: background and definition. Ergonomics 2001;44:144–63.

[21] Hong S, Dimsdale JE. Physical activity and perception of energy and fatigue in obstructive sleep apnea. Med Sci Sports Exerc 2003;35:1088–92.

[22] Youngstedt SD, O'Connor PJ, Dishman RK. The effects of acute exercise on sleep: a quantitative synthesis. Sleep 1997;20:203–14.

[23] O'Connor PJ, Breus MJ, Youngstedt SD. Exercise-induced increase in core temperature does not disrupt a behavioral measure of sleep. Physiol Behav 1998;64:213–7.

[24] Youngstedt SD, Kripke DF, Elliott JA. Is sleep disturbed by vigorous late-night exercise? Med Sci Sports Exerc 1999;31:864–9.

[25] Youngstedt SD, Perlis ML, O'Brien PM, et al. No association of sleep with total daily physical activity in normal sleepers. Physiol Behav 2003;78:395–401.

[26] Horne JA, Moore VJ. Sleep EEG effects of exercise with and without additional body cooling. Electroencephalogr Clin Neurophysiol 1985;60:33–8.

[27] Youngstedt SD, O'Connor PJ, Crabbe JB, et al. The influence of acute exercise on sleep following high caffeine intake. Physiol Behav 2000;68:563–70.

[28] Rechtschaffen A, Bergmann BM, Gilliland MA, et al. Effects of method, duration, and sleep stage on rebounds from sleep deprivation in the rat. Sleep 1999;22:11–31.

[29] Driver HS, Rogers GG, Mitchell D, et al. Prolonged endurance exercise and sleep disruption. Med Sci Sports Exerc 1994;26:903–7.

[30] Youngstedt SD. Ceiling and floor effects in sleep research. Sleep Med Rev 2003;7:351–65.

[31] Meintjes AF, Driver HS, Shapiro CM. Improved physical fitness failed to alter the EEG patterns of sleep in young women. Eur J Appl Physiol Occup Physiol 1989;59:123–7.

[32] Driver HS, Meintjes AF, Rogers GG, et al. Submaximal exercise effects on sleep patterns in young women before and after an aerobic training programme. Acta Physiol Scand 1988;133(Suppl 574):S8–13.

[33] Vitiello MV, Prinz PN, Schwartz RS. Slow wave sleep but not over-all sleep quality of healthy older men and women is improved by increased aerobic fitness. Sleep Res 1994;23:149.

[34] Naylor E, Penev PD, Orbeta L, et al. Daily social and physical activity increases slow-wave sleep and daytime neuropsychological performance in the elderly. Sleep 2000;23:87–95.

[35] Tworoger SS, Yasui Y, Vitiello MV, et al. Effects of a yearlong moderate-intensity exercise and a stretching intervention on sleep quality in postmenopausal women. Sleep 2003;26:830–6.

[36] King AC, Oman RF, Brassington GS, et al. Moderate-intensity exercise and self-rated quality of sleep in older adults. A randomized controlled trial. JAMA 1997;277:32–7.

[37] Montgomery P, Dennis J. Physical exercise for sleep problems in adults aged 60+. Cochrane Database Syst Rev 2002;4:CD003404.

[38] Singh NA, Clements KM, Fiatarone MA. A randomized controlled trial of the effect of exercise on sleep. Sleep 1997;20:95–101.

[39] Guilleminault C, Clerk A, Black J, et al. Nondrug treatment trials in psychophysiologic insomnia. Arch Intern Med 1995;155:838–44.

[40] Giebelhaus V, Strohl KP, Lormes W, et al. Physical exercise as an adjunct therapy in sleep apnea–an open trial. Sleep Breath 2000;4:173–6.

[41] Peppard PE, Young T. Exercise and sleep-disordered breathing: an association independent of body habits. Sleep 2004;27:480–4.

[42] Phillips B, Young T, Finn L, et al. Epidemiology of restless legs symptoms in adults. Arch Intern Med 2000;24:2137–41.

[43] de Mello MT, Lauro FA, Silva AC, et al. Incidence of periodic leg movements and of the restless legs syndrome during sleep following acute physical activity in spinal cord injury subjects. Spinal Cord 1996;34:294–6.

[44] de Mello MT, Esteves AM, Tufik S. Comparison between dopaminergic agents and physical exercise as treatment for periodic limb movements in patients with spinal cord injury. Spinal Cord 2004;42:218–21.

[45] Task Force on DSM-IV. Diagnostic and statistical manual of mental disorders: DSM-IV. 4th edition. Washington, DC: American Psychiatric Association; 1994.

[46] Bonnet MH, Arand DL. Activity, arousal, and the MSLT in patients with insomnia. Sleep 2000;23:205–12.

[47] O'Connor PJ, Raglin JS, Martinsen EW. Physical activity, anxiety and anxiety disorders. Int J Sport Psychol 2000;31:136–55.

[48] Perlis ML, Giles DE, Buysse DJ, et al. Self-reported sleep disturbance as a prodromal symptom in recurrent depression. J Affect Disord 1997;42:209–12.

[49] O'Neal HA, Dunn AL, Martinsen EW. Depression and exercise. Int J Sport Psychol 2000;31:110–35.

[50] Vogel GW, Buffenstein A, Minter K, et al. Drug effects on REM sleep and on endogenous depression. Neurosci Biobehav Rev 1990;14:49–63.

[51] Cartwright R, Baehr E, Kirkby J, et al. REM sleep reduction, mood regulation and remission in untreated depression. Psychiatry Res 2003;121:159–67.

[52] Horne JA, Staff LH. Exercise and sleep: body-heating effects. Sleep 1983;6:36–46.

[53] Bunnell DE, Agnew JA, Horvath SM, et al. Passive body heating and sleep: influence of proximity to sleep. Sleep 1988;11:210–9.

[54] Van Someren EJ. More than a marker: Interaction between the circadian regulation of temperature and sleep, age-related changes, and treatment possibilities. Chronobiol Int 2000;17:313–54.

[55] Gilbert SS, van den Heuvel CJ, Ferguson SA, et al. Thermoregulation as a sleep signalling system. Sleep Med Rev 2004;8:81–93.

[56] Murphy PJ, Campbell SS. Nighttime drop in body temperature: a physiological trigger for sleep onset? Sleep 1997;20:505–11.

[57] Monroe LJ. Psychological and physiological differences between good and poor sleepers. J Abnorm Psychol 1967;22:255–64.

[58] Avery DH, Wildschiodtz G, Rafaelsen OJ. Nocturnal temperature in affective disorder. J Affect Disord 1982;4:61–71.

[59] Arbisi PA, Depue RA, Spoont MR, et al. Thermoregulatory response to thermal challenge in seasonal affective disorder: a preliminary report. Psychiatry Res 1989;28:323–34.

[60] Mrosovsky N. Locomotor activity and non-photic influences on circadian clocks. Biol Rev Camb Philosoph Soc 1996;71:343–72.

[61] Edwards B, Waterhouse J, Atkinson G, et al. Exercise does not necessarily influence the phase of the circadian rhythm in temperature in healthy humans. J Sports Sci 2002;20:725–32.

[62] Van Reeth O, Sturis J, Byrne MM, et al. Nocturnal exercise phase delays circadian rhythms of melatonin and thyrotropin secretion in normal men. Am J Physiol 1994;266:E964–74.

[63] Buxton OM, Lee CW, L'Hermite-Balériaux M, et al. Exercise elicits phase shifts and acute alterations of melatonin that vary with circadian phase. Am J Physiol Regul Integr Comp Physiol 2003;284:R714–24.

[64] Baehr EK, Eastman CI, Revelle W, et al. Circadian phase-shifting effects of nocturnal exercise in older compared with young adults. Am J Physiol Regul Integr Comp Physiol 2003; 284:R1542–50.

[65] Eastman CI, Hoese EK, Youngstedt SD, et al. Phase-shifting human circadian rhythms with exercise during the night shift. Physiol Behav 1995;58:1287–91.

[66] Barger LK, Wright Jr KP, Hughes RJ, et al. Daily exercise facilitates phase delays of circadian melatonin rhythm in very dim light. Am J Physiol Regul Integr Comp Physiol 2004; 286:R1077–84.

[67] Miyazaki T, Hashimoto S, Masubuchi S, et al. Phase-advance shifts of human circadian pacemaker are accelerated by daytime physical exercise. Am J Physiol Regul Integr Comp Physiol 2001;281:R197–205.

[68] Youngstedt SD, Kripke DF, Elliott JA, et al. Exercise phase-response curves in young and older adults. Soc Res Biol Rhythms 2002;8:110.

[69] Benloucif S, Bangalore S, Orbeta L, et al. Duration of light exposure and time of sleep/wake affect the phase of circadian rhythms in humans. Soc Res Biol Rhythms 2002;8:31.

[70] Mrosovsky N. Double-pulse experiments with nonphotic and photic phase-shifting stimuli. J Biol Rhythms 1991;6:167–79.

[71] Youngstedt SD, Kripke DF, Elliott JA. Circadian phase-delaying effects of bright light alone and combined with exercise in humans. Am J Physiol Regul Integr Comp Physiol 2002;282: R259–66.

ELSEVIER
SAUNDERS

Clin Sports Med 24 (2005) 367–380

CLINICS
IN SPORTS
MEDICINE

Jet Lag and Air Travel: Implications for Performance

Thomas Reilly, BA, MSc, PhD, DSc, FErgS, FIBiol, DHC*,
Jim Waterhouse, DPhil, Ben Edwards, BSc, MSc, PhD

*Research Institute for Sport and Exercise Sciences, Liverpool John Moores University,
Henry Cotton Campus, 15–21 Webster Street, Liverpool L3 2ET, England*

Sport at an elite level is now a major industry that transcends continental boundaries. Championships and major tournaments tend to rotate across the globe. For example, the Winter Olympics have been held in Lillehammer (Norway), Nagano (Japan), Salt Lake City (United States), and Turin (Italy) over the most recent cycles. Corresponding venues for men's World Cup soccer have been the United States, France, Korea and Japan, and Germany. These examples and the competitive schedules of golf and tennis players provide good illustrations of travel stress [1]. Many sports-governing bodies use training camps in other parts of the world for purposes of warm-weather training or gaining physiologic adjustments to altitude. The frequency of such trips may in itself be disruptive unless the stresses associated with travel are managed appropriately.

International travel presents a potential problem for the serious athlete because the physiologic disturbances caused and the travel stresses implied can interfere with training and preparation for competition. Unless the personal disruptions are minimized, exercise performance or the quality of training may be adversely affected. The health of the traveler can be a concern, including the likely transient increase in injury risk. There have been various sets of guidelines to help traveling athletes adjust quickly to new locations, based on chronobiological principles and an understanding of how the "body clock" operates [2]. Before considering these, the causes of biological disturbances linked with travel and a description of the body clock are presented.

* Corresponding author.
E-mail address: T.P.Reilly@livjm.ac.uk (T. Reilly).

0278-5919/05/$ – see front matter © 2005 Elsevier Inc. All rights reserved.
doi:10.1016/j.csm.2004.12.004
sportsmed.theclinics.com

Travel fatigue and jet lag

Long journeys cause tiredness. Apart from the cramped conditions on board the aircraft, stresses may be compounded by transport arrangements at departure and arrival and the control checks associated with crossing national borders. Travelers may become dehydrated as a result of the dry air they inhale on board the plane, and whole-body stiffness can result from the relative inactivity while traveling. Mood states may be negatively affected by the uncertainties associated with the trip and arrival. These symptoms constitute travel fatigue and can be reversed quickly once destination is reached.

A particular malaise is evident when the journey entails crossing multiple time zones rather than covering a similar distance in a northerly or southerly direction. Among the symptoms are an inability to sleep at the correct local time, bowel irregularities, transient disorientation, poor mental concentration, increased incidence of headaches, and irritability [3]. Symptoms vary during the day, are more severe with the number of meridians crossed, and are worse after flying eastwards compared with westwards. The symptoms are referred to as jet lag [4] and have been monitored in a range of athletes [5]. They cannot be attributed to exposure to an unfamiliar culture, excitement, or apprehension because symptoms return after the journey home.

Jet lag is caused by a desynchronization of the body's circadian system as the normal diurnal rhythm is out of harmony with the new local time. The natural urge to sleep is displaced by local time to earlier in the day after a westward flight and later in the day when the journey is eastwards. Following a westward journey, a circadian phase delay is required for adjustment to the new time zone, and following an eastward journey, normally a phase advance is needed. Traditionally, the rate of adjustment was deemed to be 1 day for each time zone crossed, but there seems to be great interindividual variation in this rate. For athletes, there is a question of how performance might be affected by jet lag. Its consideration requires an explanation of the biologic basis of circadian rhythms and the evidence for a circadian rhythm in exercise performance.

The circadian rhythm in performance

Circadian rhythms refer to fluctuations in physiologic functions over the solar day, corresponding to the daily light–darkness cycle. The classical circadian rhythm is characterized by a cosine wave, the daily change in core temperature being one example. The acrophase refers to the time of peak of the cosine wave fitted to the rhythm (Fig. 1A). The rhythm may be influenced not only by the biological clock (the endogenous component) but also by exogenous factors, such as habitual activity, diet, exercise, heat, and other environmental variables.

The suprachiasmatic nuclei within the hypothalamus regulate the body's circadian system. The cells have receptors for melatonin, a hormone secreted by the pineal gland. The retinohypothalamic tract affords a direct neural pathway from the retina to the suprachiasmatic nuclei, with the intergeniculate leaflet being another input pathway [4]. For light to be effective in synchronizing the body clock to the environment, it has to be relatively bright and sustained. It is likely that the visual receptors that achieve this are independent of the classical rods and cones, and act to assess the time of dawn and dusk according to several aspects of the quality and quantity of light. As darkness falls, melatonin is secreted and its vasodilatory effect causes body temperature to fall and other physiologic functions to slow down in preparation for sleep (Fig. 1B). Light inhibits the release of melatonin so that the natural alternation of light and darkness is linked directly to the body's chronobiologic system. There are rhythms also apparent in local tissues, probably entrained by the timekeeping cells of the suprachiasmatic nucleus (SCN), which can exert their effects on peripheral tissues by means of core temperature, hormones, and the sympathetic nervous system, for example.

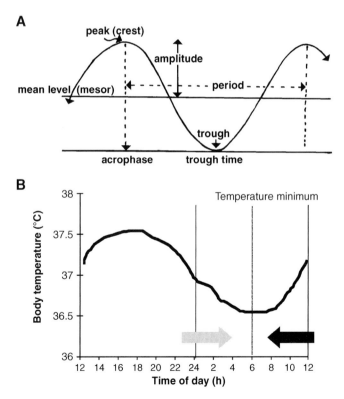

Fig. 1. The circadian rhythm represented as a cosine function (*A*), measured in rectal temperature (*B*), for self-chosen exercise intensity (*C*), and for whole-body flexibility (*D*). (*Data from* Reilly T, Waterhouse J. Sport, exercise and environmental physiology. Edinburgh, Scotland: Elsevier; 2005 [panels *C, D*].)

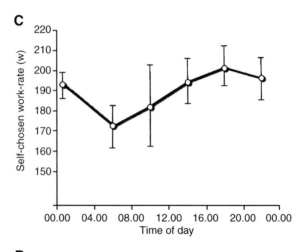

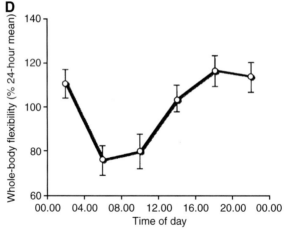

Fig. 1 (*continued*).

Many aspects of exercise performance display circadian rhythms closely synchronized with the rhythm in core body temperature. These include peak force of leg and back muscles [6], arm muscles [7], anaerobic power output, and performance in broad and vertical jumps [8]. The self-chosen work-rate, which is the level at which individuals pace more sustained efforts, also exhibits a circadian variation—one that mirrors the body temperature curve. Peak performance was found to occur at 18:00 hours, the same timing observed for muscle strength and flexibility (see Fig. 1). Although these variables comprise components of performance rather than outcomes in competition, performance in simulated contests or time trials corroborates the existence of circadian rhythms; this applies to swimming [9,10], cycling [11], football skills [12], tennis skills [13], and badminton [14].

Several studies provide evidence of an endogenous component to the circadian rhythm in performance [15]. Extraneous (exogenous) factors such as warm up, diet, sleep disturbance, habits, and chronotype cannot explain the circadian variations observed in well-controlled studies conducted under quasi-constant routines. The circadian variations include physiologic responses to exercise, such as heart rate [16], minute ventilation [17], blood lactate [18], and body temperature [19]. Because these rhythms are relevant to exercise performance and contain an endogenous element, their disturbance following time-zone transitions is likely to impact on sports performance.

Observations in elite athletes

Elite athletes suffer from jet lag after flights to the west [20] and east [21]. Athletes traveling from the United Kingdom to Florida demonstrated a shift in performance variables that was in phase with alterations in intra-aural temperature [20]. These measures included simple and choice reaction times and grip, back, and leg strength. The average rate of adjustment to the new time zone was about 5 days and equal to the number of time zones crossed. Only after the sleep–wake cycle was restored and the acrophase of body temperature re-established did the performance curves return to reference values.

Retrospective analysis of American Football matches demonstrated adverse effects on results when teams had to travel coast-to-coast for matches [22]. The decrement tended to be worse after eastward than westward travel, because the body clock adjusts less easily to a shortening than a lengthening of the day, its endogenous rhythm being in excess of 24 hours. Moreover, decrements were more marked if matches were played at times close to nighttime according to the visitors' home time. Changing training times for a few days before departure to reflect the timing of the forthcoming game in the other time zone benefited the players.

Circadian disruptions were also observed when Olympic athletes and sedentary subjects were monitored on travelling eastwards from the United Kingdom to Australia [5]. Some travelers adjusted by a phase delay, others by a phase advance, following the transition over ten meridians. The study highlighted the importance of individual coping mechanisms and benefits of experience in overcoming the worst symptoms.

Some studies have not shown evidence for a decrement in athletic performance after time zone transitions, but the experimental design has been inadequate. For example, swimmers traveling between mainland United States and Hawaii were reported to show no change in performance [23]. The research design did not account for the rhythmic characteristics of the functions being assessed. A one-off set of observations at one time point in the day is inadequate because several time points are needed to establish the phase of a circadian rhythm. For example, a single time point taken at 12:00 local time might be before the acrophase before travel and yet close to peak performance (about 17:00 hours) after a journey westwards across five time zones. The same limitation applies to a related study of female soccer players (although three separate journeys were considered) where the results indicated a significant effect of jet lag on anaerobic power [24], and to a study involving military personnel where decrements in arm strength and sprint times were reported up to 5 days postflight across six time zones eastwards [25]. Although circadian studies require more than one test event per day (preferably evenly spread throughout the 24 hours, at 4-hour intervals or less), repeated all-out tests at different times of the same day are likely to contain residual fatigue effects and therefore pose another problem [26].

Some of these difficulties were overcome by focusing on components of performance in Rugby League players and recording measurements in the morning and in the evening [27]. Performance measures were depressed for 5 days having crossed ten time zones eastwards. Only after this time was the evening performance in muscle strength superior to that in the morning and it was estimated that at least another 2 to 3 days were needed for the normal circadian rhythm to be restored.

Health consequences

One of the major health risks associated with long-haul flights, deep vein thrombosis, is caused by remaining in a restricted posture for the duration of the journey. Prevention entails becoming periodically active (once every 90–120 minutes), such as walking about the plane, doing isometric exercises while seated, or performing gentle stretches. Use of compression stockings can prevent the pooling of blood in the legs.

The hypoxia in pressurized cabin air may also be a factor in travel fatigue. Coste and colleagues [28] provided evidence of sleep disturbances following a simulated 8-hour flight in a hypobaric chamber. The evening decline in body temperature was delayed with a knock-on consequence for sleep latency. They concluded that the results explain in part the frequent complaints of fatigue after long flights, even when no time zones are crossed.

Long-haul flights have been associated with increased risk of infection. Guidelines are provided by the World Health Authority on health and sanitation in aircraft and the quality of air circulated. Changes in immune function accompany sleep disruption, and an increased risk of infection is caused by reduced defense rather than just increased exposure.

Severity of jet lag seems to be similar in men and in women, but women may experience particular effects. The interaction of melatonin and estrogens released during the menstrual cycle has been linked with secondary amenorrhea in habitual female travelers [29] and dysmenorrhea is common in flight attendants.

A common experience of travelers, including athletes, is gastrointestinal disturbance. The wrong choice of local foods or poor hygiene is often the cause.

When the digestive upsets lead to diarrhea, the individual must be careful to adopt a rehydration regimen. Loss of appetite, hard stools (or constipation), and disruption of the normal eating pattern are characteristics of jet lag.

The managers, technical staff, and mentors of individual athletes and sports teams should also be considered, as performance in their occupational tasks is likely to be affected by jet lag. The support personnel may be at greater health risk than the athletes, especially from cardiovascular disorders. Maximal muscular efforts provide a greater shock to the cardiovascular system early in the morning compared with other times of the day, as indicated by changes in blood pressure [30]. It also seems that by the time body temperature has readjusted to the new time zone, blood pressure responses have not returned to normal [31]. Vulnerable individuals need to be cautious when maintaining their habitual activity programs during their sojourns while circadian rhythms are in the process of resynchronization.

Coping with jet lag

The behavioral approach

The issue of coping with jet lag syndrome has been dominated by problems with the sleep–wake cycle. The questions then arise as to how nocturnal sleep and waking performance can be improved, the cause of sleep disturbances removed, and adjustment of the body clock promoted. A behavioral strategy for coping with jet lag should incorporate activity preflight, during the trip, and following arrival. The journey should also be planned so that the optimal itinerary is chosen to minimize travel fatigue.

For example, a strategy used by the national soccer team of Wales when playing Azerbaijan in a World Cup qualifying match in September, 2004, was to stay on home time for the duration of the short trip. In this instance, the kick-off time of 21:00 hours (17:00 hours on home time) would have suited the strategy. Such an approach is useful if the stay in the new time zone is 3 days or less and adjustment of circadian rhythms is not essential. It also requires the time of competition to coincide with daytime on home time. If this is not the case, then adjustment of the body clock is required. Thus, a European team that is to compete in the morning in Japan or in the evening in the United States would require clock adjustment.

The sleep–wake cycle might be altered for some days before departure with a view toward starting the resynchronization process early. This maneuver (3-, 4-, and 5-hour shifts in delay and advance modes) was only partially effective in altering the circadian phase, because of the difficulty in adjusting the exposure to light [32]. Meanwhile, performance in a range of activity tasks was adversely affected, thereby compromising the quality of training attempted. In general, therefore, itineraries should be arranged to arrive in sufficient time for the body clock to adjust before competitive engagements. Nevertheless, an advance of 1 to 2 hours for 1 to 2 nights before a long-haul flight eastward would be acceptable when a phase-advance strategy is chosen to promote adjustment.

Attention to in-flight activity would focus on meals (eg, which ones to take and which ones to miss), fluid ingestion over and above normal intake, means of obtaining some physical activity periodically, and the timing of attempts to sleep. Because the body clock is in transit between home and the local time at destination, such an attempt is best planned in conjunction with local time at destination. Even though the duration of sleep on board may help the traveler by reducing the time spent awake and idle, it does not seem to speed adjustment after disembarkation [33].

A feeding program in which the macronutrient content of the diet is manipulated may promote circadian resynchronization. The theory is that a breakfast high in protein raises plasma tyrosine levels and their uptake into the brain, thereby stimulating the synthesis and release of dopamine and norepinephrine. This effect activates the body's arousal system, making the individual feel more alert. An evening meal high in carbohydrate would raise plasma tryptophan levels because raised insulin levels promote the cellular uptake of tyrosine rather than tryptophan by the body, thereby increasing the plasma tryptophan/tyrosine ratio and promoting the synthesis and release of serotonin. Serotonin is a neurotransmitter of the raphe nucleus (important in the regulation of sleep) and a precursor of melatonin. As a result of this high-carbohydrate meal, the individual would feel drowsy and inclined toward sleep. Evidence to support the feeding hypothesis is not strong, and indications are that the timing rather than the type of meal is more likely to help readjust the body clock [3].

There are suggestions that exercise adjusts the body clock. The original evidence emerged from studies of rodents undergoing long exercise sessions whose equivalent could not be employed by athletes in practice. Exercise may have some value in phase delays, but its role in phase advances is more uncertain [34]. It may help indirectly by securing a pattern to the habitual activity in the new time zone, linking with social factors and eating habits to restore daily activity to normality. Exposure to light by engaging in activity outdoors and relaxing indoors in dim light can also be part of an adjustment strategy. Light in the 6-hour window before the temperature trough promotes a delay of the body clock, and promotes a phase advance in the 6-hour window after this trough. In practice, exposure to natural light after a flight westwards promotes adjustment of the body clock (Table 1); after a flight to the east, bright light exposure should be avoided until the afternoon [4].

The pharmacologic approach

Various drugs have been used in attempts to ease the effects of jet lag and hasten adjustment to new time zones. Among these are drugs that increase alertness after waking and sustain mental performance during extended periods

Table 1
Recommendations for the use of bright light to adjust the body clock after time zone transitions

Time zones to the west (h)	Bad local times for exposure to light	Good local times for exposure to light
	Local time	Local time
3	02:00–08:00[a]	18:00–24:00[b]
4	01:00–07:00[a]	17:00–23:00[b]
5	24:00–06:00[a]	16:00–22:00[b]
6	23:00–05:00[a]	15:00–21:00[b]
7	22:00–04:00[a]	14:00–20:00[b]
8	21:00–03:00[a]	13:00–19:00[b]
9	20:00–02:00[a]	12:00–18:00[b]
10	19:00–01:00[a]	11:00–17:00[b]
11	18:00–00:00[a]	10:00–16:00[b]
12	17:00–23:00[a]	09:00–15:00[b]
13	16:00–22:00[a]	08:00–14:00[b]
14	15:00–21:00[a]	07:00–13:00[b]
15	14:00–20:00[a]	06:00–12:00[b]
16	13:00–19:00[a]	05:00–11:00[b]

Time zones to the east	Local time	Local time
3	24:00–06:00[b]	08:00–14:00[a]
4	01:00–07:00[b]	09:00–15:00[a]
5	02:00–08:00[b]	10:00–16:00[a]
6	03:00–09:00[b]	11:00–17:00[a]
7	04:00–10:00[b]	12:00–18:00[a]
8	05:00–11:00[b]	13:00–19:00[a]
9	06:00–12:00[b]	14:00–20:00[a]
10	Can be treated as 14 h to the west[c]	
11	Can be treated as 13 h to the west[c]	
12	Can be treated as 12 h to the west[c]	

[a] Denotes promotion of a phase advance.
[b] Denotes a delay of the body clock.
[c] Reflects that the body clock adjusts to large delays more easily than to large advances.

without sleep. The drugs include amphetamines, pemoline, and modafinil. Use of these drugs is unacceptable for traveling athletes because they are on the list of drugs banned by the International Olympic Committee. However, patients who use prescribed stimulants (eg, for narcolepsy, attention deficit disorder) are allowed to persist with their medication. Modafinil showed up in positive tests on two prominent competitors (subsequently banned for illegal use) following the 2003 World Athletics Championships in Paris.

Soporific drugs or hypnotics that induce drowsiness and promote sleep, and chronobiotics that exert a direct shifting effect on the SCN, should be useful. Among these drugs are the benzodiazepines or minor tranquilizers. No beneficial effects of temazepam were evident in the athletes traveling five time zones to the west from the United Kingdom to Florida because arrival at destination in the late evening local time helped subjects get to sleep without needing any drug assistance [20]. Diazepam has a longer half-life and would be unsuitable for use by athletes because of residual effects on alertness and psychomotor performance. Hangover effects of loprazolam have been found on a range of physical performance tasks 10 hours after administration [35]. Zolpidem, zopiclane and zaleplon have shorter half-lives than temazepam and affect short-term memory less than other benzodiazepines. Daurat et al [36] found no difference between zopiclane (7.5 mg) and placebo on jet-lag scores after a flight across five time zones between France and Martinique. Zopiclane seemed to accelerate readjustment of the rest–activity rhythm and help restore the phase relationship between sleep and the temperature rhythm.

Although some authorities have advocated the use of hypnotic drugs [37], this view is not universal. In its position statement on use of sleeping pills and melatonin, the British Olympic Association concluded that use of sleeping pills was unnecessary for its athletes and support staff, and counseled against use of these substances [38]. The association acknowledged, however, that individual athletes may have confidence in the effects of these substances from previous personal experience and that physicians may choose sleeping pills to treat persistent insomnia in special cases.

Melatonin has hypnotic and chronobiotic properties. When taken before going to sleep, it induces drowsiness and has no hangover effects on performance the morning after [39]. Melatonin reduces subjective symptoms of jet lag after real or simulated flights and improves sleep in the laboratory environment [4], and therefore might be a valuable palliative. Its chronobiotic function is less clear, as its phase-response curve means that the timing of ingestion is critical and can be inconvenient after certain time-zone transitions [40]. If taken before the trough in body temperature, it would promote a phase advance, and if taken afterwards it would promote a phase delay. Ingestion at all times induces fatigue. Although there are several positive reports for melatonin in treating jet lag, its use was ineffective in ameliorating symptoms in travelers between the United Kingdom and Australia, where the responses were similar to a placebo group for the first week in the new time zone (Fig. 2) [21]. Melatonin may help induce sleep in the evening, even if a phase-shifting effect is absent [4], and any chronobiotic function is separate from its hypnotic and temperature-lowering properties [41].

Caffeine is a central nervous system stimulant that increases alertness and therefore would be appropriate for administration in the mornings after arrival. It can also modify the endogenous secretion of melatonin by inhibiting adenosine receptors $\alpha 2b$ of the pineal cells. The usefulness of slow-release caffeine (administered in the morning) and melatonin (administered in the evening) was compared with a placebo in volunteers undertaking an eastbound trip across seven time zones [42]. Performance was recorded twice each day in the form of grip strength, squat jump, and a multiple jump test that took 15 seconds. Subjects in the placebo group showed a decrease from reference values for the first four mornings in the new time zone, confirming the negative impact of jet lag on human performance. Slow-release caffeine and melatonin maintained a satisfactory level of performance but only in grip strength of the dominant hand. Results

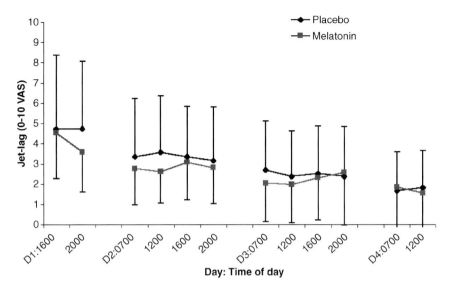

Fig. 2. No effect of melatonin ingestion on jet lag ratings following a 10-hour time zone transition eastwards. (*From* Edwards BJ, Atkinson G, Waterhouse J, et al. Use of melatonin in recovery from jet-lag following an eastward flight across 10 time-zones. Ergonomics 2000;43: 1501–13; with permission.)

in the dynamic tests were variable. In a related report from the same study, caffeine reduced daytime sleepiness for a few days but had unwanted effects on recovery sleep [43]. Although the investigators concluded that both drugs may have value in alleviating some symptoms related to jet lag combined with sleep deprivation, their observations did not provide convincing evidence to support the claim.

Combined behavioral and pharmacologic manipulations have been used. Cardinali et al [44] controlled the environment to which the Boca Juniors team was exposed when traveling from Argentina to Japan for the intercontinental club's soccer championship. They reported successful results from a manipulation of the environmental light–dark cycle that commenced on boarding the flight and was complemented by use of melatonin. The claims for a complete adjustment have not been replicated in other comparable studies, notably when temazepam [20] and melatonin [21] have been administered as putative chronobiotics.

Things to avoid

In a new time zone, some degree of mental toughness is required to get through the periodic episodes when effects of jet lag or drowsiness may become difficult to overcome. During the period of adjustment, a prolonged nap anchors sleep in the rhythm of the zone departed [45]. It is not known if a short "power nap" has any adverse effects on athletes' adjustment, but it seems that a 20-minute nap (which does not induce sleep inertia) is acceptable early within the first day to recuperate from sleep deprivation [3].

Alcohol is best avoided by athletes and mentors during the adjustment period. As a diuretic, it could interfere with hydration strategies, especially if there are other environmental stresses such as heat or altitude acting in combination. Furthermore, alcohol may help in inducing sleep but cause awakenings during the night for micturition [46].

It is accepted practice that strenuous training is avoided for the first few days in a new time zone. Lapses in concentration may cause errors in complex and risky physical routines and lead to injury. Although such lowering of the exercise intensity is adopted as good practice, there are no reliable published statistics that show an increase in injuries following long-haul flights. However, a causal link between jet lag and accidents has been shown in occupational settings, and is therefore assumed to also apply to sports training contexts [47]. Nevertheless, light-intensity exercise and moderate activity are recommended to aid resynchronization, although training in the morning should be eschewed after long-haul flights eastwards when a phase delay is undesirable and light exposure should be avoided.

Breaking up the journey with a stopover could reduce the severity of jet lag symptoms and hasten readjustment [48]. Flying from the United Kingdom to Australia with a 2-day stopover in Singapore decreased the severity of jet lag compared with that typically reported by other travelers going the same route without a stopover [49]. However, a break in the journey is not popular with individual athletes who prefer to have minimal disruption to their training. Furthermore, the logistics involved with traveling teams makes stopovers impractical, unless an exhibition or friendly match is built into the schedule.

Summary

The effects of jet lag are transient and should not entail cessation of athletic training. Symptoms will not cause performers to desist because of exhaustion, as might occur with heat stress, but can hinder quality of training and performance. Rehydration is important, particularly if the ambient temperature in the new time zone is high, as heat stress may be compounded by fluid losses incurred during flight. Behavioral means of coping with jet lag should be sufficient provided the travelers arrive in time to allow the body clock to adjust by the first competition. Because pharmacology has not provided a panacea for overcoming jet lag, a behavioral strategy can be implemented by raising awareness of the issues and by setting guidelines as to the actions required on specific trips and the things to avoid. The educational program should be extended to support staff in addition to the active members of the traveling team. With this background information, the physician can tailor a coping program to the needs and characteristics of an individual athlete.

References

[1] Reilly T, Atkinson G, Waterhouse J. The traveling racket sports player. In: Lees A, Maynard I, Hughes M, et al, editors. Science and racket sports II. London: E&F N Spon; 1988. p. 97–106.

[2] Reilly T, Atkinson G, Waterhouse J. Biological rhythms and exercise. Oxford, England: Oxford University Press; 1997.

[3] Reilly T, Waterhouse J. Sport, exercise and environmental physiology. Edinburgh, Scotland: Elsevier; 2005.

[4] Waterhouse J, Reilly T, Atkinson G. Jet-lag. Lancet 1997;350:1611–6.

[5] Waterhouse J, Edwards B, Nevill A, et al. Identifying some determinants of "jet lag" and its symptoms: a study of athletes and other travellers. Br J Sports Med 2002;36:54–60.

[6] Coldwells A, Atkinson G, Reilly T. Sources of variation in back and leg dynamometry. Ergonomics 1994;37:79–86.

[7] Gauthier A, Davenne D, Martin A, et al. Diurnal rhythm of the muscular performance of elbow flexors during isometric contractions. Chronobiol Int 1996;13:135–46.

[8] Reilly T, Down A. Investigation of circadian rhythm in anaerobic power and capacity of the legs. J Sports Med Phys Fitness 1992;32:343–7.

[9] Baxter C, Reilly T. Influence of time of day on all-out swimming. Br J Sports Med 1983;17:122–7.

[10] Reilly T, Marshall S. Circadian rhythms in power output on a swim bench. J Swim Res 1991;7(2):11–3.

[11] Atkinson G, Todd C, Reilly T, et al. Diurnal variation in cycling performance: influence of warm-up. J Sports Sci, in press.

[12] Reilly T, Fairhurst E, Edwards B, et al. Time of day and performance tests in male football players. In: Reilly T, Cabri J, Araujo D, editors. Science and football V. London: Routledge, in press.

[13] Atkinson G, Speirs L. Diurnal variation in tennis service. Percept Mot Skills 1998;86:1335–8.

[14] Edwards BJ, Lindsay K, Waterhouse J. Effect of time of day on the accuracy and consistency of the badminton serve. Ergonomics, in press.

[15] Drust B, Waterhouse J, Atkinson G, et al. Circadian rhythms in sports performance: an update. Chronobiol Int, in press.

[16] Reilly T, Brooks GA. Investigation of circadian rhythms in metabolic responses to exercise. Ergonomics 1982;25:1093–107.

[17] Reilly T. Circadian variation in ventilatory and metabolic adaptations to submaximal exercise. Br J Sports Med 1982;16:115–6.

[18] Forsyth JJ, Reilly T. Circadian rhythms in blood lactate concentration during incremental ergometer rowing. Eur J Appl Physiol 2004;92:69–74.

[19] Aldemir H, Atkinson G, Cable T, et al. Comparison of the immediate effects of moderate exercise in the late morning and late afternoon on core temperature and cutaneous thermoregulatory mechanisms. Chronobiol Int 2000;17:197–207.

[20] Reilly T, Atkinson G, Budgett R. Effect of low-dose temazepam on physiological variables and performance tests following a westerly flight across five time zones. Int J Sports Med 2001; 22:166–74.

[21] Edwards BJ, Atkinson G, Waterhouse J, et al. Use of melatonin in recovery from jet-lag following an eastward flight across 10 time-zones. Ergonomics 2000;43:1501–13.

[22] Jehue R, Street D, Huizenga R. Effect of time zone and game time changes on peak performance: National Football League. Med Sci Sports Exerc 1993;25:127–31.

[23] O' Connor PJ, Morgan WP, Koltyn KF, et al. Air travel across four time zones in college swimmers. J Appl Physiol 1991;70:756–63.

[24] Hill DW, Hill CM, Fields KL, et al. Effects of jet lag on factors related to sports performance. Can J Appl Physiol 1993;18:91–103.

[25] Wright JE, Vogel JA, Sampson JB, et al. Effects of travel across time zones (jet-lag) on exercise capacity and performance. Aviat Space Environ Med 1983;54:132–7.

[26] Reilly T, Bambaeichi E. Methodological issues in studies of rhythms in human performance. Biol Rhythm Res 2003;34:321–36.

[27] Reilly T, Mellor S. Jet lag in student Rugby League players following a near-maximal time zone shift. In: Reilly T, Lees A, Davids WJ, et al, editors. Science and football. London: E&FN Spon; 1988. p. 249–56.

[28] Coste O, Beaumont M, Batejat D, et al. Prolonged mild hypoxia modifies circadian core temperature and may be associated with sleep disturbances. Chronobiol Int 2004;21:419–33.

[29] Suvanto S, Harma M, Ilmarinen J, et al. Effects of 10 h time zone changes on female flight attendants' circadian rhythms of body temperature, alertness, and visual search. Ergonomics 1993;36:613–25.

[30] Cabri J, De Witte B, Clarys JP, et al. Circadian variation in blood pressure responses to muscular exercise. Ergonomics 1988;31:1559–66.

[31] Lemmer B, Kern RI, Nold G, et al. Jet lag in athletes after eastward and westward time-zone transition. Chronobiol Int 2002;19:743–64.

[32] Reilly T, Maskell P. Effects of altering the sleep-wake cycle in human circadian rhythms and motor performance. Proceedings of the First IOC World Congress on Sport Science, Colorado Springs, CO: U.S. Olympic Committee; 1989. p. 106.

[33] Carvalho Bos S, Waterhouse J, Edwards B, et al. The use of actimetry to assess changes to the rest-activity cycle. Chronobiol Int 2003;20:1039–59.

[34] Edwards B, Waterhouse J, Atkinson G, et al. Exercise does not necessarily influence the phase of the circadian rhythm in temperature in healthy humans. J Sports Sci 2002;20:725–32.

[35] Grobler LA, Schwellnus MP, Trichard C, et al. Comparative effects of zopiclone and loprazolam on psychomotor and physical performance in active individuals. Clin J Sport Med 2000;10:123–8.

[36] Daurat A, Benoit O, Buguet A. Effects of zopiclone on the rest/activity rhythm after a westward flight across five time zones. Psychopharmacology (Berl.) 2000;149:241–5.

[37] Stone BM, Turner C. Promoting sleep in shiftworkers and intercontinental travelers. Chronobiol Int 1997;14:133–43.

[38] Reilly T, Maughan R, Budgett R. Melatonin: a position statement of the British Olympic Association. Br J Sports Med 1998;32:99–100.

[39] Atkinson G, Buckley P, Edwards B, et al. Are there hangover-effects on physical performance when melatonin is ingested by athletes before nocturnal sleep? Int J Sports Med 2001; 22:232–4.

[40] Lewy AJ, Ahmed S, Jackson JM, et al. Melatonin shifts human circadian rhythms according to a phase-response curve. Chronobiol Int 1992;9:380–92.

[41] Waterhouse J, Reilly T, Atkinson G. Melatonin and jet lag. Br J Sports Med 1998;32:98–9.

[42] Lagarde D, Chappuis B, Billaud PF, et al. Evaluation of pharmacological aids on physical performance after a transmeridian flight. Med Sci Sports Exerc 2001;33:628–34.

[43] Beaumont M, Batejat D, Pierard C, et al. Caffeine or melatonin effects on sleep and sleepiness after rapid eastward transmeridian travel. J Appl Physiol 2004;96:50–8.

[44] Cardinali DP, Bortman GP, Liotta G, et al. A multifactorial approach employing melatonin to accelerate resynchronization of sleep-wake cycle after a 12 time-zone westerly transmeridian flight in elite soccer athletes. J Pineal Res 2002;32:41–6.

[45] Minors DS, Waterhouse JM. Anchor sleep as a synchronizer of rhythms on abnormal routines. Int J Chronobiol 1981;7:165–88.

[46] Reilly T. Alcohol, anti-anxiety drugs and sport. In: Mottram DR, editor. Drugs in sport. London: Routledge; 2003. p. 256–85.

[47] Samel A, Wegmann HM, Vejvoda M. Jet lag and sleepiness in aircrew. J Sleep Res 1995; 4(Suppl 2):S30–6.

[48] Tsai TH, Okumura M, Yamasaki M, et al. Simulation of jet lag following a trip with stopovers by intermittent schedule shifts. J Interdiscipl Cycle Res 1988;19:89–96.

[49] Reilly T. Chronobiology and sports performance. Pre-Olympic Scientific Conference, Thessaloniki, Greece, August 6–11, 2004.

CLINICS
IN SPORTS
MEDICINE

Clin Sports Med 24 (2005) 381–413

ELSEVIER
SAUNDERS

Circadian Phase Shifting, Alerting, and Antidepressant Effects of Bright Light Treatment

Teodor T. Postolache, MD[a,b,*], Dan A. Oren[c]

[a]Department of Psychiatry, University of Maryland School of Medicine, 685 West Baltimore Street, Baltimore, MD 21201, USA
[b]Institute for Sports Chronobiology, 2423 Pennsylvania Avenue, NW, Washington, DC 20037, USA
[c]Department of Psychiatry, Yale University School of Medicine, P.O. Box 5078, Woodbridge, CT 06525, USA

As our planet rotates around the Sun, a world of darkness alternates with a world of light. Because the axis of Earth is shifted, the northern and southern hemispheres come under the influence of seasonal changes in the duration of day length as it revolves around the Sun. Living organisms have developed mechanisms to track changes in environmental light in order to be active and engage their environment during a specific temporal niche (eg, diurnal, nocturnal, crepuscular species) and to retreat at other times to a burrow for rest and sleep. Many species have also developed mechanisms to track day length in anticipation of changes in seasons and manifest certain marked seasonal behavioral changes, such as those associated with reproduction, rearing of the young, pelage, nest building, hibernation, and migration—seasonal rhythms that find the best species-significant alignment between seasonal environmental resources and energetic demands, considering food and water supply and reproductive cycles.

Our ancestors lived with brighter days, darker and longer nights, and did not travel across time zones. Our physiology is anchored in ancestral evolutionary conditions rather than our current, relatively shielded microclimate, with artificial light and temperature control.

Like plants, insects, fishes, birds, and mammals, humans have body clocks that maintain endogenous rhythms in constant conditions and adjust their inter-

* Corresponding author. Department of Psychiatry, University of Maryland School of Medicine, 685 West Baltimore Street, Baltimore, MD 21201.
   E-mail address: tpostolache@psych.umaryland.edu (T.T. Postolache).

nal time to the external time by way of light input through the retina. For all of these organisms, light is not just a vehicle for vision but also the main synchronizer between circa 24-hour rhythms in physiologic states and 24-hour fluctuations in environmental conditions.

The role of light in entrainment and phase shifting

Light as a zeitgeber

The "master" circadian oscillator is situated in the suprachiasmatic nuclei (SCN) of the hypothalamus. The article by Stiller and Postolache elsewhere in this issue further discusses this topic.

The SCN drives oscillations in electrophysiological neuronal activity and hormonal rhythms that convey information to "slave" oscillators dispersed at diverse levels of the organism. The circadian rhythms are endogenous and continue "free-running" in constant conditions with a period slightly different from 24 hours. For some organisms where the period is shorter than 24 hours, phase advances of circadian rhythms are evident (ie, certain physiologic and behavioral rhythms tend to occur at an earlier time each day), and in others where it is longer, phase delays in circadian rhythms occur (ie, certain physiologic and behavioral rhythms tend to occur at a later clock time each day).

Although the SCN generates circadian rhythms, it also adjusts the timing of circadian rhythms to the environment. The most important aspect of this external synchronization is the entrainment of the circadian rhythms to the 24-hour period of the day and night alternation. For this purpose, the SCN uses "zeitgebers" or "time givers," which represent environmental entrainment agents that cue a 24-hour period.

In many species, light is the main entrainment agent. Early human experiments incorrectly suggested that the primary entrainment agent for humans was social interaction [1]. Methodological inadequacies, such as self-selection of lighting schedules are now considered to have contributed to this false impression. At this point it is unequivocally known that light cycles are the primary entrainment agent for human circadian rhythms [2–4].

Light as a circadian phase shifting agent

Several studies have shown that timed single pulses of light can delay or advance circadian rhythms in humans and other mammals [5–14]. Certain studies have applied two bright light stimuli during two different circadian phases, demonstrating phase-dependent phase-shifting with light [5,9,15].

The most comprehensive analysis of the phase response to light is achieved by deriving a phase response curve (PRC), in which the relationship between the timing of the administration of light stimulus (graphically represented on the *x*-axis) and the direction and magnitude of a shift (graphically represented on the *y*-axis) is quantified.

To date there have been six reported studies on PRC to light in humans. The earliest study, which was discordant with other empirical and laboratory studies [16], revealed a PRC without a phase-delaying portion. This study, in addition to several others that followed [17], suffered from gaps in the PRC for periods as long as 11 hours, with the phase-delaying portion of the curve poorly defined. Further problems with these initial PRCs were that they did not use a constant routine protocol to minimize the masking effects of sleep–wake, posture, and food and water intake on temperature minimum. Constant routine consists of prolonged wakefulness in a semirecumbent position of 30 to 50 hours, often of 40 hours, enforced by an attending technician, in a room lit with dim light. Food, water, and any medications (if any) are distributed throughout day and night, at equal short intervals to minimize possible masking influences on circadian rhythms. The effect of duration of wakefulness is eliminated using mathematical models, before the circadian effects are analyzed by fitting a cosine function. A retrospective analysis [18] was weakened by insufficient data points (only 11). In that study, the light-pulse duration was variable, lasting from 4.2 to 6.2 hours. One well-designed study used a bright light stimulus of 7,000 to 12,000 lux for 5 hours, followed by a 7- to 8-hour sleep episode in total darkness 12 hours later, and repeated this cycle for three consecutive days before its effect on circadian phase was determined. This strong or type 0 PRC resulted in shifts as large as 6 to 12 hours when light was administered at a critical time around the minimum core body temperature [19]. The type 0 PRC may be characteristic in humans, with the first exposure decreasing the rhythm amplitude and making the circadian system more sensitive to the second exposure, resulting in significantly large phase shifts. Van Cauter et al [20] used well-controlled conditions in a constant routine protocol with an administration of a single pulse of 3 hours and 5000 lux of light to describe the phase-advance and phase-delay portion of the human PRC as similar to the PRC to light in most mammals. This weak or type 1 PRC has been replicated in highly controlled laboratory conditions by Khalsa et al [21], who reported a peak to trough PRC of 5.2 hours, with delays occurring when the stimulus was administered before the temperature minimum (ie, at the critical phase or the inflection point on the PRC) and delays occurring when the light stimulus was administered after the temperature minimum (Fig. 1). The amplitude of the delays (up to 3 hours) was greater than the amplitude of the advances (up to 2 hours). This type 1 PRC has two inflection points: one nocturnal, when the phase-delaying region converts into the phase-advancing region at the temperature minimum; and the second when the phase-advancing region converts into the phase-delaying region 10 hours after the temperature minimum (Fig. 1). It is also relevant that the maximum phase advances and delays tend to occur between 2 and 6 hours before (phase delay) and after (phase advance) the temperature minimum. In contrast to a type 0 PRC, where phase shifts as large as 12 hours have been reported, the type 1 PRC phase shifts are near zero when light is administered close to temperature minimum.

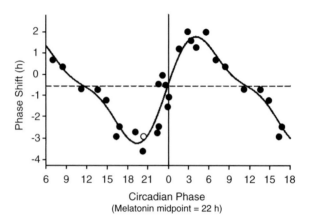

Fig. 1. PRC to the bright light stimulus using melatonin midpoints as the circadian phase marker. Phase advances (positive values) and delays (negative values) are plotted against the timing of the center of the light exposure relative to the melatonin midpoint on the prestimulus circadian rhythm (defined as 22 hours), with the core body-temperature minimum assumed to occur 2 hours later at 0 hours. Data points from circadian phases 6 to 18 are double plotted. The filled circles represent data from plasma melatonin, and the open circle represents data from salivary melatonin in subject 18K8 from whom blood samples were not acquired. The solid curve is a dual harmonic function fitted through all of the data points. The horizontal dashed line represents the anticipated 0.54-hour average delay drift of the pacemaker between the pre- and poststimulus phase assessments. (*From* Khalsa SB, Jewett ME, Cajochen C, et al. A phase response curve to single bright light pulses in human subjects, J Physiol 2003;549:945–52; with permission.)

Wavelength considerations

Although the resetting response to bright light has been shown to depend on duration intensity, timing, and number of exposures [22], the effects of the wavelength are less clearly known. Blue light appears to have stronger circadian effects than red light. For instance, in a recent study, exposure to 6.5 hours of monochromatic light at 460 nm induced a two-fold greater phase delay, and twice the amount of melatonin suppression than exposure to light at 555 nm of equal duration and photon density [23]. This finding is consistent with that of Rea et al [24], who reported that short-wavelength light (420–520 nm) dominates melatonin suppression over broad-spectrum distribution, and with that of Figueiro et al [25], who reported that blue light-emitting diodes suppress melatonin more effectively than mercury vapor lamps of greater illuminance.

Lockley et al [23] reported an interaction between the wavelength and the duration of melatonin suppression. Short-wavelength light resulted in a prolonged, uninterrupted signal that caused continuous melatonin suppression for at least 6.5 hours. Long-wavelength light also suppressed melatonin in a majority of subjects, but the suppressive effect disappeared earlier than with shorter wavelength.

The exact molecular mechanism of these effects remains unknown. The three-cone photopic system used for image forming is not the primary mediator of circadian responses to light. Normal circadian shifting and melatonin suppression persist in red–green color-blind individuals [26], as in blind individuals [27,28]. Research in nocturnal animals suggests that conventional rod and cone–mediated photoreception that mediates sight is not required for non–image-forming ocular responses [29–31]. Two candidate molecules have received the most recent attention. Greatest interest has been shown in melanopsin, an opsin that is present in the majority of retinal ganglion cells that project to the SCN [32–36]. Melanopsin-containing cells in rats [36] are directly photosensitive to short-wavelength light, and are also present in human retinae [37]. Recent studies on knockout mice lacking melanopsin have shown attenuation of circadian responses [38,39]. Although they likely play some role in the mammalian time-keeping apparatus, there is lesser support for the idea that cryptochromes—flavoproteins used for blue light detection, including circadian responses in plants and lower organisms—are also mammalian circadian photoreceptors [40].

A potential greater effectiveness and energy-efficiency of shorter-wavelength as compared with higher-energy polychromatic white light for circadian phase-shifting may be applicable to the treatment of circadian rhythm sleep disorders, including jet lag, shift work, and delayed or advanced sleep phase. Reduction in overall intensity of light and possibly duration of light treatment could result in improvement in certain adverse effects of light, such as headaches, visual discomfort, glare, and nausea. The greater potential of retinal damage with shorter wavelengths could be offset by a lower illuminance and duration of exposure required to produce an effect.

For future clinical applications, research, and lighting industry standards, it may be very important to include considerations of wavelength in addition to irradiance, timing, duration, and pattern of exposure [23].

Light treatment for jet lag

Jet lag represents a frequent problem for individual athletes and teams. Because the sports-specific aspects of jet lag are discussed in the review by Reilly et al found elsewhere in this issue, they will only be discussed here in terms of the use and avoidance of light.

Performance decrements result from at least three processes: (1) desynchronization between the timing of peak performance (ie, mental and physical resources) and environmental demands, specifically with respect to athletes' timing of competition or training; (2) sleep loss and sleep debt (ie, impaired sleep initiation after westward flights versus premature awakening after eastward flights [41]); and (3) sickness, which might be an expression of internal de-synchronization between the SCN and peripheral oscillators [42]. The effects of sleep debt are described elsewhere in this issue by Dement.

Many people equate jet lag with the effects of sleep loss as a result of an inability to fall asleep or to maintain sleep at the destination's local time. However, a laboratory experiment comparing the securing of sleep duration with the realignment of circadian rhythms showed that even partial (ie, incomplete) realignment, achieved using bright light exposure, melatonin, and sunglasses out-doors, resulted in better cognitive performance on a neurobehavioral assessment battery, mood, and subjective alertness than maintaining a reasonable sleep du-ration only [43].

As more time zones are crossed, misalignment increases and the severity of symptoms and duration of the jet lag worsen. Jet lag is typically worse when traveling east than when traveling west [44]. There are at least three explanations why it is more difficult to adjust for travel east. One explanation is that the circadian clock has a period slightly longer than 24 hours [45], thereby having a natural tendency to phase delay, which may explain why phase delays proceed more rapidly than phase advances. Another explanation is that the amplitude of phase delays is greater than phase advances on the light PRC (see Fig. 1). Finally, the risk of antidromal re-entrainment is greater in traveling five to ten time zones west than five to ten time zones east.

Antidromal re-entrainment represents re-entrainment by phase-shifting in the opposite direction of the shortest shift between the time of origin and destination. For instance, traveling from New York to Paris requires a phase advance of 6 hours to synchronize internal rhythms to the external clock. An equivalent result would be achieved, however, with a phase delay of 18 hours (24 minus 6 hours). This delay would take significantly longer. There is, however, the exception of transmeridian travel of approximately 12-hours (anywhere from 10–14 hours), where adjusting antidromally would be similar, and in certain situations even faster (given the greater magnitude of phase delays), than adjusting in the direction of the shift in external time. In fact, Waterhouse et al [46] recommended adjustment using phase delays in eastward flights crossing nine or more meridians, consistent with phase delays being more easily achieved than phase advances.

Takahashi et al [47] reported that among six travelers who traveled east across eight time zones, one traveler did not shift at all and one showed an antidromal shift after 5 days at destination. With a ten time-zone flight, 11 of 12 travelers phase delayed rather than phase advanced [48]. Similarly, after an 11 time-zone eastward flight, seven of eight participants phase delayed, instead of phase advancing, and only one phase advanced [49]. The probability of antidromal re-entrainment following eastward travel increases with the number of time zones crossed [48], especially if that number is greater than seven. The pattern of light–dark exposure during the travel and destination is crucial for the direction of entrainment.

The main cause of antidromal entrainment is exposure to light on the wrong arm of the light PRC (see Fig. 1). For instance, considering the example of traveling from New York to Paris, assume that someone arrives at 8 AM in Paris. At this point, there is a 6 hour lag between the internal circadian rhythms and the external clock time in Paris. At that time the sun is relatively oblique and, unless conditions are cloudy or it is during late fall/early winter, creates the condition of bright light exposure. This bright light is not stimulating the SCN at 8 AM (as Paris time) but at 2 AM (the internal time). If one looks at the PRC, this may be the region of the light PRC where maximum phase delays occur. Therefore, at the end of the light exposure, one could consider that, by way of phase delays, instead of a 6-hour jet lag, there is now an 8-hour jet lag. To avoid this effect, one would have to avoid or minimize light exposure before the temperature minimum, between 10 AM and 11 AM Paris time. Afterwards, bright light exposure is highly recommended, as it will hit the phase-advancing portion of the PRC.

One common mistake travelers make is to follow the wrong advice that indiscriminate exposure to light at destination hastens the adaptation to the new time zone. In fact, avoidance of light at certain times is important to prevent worsening of the internal–external desynchrony and jet lag. Appropriately timed light exposure and light avoidance in the new destination may hasten adaptation to the new time zone [46,50]. Although it was initially believed that only bright light effectively suppresses melatonin in humans, it is now known that even intensities commonly encountered in real-life situations are potent phase shifters and melatonin suppressors [51]. A study of 15 healthy young men in a laboratory simulation of a trip from Montreal to London (ie, an eastward flight across five time zones), using a schedule of exposure to the indoor room light to which urban dwellers are typically exposed, found that exposure to room light during the advancing portion of the PRC (see Fig. 1) was effective in synchronizing the biological night and day to the sleep–wake rhythms in the new destination [52]. In contrast, individuals exposed to 6 hours of room light during the delaying portion of the PRC had their biological night and day synchronized with the sleep–wake cycles of the point of departure.

Light avoidance is an effective circadian shifter. For instance, in laboratory conditions, darkness or sleep in the afternoon resulted in a 1-hour phase advance of melatonin onset [53]. Darkness can be simulated by the use of eye shades, window shades (in an airplane or hotel), or sunglasses to block the lateral light that could stimulate the nasal portion of the retina. Sunglasses with a low light transmission, such as those with dark lenses that have a transmission of 2%, should not be used by drivers, as the limited light transmission poses a risk for accidents [54]. Sunglasses with a higher light transmission (eg, 15%) can be used for nighttime blocking of blue-green light.

If logistically feasible, there is merit to initiating a preflight circadian adjustment. For instance, for an eastward flight over at least five time zones, it is useful to shift the rhythms preflight, thereby avoiding the exposure to natural light during the phase-delaying portion of the PRC on arrival. In this example (applicable for a flight from the east coast of the United States to London), the temperature minimum for most people, occurring between 4 and 5 AM on the East Coast, will occur between 9 AM and 10 AM in London. Because many flights land well before 9 AM, exposure to light after arrival hits the PRC in the vicinity of its maximum phase-delaying inflection. Moreover, many people spend their phase-advancing portion of the PRC in dimmer environments, such as hotels or gyms. With a maximum 2-hour delay, the difference between the internal time and the external time will therefore not be 5, but 7 hours, which will move the inflection point in the wrong direction, and the next day the inflection point will be at 11 AM. Therefore, light before 11 AM will further move the PRC in the wrong direction, accentuating the abnormalities and worsening symptoms.

If someone, however, was able to advance 2 to 3 hours before departure, the natural light exposure on arrival at the airport or during the travel from the airport to the hotel would occur during the phase-advancing portion of the PRC, and concerns about antidromal phase shifting would be greatly reduced. A 2-hour advance would reduce the risk of antidromal adaptation in travelers who arrive in the new time zone in the morning. For instance, for a journey from New York to Paris (a 6-hour eastward flight) arriving at 8 AM, the estimated temperature minimum would be between 10 AM and 11 AM. Therefore, light should be avoided (eg, using sunglasses) before 11 AM so to not worsen jet lag. This might be difficult, given the exposure in the airport and the travel from the airport to the city. Thus, a 2-hour advance should be sufficient to reduce the interval that would favor antidromal adaptation. If the flight takes place during summertime (with its early sunrise), the traveler should avoid looking at the morning sky through the windows of the airplane.

Moving the timing of bright light administration along the PRC of light assures that bright light administration occurs at a more optimal time for the intended time shift. Appropriately timed bright light acts like a broom, sweeping the rhythms in the desired direction [54]. Inappropriately timed bright light sweeps the rhythms antidromally. For tables on the recommended timing to avoid or seek light, see the article by Reilly et al elsewhere in this issue.

Alerting and antidepressant effects of light

Immediate alerting effects of bright light

Through circadian phase shifting, light may have a very pronounced effect on the alertness/sleepiness rhythms of the following day or days. Light also has direct alerting effects [55] especially in adverse circadian or homeostatic conditions. Circadian adversity refers to an unfavorable internal time when the individual or team may need to perform. It includes the biological night, as discussed by Stiller and Postolache elsewhere in this issue, especially in the temporal vicinity of the temperature trough, and the postprandial dip, as discussed by Monk elsewhere in this issue. Homeostatic adversity refers to sleep debt, or an unfavorable demand for performance (eg, competition, practice) in conditions of insufficiently satisfied appetite for sleep.

Bright light effects on alertness and performance in conditions of circadian adversity

In certain sports, many competitions start and may continue until late in the evening and night (eg, figure skating, baseball, football, soccer). Alertness diminishes abruptly 1 to 2 hours after the onset of nocturnal melatonin se-cretion [56]. In baseball, because a great number of games extend late into the evening, circadian rhythms may be phase-delayed and, as an adaptation occurs, the circadian adversity may not be as big as in sports such as figure skating or football, where training and the majority of games occur at a much earlier time and the frequency of games is smaller compared with baseball. Light administered late in the evening, in the early "biological night" after melatonin starts being secreted, immediately reduces sleepiness [57]. This ele-vation in alertness appears proportional to melatonin suppression [58], and occurs at rest and during a stimulating mental task [59]. These results are con-sistent with other studies that indicate an alerting effect of light during internal night [60–63].

When performance is measured throughout the night, dissociation between alertness/reaction time and accuracy of performance has been reported. For instance, Babkoff et al [64] reported that bright light exposure of 1 hour at approximately 3000 lux, as compared with dim light, improved subjective alertness and reaction time, but worsened error rate in a simulated nightshift in the lab. In that study, the most effective intervention, with better outcome than bright light or caffeine alone, was the combination of 1 hour of bright light with 200 mg of caffeine, which maintained alertness and performance from 1:30 AM to 8:30 AM. Wright et al [65] achieved similar results.

Bright light appears to be difficult to tolerate for some subjects, especially those who are sleep-deprived. An alternative might be lower-intensity light, especially using shorter wavelengths that have more potent melatonin-suppressor and phase-shifting effects. For instance, a study by Horne et al [66] suggests that low-intensity bright green light improves alertness and performance during nighttime, independent of a circadian-shifting mechanism.

Another circadian vulnerability, the postprandial dip in subjective alertness and cognitive performance, affects a sizable number of individuals (especially morning types, according to the article by Monk elsewhere in this issue) and also improves with bright light administration [67]. The improvement is most potent when light is associated with caffeine intake and face washing after a short nap.

There are few field studies on the immediate alerting effects of light compared with laboratory studies. Landstrom et al [68] reported that 30 minutes of exposure to bright light during a break did not improve subjective reported alertness in sleep-deprived drivers during a 9-hour drive. However, in another field study, night workers reported significant improvement in alertness when exposed dur-ing breaks to 2500 lux compared with routine light conditions.

What might be the neurocircuitry responsible for the increase in alertness immediately following exposure to bright light at night? Perrin et al [69] measured regional cerebral blood flow in 13 subjects exposed to light during the biological night. As light suppressed melatonin and enhanced alertness, a large-scale activation of the occipitoparietal attention network, including the right intraparietal sulcus.

Bright light effects on alertness and performance in conditions of homeostatic adversity

Athletes may accumulate acute and chronic sleep debt for many reasons, including occasional acute insomnia associated with competition anxiety; inability to cool down after games or qualifiers; or remnants of or antidromal adjustment to jet lag, noise, or unfamiliar environments during travel. Sleep debt affects daytime reported alertness and performance even on simple reaction-time tests, as discussed by Dinges et al elsewhere in this issue.

Although the effects of bright light on impairment of alertness in circadian adverse conditions have been reported consistently, effects of bright light on alertness in circadian neutral conditions have been reported inconsistently. For instance, Badia et al [70] found that although the difference between bright and dim light increases with increased homeostatic sleep pressure, it is only significant during adverse circadian conditions (specifically nighttime).

In contrast, Phipps-Nelson et al [71] used a thorough design (ie, a constant routine) to study subjects who accumulated sleep debt by sleeping 5 hours for two nights, and reported that bright light during daytime, compared with dim light, reduced subjective sleepiness and increased performance. Therefore, contrary to the opinion that the immediate effect of bright light is caused by melatonin suppression, at least two studies [67,71] reported an alerting effect in the absence of a melatonin-suppressing effect.

In another laboratory study, bright light did not to enhance subjective alertness in conditions of sleep debt compared with dim red light [72]. A faster reaction time in the bright light condition was offset by a greater error rate.

Studies in athletes

Given the importance of alertness in sports, the general relationship between alertness and bright light exposure, especially in conditions of sleep debt during an adverse circadian phase, and the relatively predictable exposure of athletes to variable indoor/outdoor light conditions, direct comparisons of sports performance between diverse light conditions are necessary.

In one study, O'Brien and O'Connor [73] exposed 12 competitive male cyclists to three intensities of light during daytime using sunglasses that provided high-, medium-, and low-light filtration. The investigators found no significant differences among the conditions in alertness, leg muscle pain, perceived exertion, heart rate, oxygen consumption per unit time, or mood responses to the exercise between 1411 lux (274.9 ± 21.8 W), 2788 lux (274.4 ± 20.5 W), and 6434 lux (270.3 ± 19.8 W) conditions. However, this was a comparison between three relatively intense light conditions with no dim light controls, and not during some adverse circadian times or sleep debt when the effects of bright light are greatest.

In conclusion, light has alerting properties especially in conditions of sleep debt and adverse circadian conditions, which in athletes include competing in the late evening/early night and during the early-afternoon postprandial dip. The alerting effects of light are magnified if light is combined with timed naps and caffeine. Caution should be taken, however, when extrapolating from laboratory and field studies on nonathletes to athletes. We recommend a highly individualized approach to extrapolation of data to athletes who perform at a competitive, professional, or elite level, where schedules and physiological responses tend to show a large interindividual variation.

Antidepressant effect of bright light

In seasonal depression

Seasons are caused by changes in the duration of day length resulting from the Earth's movement around the Sun on a tilted axis. These changes result in rhythms in day length (ie, photoperiod) with a period of one year. The magnitude of photoperiodic changes and climatic seasonal changes (eg, temperature, humidity, sky cover, rainfall) is related to latitude, which is more pronounced farther away from the equator. Numerous species manifest marked seasonal changes in physiology and behavior and use specialized neuronal circuits to detect, store, anticipate, and respond to information regarding day length. Photoperiodic organisms use absolute measures of day length and direction of day length change to regulate seasonal changes [74].

Certain seasonal behavioral changes in humans, which include sleepiness and changes in appetite, interest in socializing, assertiveness, approach behavior, and sexual activity, resemble those found in photoperiodic mammals (mammals that display marked seasonal behavioral changes in response to changes in day length). Although no seasonal changes in mood and behavior are reported in most people, mild changes occur in 10% to 20% of the adult population in the United States. A minority of the population (1%–4%) has seasonal affective disorder (SAD), which consists of episodes of major depression in fall and winter with spontaneous remissions in spring and summer [75]. This interindividual variation is not uncommon even in species that experience more drastic and uniform behavioral changes in response to photoperiodic changes than humans, with certain individuals of photoperiodic species not responding at all to changes in photoperiod [76,77].

The prevalence of SAD in professional athletes is unknown. Seasonality in athletes may have more to do with seasonality of competitions and schedules than with internal ancestral photoperiodic processes. See the article by Atkinson et al elsewhere in this issue for further discussion of this topic. We will develop aspects of seasonality that are related to photoperiodic considerations and light treatment for winter depression. However, the article by Atkinson et al should be consulted for other important aspects involving seasonality of exercise.

In 1946, the German physiologist H. Marx first described the "hypophyseal insufficiency associated with lack of light," [78] which represented the first scientific description of SAD. Marx also hypothesized that light affected patients' behavior by way of the retinohypothalamic tract, which he termed "the hypothalamic root of the optic nerve" [79].

Duration of melatonin secretion mediates photoperiodic changes in animals. The report that bright light suppresses melatonin in humans [80] was followed somewhat serendipitously by the first modern description of bright light improving symptoms of SAD [81]. Rosenthal et al [75] reported the first categorical description of the syndrome and controlled trials of light treatment. Further controlled trials confirmed the efficacy of light treatment, including those conducted by Eastman et al [82] and Terman et al [83] in 1998. Wehr and colleagues [84] showed that patients who have SAD, and not matched controls, have a longer duration of active melatonin secretion in winter than in summer, similar to melatonin-duration changes in animals.

Ethnicity plays a role in the vulnerability and resilience to SAD. For instance, Icelanders are relatively protected from winter depression [85], with this resilience confirmed in their Canadian descendants [86]. Whereas Chinese and Japanese tend to be relatively resilient to winter depression and more vulnerable to summer depression [87–89], African Americans [90], for instance, are likely to be as vulnerable to changes in seasons as the general population with Caucasian dominance.

Although initial reports suggested a strong relationship between latitude and prevalence of SAD, subsequent studies, especially on clinical populations, have not confirmed that concept [91]. It is likely that the direction of the changes in photoperiod rather than absolute values of photoperiod are the trigger for seasonal mood episodes [78,84].

Age and gender are important factors in SAD, with an increased occurrence in the younger and female population [89]. Therefore, SAD may be especially relevant for female athletes and coaches.

Pathophysiology of seasonal affective disorder and mechanisms of action of light treatment

There are three general levels/mechanisms involved in SAD: genetics, neurotransmitter alterations, and chronobiological mechanisms.

Genetic considerations

A large study of 4639 adult twins from Australia found that genetic effects accounted for 29% of the variance in seasonality [92]. The inheritability of seasonality was mainly associated with the preponderance of the neurovegetative symptoms of winter depression, such as increased appetite, weight gain, and increased sleep, which are also good predictors of light therapy response [93,94]. Another study of 339 twin pairs [95] reported greater genetic effects (average 50%) with the inheritability accounting for more variance in seasonality in men (69%) than in women (45%).

Associations were reported between the rate of SAD, serotonin-related polymorphisms such as the 5-HT$_{2a}$ promoter polymorphism -1438G/A [96], and the
short allele of the serotonin transporter promoter gene [97].

*Neurotransmitter dysfunctions in seasonal affective disorder and correction by
light treatment*

A number of studies have strongly suggested a serotonin dysfunction in SAD,
and several studies suggest possible alterations in norepinephrine or dopamine
systems. Bright light treatment may work by correcting the serotonin- and
norepinephrine-related abnormalities.

Precursors and metabolites of serotonin markedly fluctuate with the seasons.
For example, the levels of L-tryptophan, the precursor of serotonin, are highest in
spring and decrease in late/early fall [98,99]. Measuring serotonin metabolites in
the jugular vein, Lambert et al [100] reported that turnover of serotonin by the
brain was lowest in winter (P = .013). In addition, the rate of serotonin
production by the brain positively correlated with luminosity, with the strongest
interval for the correlation occurring on the day of testing (ie, the relationship is
not particularly lagged). This finding suggests that bright light exposure robustly
and immediately results in serotonin synthesis in the brain.

Serotonin content in the hypothalamus has a marked seasonal variation, with
a minimal presence in the winter [101]. The major metabolite of serotonin,
5-HIAA, has its trough in springtime, which may reflect low serotoninergic activity during winter [98,102].

Tryptophan depletion, resulting in a relapse of depressive symptoms in SAD
patients remitted on light treatment [103–105], strongly suggests that light improves mood in patients with SAD by correcting a serotoninergic abnormality.

Only indirect evidence exists to suggest a dopamine involvement in SAD.
Low-resting prolactin levels were reported in SAD patients independent of
season (suggested trait marker) and interpreted as an expression of up-regulation
of D2 receptors, secondary to low activity of dopamine [106,107]. A double-
blind placebo-controlled trial of L-dopa/carbidopa did not show any benefit in
SAD patients [108].

Indirect evidence for the role of norepinephrine in SAD is suggested by a
negative relationship between depression scores in patients who have SAD and
cerebrospinal fluid levels of norepinephrine metabolites [109], by a lower plasma
norepinephrine concentration in untreated patients who have SAD than in
controls, and in untreated versus light-treated conditions [110]. After light treatment, plasma norepinephrine levels [111] and norepinephrine turnover increase
[112], but it is not known if this is the result of mechanisms associated with
the effects of bright light or if these are aftereffects of an improved mood and
activity. Neumeister et al [105] subjected patients who had SAD, remitted with
light treatment, to tryptophan and catecholamine depletion, with sham depletion
using an active placebo (benztropine) also included in the protocol. A temporary
relapse in depressive symptoms resulted from norepinephrine and serotonin

depletion, suggesting that catecholamines, not only serotonin, are involved in the effect of light treatment in SAD.

Chronobiologic dysregulation in seasonal affective disorder

There are two hypotheses of dysregulation of seasonal rhythms in patients who have SAD that suggest two distinct mechanisms of action of light treatment. The first is based on the signal that induces seasonal changes in photoperiodic mammals; namely, the seasonal difference in nocturnal melatonin secretion. The second is based on a hypothesis of delayed circadian rhythms in patients who have SAD, creating conditions for a seasonal jet lag.

In many mammals, the photoperiod signal is encoded in the duration of nocturnal melatonin secretion. In humans, as previously described in photoperiodic rodents, the nocturnal duration of melatonin secretion reflects previous exposure to photoperiod [113].

Recent studies report that only patients, and not controls, have a winter–summer difference in the duration of active melatonin secretion, showing for the first time that patients who have SAD generate a signal of change in season similar to that used by other mammals to regulate seasonal behavior [56,84].

However, previous research found that suppression of melatonin secretion is not sufficient to produce an antidepressant effect [114]. In addition, if the duration hypothesis of melatonin secretion were true, the addition of melatonin in the afternoon should have resulted in worsening of the symptoms of depression, which it did not. By contrast, a late-afternoon dose of melatonin reduces symptoms of depression [115]. Therefore, the extension of the duration of melatonin secretion is unlikely the necessary and sufficient pathophysiologic mechanism of SAD.

Circadian phase-shift hypothesis

Lewy and colleagues [116,117] hypothesized that a phase delay in circadian rhythms was conducive to SAD. The theory stated that the internal clock is lazier in patients who have SAD than in controls, including, in the original formulation of the hypothesis, patients who have nonseasonal depression. Therefore, because it would require more light to synchronize it, the internal clock is phase-delayed relative to the external clock. An elaboration of the phase-shift hypothesis is the conjectured desynchronization between the sleep–wake cycle and other biological rhythms, such as cortisol, melatonin, and body temperature, and that light would resynchronize these rhythms [117]. According to this theory, as the morning light phase advances circadian rhythms, it corrects the pathophysiologic delay in patients who have SAD. The reported improvement in depression from melatonin administered in the late afternoon, at a time when it results in a phase advance [115], further supports the SAD phase-shift hypothesis. Moreover, the antidepressant effect of melatonin administration correlated with the degree of phase advance [118]. Recently, however, Terman et al [119] did not find a positive relationship between circadian phase and severity of depression. In support of the phase-delay hypothesis, however, the authors found a correlation between the magnitude of the phase advance to morning light and improvement in depression. The ideal scheduling for light treatment according to Terman et al [119] would be according to circadian time and not sleep time, and would commence 8.5 hours after melatonin onset.

Other support for the phase-delay hypothesis comes from constant-routine studies, with patients who have SAD demonstrating phase-delayed dim-light melatonin onset (DLMO, in saliva), core temperature, and cortisol rhythm, and these abnormalities being corrected by light treatment [120].

There is also experimental evidence against the phase-delay hypothesis, such as the response of SAD to evening light. To support the phase-delay hypothesis, according to the previously described PRC to light, the morning light would have to improve and the evening light to worsen depression. Direct comparisons and most meta-analysis show that morning light is a more potent antidepressant than evening light [83,115,121,122]. However, there are studies that found evening light to be as, or almost as, effective as morning light in reducing depression [82,123,124]. Most of all, even as evening light was less effective than morning light, it was more effective than placebo and certainly not detrimental, as the phase-delay theory predicts.

Another strong argument against the phase-delay hypothesis is the absence of observed delayed circadian rhythms (using melatonin and temperature markers) in patients who have SAD who undergo a "forced desynchrony" protocol, the gold standard circadian intervention to separate the sleep–wake cycle from circadian rhythms without changing the ratio between sleep and wakefulness and without depriving patients of sleep. The principle is that although the circadian pacemaker is able to alter the duration of internal night or day to match naturally occurring changes in duration of the environmental night or day, it is unable to match drastically reduced or extended periods of imposed light–dark and rest–activity cycles. Consequently, while subjects sleep and are awake on these very short (eg, 20 hours) or very long (28- to 30-hours) days, the SCN continues to pace with a period of approximately 24 hours. The procedure's intention is to have the subjects sleep and be awake at different circadian periods. Using such a protocol (20-hour days), Koorengevel and colleagues [125,126] found no difference in circadian phase between patients who have SAD and controls. Therefore, similar to the melatonin duration hypothesis, "one would conclude that phase advance is neither necessary nor sufficient for the therapeutic effect" [119].

In conclusion, there is no consensus regarding the chronobiologic abnormality in SAD and the primordial chronobiologic mechanism by which light exerts its positive effect in SAD. It is relatively clear, however, that light is an effective and safe treatment for SAD, and that morning light appears to be more effective than evening light.

Bright light treatment for seasonal depression has been recognized by the Clinical Practice Guidelines issued by the US Department of Health and Human

Services [127] and appears in the American Psychiatric Association's *Treatments of Psychiatric Disorders* [128]. However, light treatment in the winter, although effective, does not make patients feel as well as they do in summer [129], and therefore other modalities such as cognitive behavioral therapy [130], antidepressant medication, or travel to the south should also be considered.

Less is known about the effectiveness of light in treating subsyndromal SAD. Most patients who have subsyndromal SAD experience marked changes in atypical symptoms and a significant increase in appetite, weight, sleepiness, and sleep duration. A form of subsyndromal SAD is more common and frequently encountered in athletic settings than is full-blown SAD. Kasper et al [131] found that patients who had subsyndromal SAD, and not healthy controls, responded to light treatment, consistent with the findings of Barbini and Colombo [132]. In 44 subjects, Levitt et al [133] found similar response rates to bright light treatment in patients who had SAD (62%–69%) and those who had subsyndromal SAD (40%–67%). Lam et al [134], in an open-label design, found a higher response rate in subsyndromal SAD patients (N = 32, response rate 78%) than in SAD patients (N = 113, response rate 66%).

Could light administered early in the fall prevent the emergence of a full-blown winter SAD syndrome? Meesters et al [135] showed that if light is administered before the onset of any depressive symptoms, it will not block the onset of depression. On the other hand, the same group reported that if light is given after the onset of the very first depressive symptoms, even for only 5 days, it will effectively prevent the development of severe winter depression [136].

Nonseasonal depression

Nonpharmacologic treatments of depression are of particular relevance for the depressed athlete whose performance may suffer as the result of adverse effects of medication.

According to Kripke and colleagues [137], light treatment is as beneficial in nonseasonal depression as in seasonal depression. However, an ongoing Cochrane Review analysis of 20 randomized controlled trials comparing bright light with inactive placebo treatments for nonseasonal depression states that because of limited data and the heterogeneity of studies, the results need to be interpreted with caution, and that "light therapy offers modest though promising antidepressant efficacy, especially when administered during the first week of treatment" [138]. The authors also found an increased incidence of hypomania in the light treatment group.

Because the antidepressant effect of bright light has a faster onset than that of most antidepressant pharmacologic agents, bright light could be used to hasten the response of antidepressant drugs. For instance, Benedetti and colleagues [139] reported faster responses to a combination of citalopram and low-intensity green light than citalopram and placebo.

Functional neuroimaging of the antidepressant effect of bright light treatment

From a functional neuroimaging perspective, antidepressant agents act in two ways. First, they may reduce activity in regions involved in the production of depressive symptoms, such as amygdala. In those regions, activity tends to increase during depressed states and persist to some degree when the depressed state has been remitted. The functional activity in those regions tends to positively correlate with depressive affect. Second, antidepressant agents may increase activity in regions that are involved in the modulation of the depressive affect, such as the orbitofrontal cortex and ventrolateral prefrontal cortex. In those regions, activity tends to increase only in the depressed state and negatively correlates with depressive affect. Increasing activity in those regions represents activation of compensatory mechanisms in depression [140].

Neuroimaging studies on small samples of subjects with SAD who responded to light treatment showed that a full course of light treatment was associated with increased glucose use in the superior frontal cortex [141] and increased perfusion in the frontal and cingulate cortices (normalized to cerebellar perfusion) [142] in posttreatment compared with pretreatment scans. Because these studies involved subjects whose depression improved during treatment, it remained unclear whether the observed changes reflected neurophysiologic correlates of symptom resolution, or direct effects of light. The observation that SAD subjects show a certain degree of mood improvement after 1 hour of bright light exposure, to an extent that correlates with subsequent relevant responses to a full light-treatment course [94], suggests that one can study mechanisms of mood improvement after one session of light treatment.

We have recently reported the results of the first study on the acute administration of light in subjects who had SAD [143] and normal individuals [144]. Cerebral blood flow was measured using ^{15}O water and positron emission tomography with arterial input functions in 15 depressed subjects who had SAD and 15 matched healthy controls. Nine scans were performed at 12-minute intervals. Three scans were performed at baseline (dim light). The subsequent six scans alternated between the "on-light" (three scans) and "postlight" (three scans off-light) conditions. Light was administered with a light device suspended above the scanner delivering approximately 8200 lux at the level of the eye. The average cumulative duration per light scan was 29.7 minutes. Differences between depressed patients and controls, and effects of light on regional cerebral blood flow (rCBF) were assessed by comparing normalized blood flow in the on-light and postlight conditions relative to the baseline condition using SPM 99 (The Institute of Neurology, University College, London, United Kingdom). Subjects rested with eyes open, maintaining eye gaze toward the center of the lightbox. Mood was rated after each scan using the National Institute of Mental Health (NIMH) Mood Scale.

Global cerebral blood flow did not differ between subjects and comparison controls, but the subjects demonstrated increased rCBF in the ventrolateral prefrontal cortex (VLPFC) bilaterally, right orbitofrontal cortex, left ventral striatum, right globus pallidus, and in the vicinity of the right hypothalamus and posterior cingulate (uncorrected $P<.001$). Increased neurophysiological activity has been reported in these regions with major depressive disorder. There were no regions where rCBF was significantly lower in subjects than in the controls. After bright light treatment, mood improved in subjects and was unchanged in controls. A significant activation was found postlight versus baseline in the ventrolateral prefrontal cortex bilaterally and deactivation in the cerebellum ($P<.001$) in subjects and controls. In addition, in subjects who only had SAD, a significant activation was identified in the brainstem (pons) in the vicinity of the raphe, and deactivation found in the vicinity of the infralimbic area ($P<.001$).

With regards to the literature [145] on hemispheric laterality in emotional regulation and dysregulation, we also compared the effects of bright light treatment on hemispheric laterality in patients versus controls and in baseline versus postlight conditions. In regions where we have previously reported baseline differences between patients with SAD and controls and regions where bright light induced changes in patients and controls, the cerebral asymmetry indexes $(R - L)/(R + L)$ in rCBF were compared between the baseline and postlight and between patients and controls using two-way repeated measures analyses of variance.

After light treatment, the activity of the VLPFC increased more on the left side than the right side in subjects and controls ($P<.01$). There were no changes in laterality in other regions in either patients or controls [146].

In conclusion, the acute mood-elevating effects of bright light may be explained by an activation of brain regions involved in the modulation of the behavioral expression of depression (eg, VLPFC), rather than the deactivation of regions involved in mediating depressive affect and behavior (eg, amygdala) that is the primary mechanism of action of antidepressant drugs. Thus, bright light alters the balance between the activity in the prefrontal cortex and the amygdala (regions sending reciprocal inhibitory connections) in favor of the prefrontal cortex. Bright light also appears to shift the balance between the activity of the left and right prefrontal cortex toward the left, previously described to be associated with brighter mood, optimism, and approach behavior [145]. Mood improved only in depressed individuals, not in healthy controls. However, the balance shifts between the VLPFC and limbic system and between the left and right VLPFC took place in both controls and patients, and are therefore independent of mood changes. To understand this puzzling fact, one has to envision the role of activating the VLPFC as a brake applied on amygdala activity, as projections from the VLPFC inhibit amygdala activity (eg, when a vehicle is not moving, pressing the break does not produce any visible effects). How could these findings be extrapolated to athletes? First, bright light is not expected to improve mood acutely in euthymic athletes. However, when demoralization, lack of self-esteem/confidence, adjustment to loss with depressed mood, or major depression occurs in an athlete, exposure to bright light could activate areas of the brain that could inhibit regions that mediate depression. At the same time, increasing the left/right activity ratio in the prefrontal cortex could promote confidence, optimism, and approach behavior. Bringing these thera-peutic considerations into the athletic arena would require testing of these hypotheses in experimental settings before general recommendations could be made.

Administration of light

Natural light

Outdoor light

Arnold Rikli, referred to as "Der Sonnendoctor," or "The Sundoctor," pro-posed that "...anything indispensable for the preservation of health is a natural remedy for its restoration. [Healthy] air, light, water, nourishment, and exercise are indispensable to health; they should always be considered the first remedies to be resorted to in disease. The worst place for a patient to be cured is in his bed" [146]. After experiencing injury, elite athletes often simultaneously experience lost ability, diminished competence and self-worth, and, environmentally, an abrupt decrement in light exposure (due to reduction in outdoor training) and exercise. In vulnerable individuals this may contribute to the development of a depressive syndrome. We recommend that after trauma or athletic losses (which often result in self-seclusion) the athletes continue to be exposed to bright light, natural or artificial.

Natural light is associated with other factors that promote health, such as walking outdoors, contemplation, and companionship. Exposure is free. Outdoor light (5000–100,000 lux) is two to three orders of magnitude greater than normal 50 to 500 lux indoor light and one order of magnitude brighter than commercial light-treatment lamps (5,000–10,000 lux) [147,148].

Though natural sunlight is a key stimulant for vitamin D production and contains the blue-green wavelengths that might be optimal for the chronobiologic effects of light, the disadvantages of sunlight include exposure to ultraviolet radiation that can promote skin cancer or cataracts and blue wavelengths of visual radiation that can promote retinal damage. A hat, sunscreen, UV-blocking sun-glasses, and wearing long sleeves, long pants, and light colors may decrease ultraviolet exposure. To minimize the risk of melanoma, the duration of exposure should not be increased even after application of sunscreen. Choosing the right pair of sunglasses is a difficult task; certain UV-blocking sunglasses will not block blue and blue-green light, which may still damage the retina.

What is the evidence that outdoor bright light is effective? Wirz-Justice et al [148] reported that a 1-hour outdoor morning walk for 1 week significantly reduced depressive symptoms in patients who had winter depression, with no significant relapse after withdrawal. The response rate (65%) was similar to pre-vious studies of the same group using artificial bright light treatment [123]. The morning walk advanced the mean wake-up time by 40 minutes.

Bright light treatment administration

Devices for light treatment

Devices for bright light administration include light boxes, light visors, dawn simulators, sunrise clocks, and face masks.

The light box is a tabletop or free-standing bright light source typically consisting of a metal container housing ordinary or full-spectrum white fluorescent light, often positioned toward the eye at an angle permitting the light to enter the eyes. It has a plastic diffuser to filter ultraviolet radiation, and is the most commonly used device for light treatment (Fig. 2A). There are also models that combine a light box with a bright desk lamp (Fig. 2B). A light box can also be adapted for use during exercise (Fig. 2C). Another important feature of a light device for athletes is its mobility, and portable light boxes have become commercially available (Fig. 2D). Even more portable, the light visor is a head-mounted device with bright light directed at the eye (Fig. 2E). Mini light boxes are small, portable devices, not larger than a small book, that use light emitting diode (LED) technology and are convenient for travel (Fig. 2G). Whereas the traditional bright light treatment devices have produced white cool (Fig. 2A) or full spectrum light (Fig. 2C), narrower-spectrum, shorter-wavelength blue-green (Fig. 2F) and blue (Fig. 2G) light devices are currently commercially produced. These devices provide more potent melatonin suppression and circadian shifting, thus allowing lower light intensities or shorter periods of exposure. A "dawn simulator" is a bedroom illumination system that simulates a summer dawn lasting from 1 to 2 hours. A dawn simulator may be attached to a regular lamp. Dawn simulators can be plugged into any incandescent light and are therefore very portable. A "SunRiser Clock" is an alarm clock that produces indoor light

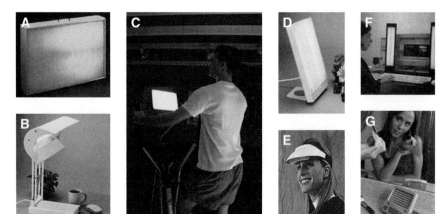

Fig. 2. Light treatment devices: (*A*) Standard light box; (*B*) Light box combined with bright desk lamp; (*C*) Full spectrum light box with capability to be used for exercise, practice, and reading; (*D*) Portable light box; (*E*) Visor; (*F*) Low-intensity, lower-wavelength green light device; (*G*) Portable, low-wavelength blue-light LED device.

in slow increments. The "light mask" is a sleep mask that delivers a dawn signal and bright light through closed eyelids during sleep.

Treatment parameters

Duration and illuminance. Insufficient data are available on dose response [137]. It had been suggested that a critical dose of 5000 lux per hour would have the highest efficacy in SAD, which would translate to parameters ranging from 30 minutes of 10,000 lux at eye level to 60 minutes of 5000 lux [149]. This initial prediction found support from a recent study using 5000 lux that reported an optimal exposure of 45 to 60 minutes [133]. However, well-controlled randomized fixed duration studies are necessary to find an optimal dose/duration of light.

Full spectrum versus cool white. Lee et al [150] conducted a meta-analysis on the spectrum of lamps used in light therapy trials and found that there was no difference between full spectrum and cool white bulbs. The presence of ultraviolet light in some full spectrum lamps may increase the risk of skin cancer and cataracts unless they are used with ultraviolet shielding.

Timing. Timing of light administration is crucial for treatment of jet lag and shift work. Iatrogenic phase advances and delays may occur with light treatment and might be appropriately treated by changing the timing of light administration.

From a clinical standpoint, it is important to monitor sleepiness versus alertness and difficulty in falling asleep versus maintaining sleep. Patients who have problems falling asleep who wake up early in the morning would more likely benefit from exposure to light in the morning as soon as they wake up or even 30 minutes earlier than their wake-up time. Patients who feel sleepy or fall asleep too early in the evening and who suffer from early awakening would benefit most from light in the evening.

Position of the lightbox. Clinical experience suggests that looking directly at the light source is not more beneficial than keeping the light source in the peripheral vision, and only occasionally glancing at the light box. This allows the patient the convenience of eating, reading, or watching television with a light source slightly to the side of the center of focus [137]. Maintaining the manufacturer-recommended distance from the light device to the eye is essential in securing the intensity of light, which varies strongly with the distance from the source.

Prediction of response

Is it possible to predict who will respond to light and who will not? For SAD, Terman et al [151] have suggested that atypical symptoms, especially hypersomnia, afternoon or evening slump, reverse diurnal variation (evenings worse), and carbohydrate craving represent favorable predictors, whereas suicidality, depersonalization, typical diurnal variation (mornings worse), anxiety, early and late insomnia, appetite loss, and guilt are negative predictors. One report suggests that for patients who have SAD, improvement in symptoms after 1 hour of bright light predicts degree of improvement after several weeks of treatment [94]. Another important consideration is compliance with treatment, which depends on time available for light treatment, expectations, and cost of the device (which is clearly less than that of drugs, but less often reimbursed by insurance companies).

Adverse effects and reactions from use of bright light

Common adverse effects

The more frequent adverse effects of bright light treatment [152] are minor and can include "eye strain" (17%), headache (19%), nausea (7%) and feeling "wired" (14%). If the symptoms are at least moderate, we recommend a decreased duration of exposure under those circumstances. If the situation does not improve, discontinuation of light treatment is appropriate.

Unwanted shifting

Early awakening is the result of a circadian phase advance induced by the administration of bright light. It is often accompanied by late-afternoon and early-evening sleepiness. If this occurs, light administration is best divided between morning and evening exposure times, with a larger duration of light allocated to evening administration.

On the other hand, evening administration may result in sleep-onset insomnia, often associated with trouble getting up in the morning. This is often the result of a circadian phase delay, and it is appropriately treated with a longer duration of light allocated to the morning session.

Possible ocular adverse effects

Light treatment produces irradiance levels that are below or within the illuminance range of a bright sunny day outdoors [153]. Outdoor light contains more ultraviolet radiation, which is filtered by the plastic diffusing screens found on most light boxes.

Schwartz et al [154] studied 59 patients who had SAD and were treated with light for an average period of nine winters, finding no evidence of eye damage. Gallin et al [155] performed tests of visual acuity, intraocular pressure, slit-lamp biomicroscopy, direct and indirect ophthalmoscopy, color vision, visual field, fundus photography, Amsler grid, ocular motility, pupillary reactions, contrast sensitivity, stereopsis, and the macular stress test in 50 patients suffering from SAD before and after 2 to 4 weeks of bright light therapy, and again in 17 patients with a history of long-term treatment for several years and found no ocular abnormalities. However, safety of light treatment for patients who have eye disease was not established through these studies, as these patients may have been excluded.

Although clinical and research experience with light treatment does not support clinically relevant damage of the eye with bright light treatment in humans, several investigators have raised concerns. According to Reme and colleagues [153], light exposure can lead to distinct lesions of ocular structures under specific experimental and naturalistic conditions. There is consensus regarding ocular damage from blue light in nocturnal mammals. It is possible, however, that nocturnal mammals are more sensitive to the retinotoxic effects of light than diurnal humans, as there is no direct evidence of such damage in humans. Although the use of bright light for a short period would be unlikely to induce detrimental long-term adverse effects, prudence dictates that possible damage to the eyes must be considered.

Practically, we suggest asking about eye problems and photosensitizing medications and we recommend an ophthalmologic clearance before starting light treatment in patients who have significant preexisting eye conditions.

Possible considerations for malignancy

In a large case-control epidemiologic study, Davis et al [156] reported an increased risk of breast cancer in subjects who worked night shifts and found a relationship between the duration of exposure to night shifts and the magnitude of the risk. The individuals reporting not sleeping at 1 AM and 2 AM had the highest risk. The risk did not involve waking up at night and turning on the lights, although the individuals with the brightest rooms at night were at an increased risk for developing breast cancer.

The results of Davis et al were consistent with four previous studies [157–160] that reported a relationship between the risk of breast cancer and shift work.

From a different perspective, breast cancer was found to be less prevalent in individuals with visual impairment. Hahn [161] was the first to report a statistically significantly reduced risk of breast cancer in women who had profound bilateral blindness. Although an attempt to replicate this relationship in a smaller data set failed [156], the inverse association between incidence of breast cancer and visual impairment was subsequently confirmed in four other studies [162–165].

However, reviews by Poole et al [166] and Erren et al [167] describe methodological challenges that preclude a definitive conclusion on the effects of light at night on increases in tumor growth in humans. In any case, until additional research is completed, some caution is recommended when prescribing more than just very occasional light treatment during the biological night, when light might not only shift but also suppress active melatonin secretion. On the other hand, administering light after awakening and not later than 2 hours before the regular sleep onset time will not generally encounter melatonin to suppress, and may even increase nocturnal melatonin by increasing the amplitude of circadian rhythms.

Considerations for suicide

Light treatment is not excepted from the energizing effect of any effective treatment for severe depression, when a patient who has suicidal ideation but previously lacked energy or motivation to formulate or carry over a plan becomes able to make suicidal plans and execute them during their early stages of improvement. Praschak-Rieder et al [168] described two patients who attempted suicide after starting light treatment. Kripke wrote that he was "aware of one patient who committed suicide soon after commencing use of a light visor" [137]. As with other antidepressant treatments, suicide risk may become more acute early in the course of light treatment.

Several epidemiologic papers have found a relationship within the general population between sunshine intensity and the highly replicated suicide peaks in spring [169]. From a molecular standpoint, as bright light appears to manifest its antidepressant effects through serotonergic and noradrenergic pathways [170–173], and because antidepressant drugs have been associated with an increased suicide risk especially at the beginning of the treatment, it is conceivable that exposure to bright light may also increase the potential for suicide in people at risk. Thus, we recommend taking a personal and family history of suicide attempts, and closely monitoring patients who are at increased risk.

Bright light and bipolar disorder: hypomanic reactions

Hypomania and mania

The occurrence of mania and hypomania with light treatment is not known and likely infrequent, but possible, as with any antidepressant treatment. To minimize the risk it is important to explore whether there is a history of hypomania or mania, and to avoid light in patients who have bipolar I disorder and are unprotected by mood stabilizers and to closely follow patients who have bipolar II disorder. In case of hypomanic reactions, the light duration should immediately be reduced and light administration moved from morning to midday, as published observations suggest that midday administration is safer in terms of triggering hypomania [174]. If this does not reduce the hypomania and stabilize mood, the light treatment should be discontinued. A hypomanic/manic reaction is not unexpected in bipolar patients treated with light if one considers that mechanisms of action of light treatment likely affect the same neurotransmitters systems as many antidepressant drugs [170–173], and that antidepressants may precipitate hypomania/mania and increase cycling in bipolar disorder.

Some studies have suggested that patients who have bipolar disorder may be supersensitive to light [175,176], although more recent work did not support this concept [177]. Our practice has found it useful to start the treatment of bipolar patients with shorter durations of light, and to increase the duration more slowly, monitoring for symptoms and signs of activation (eg, increased psychomotor activity, speech production, decreased need for sleep, sleep disruption).

Summary

The effects of bright light depend on the intensity, wavelength, duration, and most of all, timing of its administration. Shades and sunglasses that help reduce exposure to light are important components of a circadian shifting arsenal.

To improve compliance, we always emphasize that light treatment does not steal time from patients, rather it offers 30 to 45 minutes of quality time alone for reflection, grooming, reading, and planning.

Sleep onset and offset are important considerations for timing of light treatment and monitoring circadian side effects, and in our experience, fine-tuning the circadian effects of light is a key factor in maintaining compliance. Individuals who have trouble falling asleep in the evening and waking up in the morning should be exposed to more morning light for higher efficacy. Individuals who have late afternoon/early evening sleepiness and early awakening should be exposed to more evening light. Sleep patterns may alter after starting treatment, which would call for administration of light in two sessions and a redistribution of light from morning to evening or reverse.

In reviewing the shortcomings of bright light treatment, its advantages should not be underestimated: light is the most potent circadian shifter, a potent alerting agent (together with naps, caffeine, and temperature manipulations) in conditions of circadian adversity or sleep debt, and an effective antidepressant for patients suffering from winter depression and for certain individuals who have non-seasonal depression. Bright light treatment is a generally safe and effective intervention. Bright light has been generally underused in athletes, and may represent an important addition to the arsenal of sleep medicine, especially considering that adverse effects of certain medications are particularly undesirable in athletes, and certain alerting or antidepressant pharmacologic interventions may contravene doping regulations.

Acknowledgments

The authors are indebted to Joseph Soriano for his overall assistance, and thank Dr. Julian Redditt for commenting on an advanced draft of the manuscript.

References

[1] Aschoff J, Wever R. The circadian system of man. In: Aschoff J, editor. Biological rhythms: handbook of behavioral neurobiology. New York: Plenum Press; 1981. p. 311–31.

[2] Czeisler CA, Richardson GS, Zimmerman JC, et al. Entrainment of human circadian rhythms by light-dark cycles: a reassessment. Photochem Photobiol 1981;34:239–47.

[3] Wever RA, Polasek J, Wildgruber CM. Bright light affects human circadian rhythms. Pflugers Arch 1983;396:85–7.

[4] Honma K, Honma S, Wada T. Entrainment of human circadian rhythms by artificial bright light cycles. Experientia 1987;43:572–4.

[5] Honma K, Honma S, Wada T. Phase-dependent shift of free-running human circadian rhythms in response to a single bright light pulse. Experientia 1987;43:1205–7.

[6] Kennaway DJ, Earl CR, Shaw PF, et al. Phase delay of the rhythm of 6-sulphatoxy melatonin excretion by artificial light. J Pineal Res 1987;4:315–20.

[7] Buresova M, Dvorakova M, Zvolsky P, et al. Early morning bright light phase advances the human circadian pacemaker within one day. Neurosci Lett 1991;121:47–50.

[8] Laakso ML, Hatonen T, Stenberg D, et al. One-hour exposure to moderate illuminance (500 lux) shifts the human melatonin rhythm. J Pineal Res 1993;15:21–6.

[9] Van Cauter E, Sturis J, Byrne MM, et al. Preliminary studies on the immediate phase-shifting effects of light and exercise on the human circadian clock. J Biol Rhythms 1993; 8(Suppl):S99–108.

[10] Samkova L, Vondrasova D, Hajek I, et al. A fixed morning awakening coupled with a low intensity light maintains a phase advance of the human circadian system. Neurosci Lett 1997; 224:21–4.

[11] Honma K, Hashimoto S, Endo T, et al. Light and plasma melatonin rhythm in humans. Biol Signals 1997;6:307–12.

[12] Parry BL, Udell C, Elliott JA, et al. Blunted phase-shift responses to morning bright light in premenstrual dysphoric disorder. J Biol Rhythms 1997;12:443–56.

[13] Shanahan TL, Kronauer RE, Duffy JF, et al. Melatonin rhythm observed throughout a three-cycle bright-light stimulus designed to reset the human circadian pacemaker. J Biol Rhythms 1999;14:237–53.

[14] Zeitzer JM, Dijk DJ, Kronauer R, et al. Sensitivity of the human circadian pacemaker to nocturnal light: melatonin phase resetting and suppression. J Physiol 2000;526(Pt 3):695–702.

[15] Dawson D, Lack L, Morris M. Phase resetting of the human circadian pacemaker with use of a single pulse of bright light. Chronobiol Int 1993;10:94–102.

[16] Honma K, Honma S. A human response curve for bright light pulses. Jpn J Psychiat Neurol 1988;42:167–8.

[17] Minors DS, Waterhouse JM, Wirz-Justice A. A human phase-response curve to light. Neurosci Lett 1991;133:36–40.

[18] Jewett ME, Kronauer RE, Czeisler CA. Phase-amplitude resetting of the human circadian pacemaker via bright light: a further analysis. J Biol Rhythms 1994;9:295–314.

[19] Czeisler CA, Kronauer RE, Allan JS, et al. Bright light induction of strong (type 0) resetting of the human circadian pacemaker. Science 1989;244:1328–33.

[20] Van Cauter E, Sturis J, Byrne MM, et al. Demonstration of rapid light-induced advances and delays of the human circadian clock using hormonal phase markers. Am J Physiol 1994; 266:E953–63.

[21] Khalsa SB, Jewett ME, Cajochen C, et al. A phase response curve to single bright light pulses in human subjects. J Physiol 2003;549:945–52.

[22] Czeisler CA, Wright Jr KP. Influence of light on circadian rhythmicity. In: Turek FW, Zee PC, editors. Neurobiology of sleep and circadian rhythms. New York: Marcel Dekker Inc; 1999. p. 147–80.

[23] Lockley SW, Brainard GC, Czeisler CA. High sensitivity of the human circadian melatonin rhythm to resetting by short wavelength light. J Clin Endocrinol Metab 2003;88: 4502–5.

[24] Rea MS, Bullough JD, Figueiro MG. Phototransduction for human melatonin suppression. J Pineal Res 2002;32:209–13.

[25] Figueiro MG, Bullough JD, Parsons RH, et al. Preliminary evidence for spectral opponency in the suppression of melatonin by light in humans. Neuroreport 2004;15:313–6.

[26] Ruberg FL, Skene DJ, Hanifin JP, et al. Melatonin regulation in humans with color vision deficiencies. J Clin Endocrinol Metab 1996;81:2980–5.

[27] Klerman EB, Shanahan TL, Brotman DJ, et al. Photic resetting of the human circadian pacemaker in the absence of conscious vision. J Biol Rhythms 2002;17:548–55.

[28] Czeisler CA, Shanahan TL, Klerman EB, et al. Suppression of melatonin secretion in some blind patients by exposure to bright light. N Engl J Med 1995;332:6–11.

[29] McGuire RA, Rand WM, Wurtman RJ. Entrainment of the body temperature rhythm in rats: effect of color and intensity of environmental light. Science 1973;181:956–7.

[30] Brainard GC, Richardson BA, King TS, et al. The influence of different light spectra on the suppression of pineal melatonin content in the Syrian hamster. Brain Res 1984;294:333–9.

[31] Takahashi JS, DeCoursey PJ, Bauman L, et al. Spectral sensitivity of a novel photoreceptive system mediating entrainment of mammalian circadian rhythms. Nature 1984;308:186–8.

[32] Gooley JJ, Lu J, Chou TC, et al. Melanopsin in cells of origin of the retinohypothalamic tract. Nat Neurosci 2001;4:1165.

[33] Hannibal J, Hindersson P, Knudsen SM, et al. The photopigment melanopsin is exclusively present in pituitary adenylate cyclase-activating polypeptide-containing retinal ganglion cells of the retinohypothalamic tract. J Neurosci 2002;22:RC191.

[34] Hattar S, Liao HW, Takao M, et al. Melanopsin-containing retinal ganglion cells: architecture, projections, and intrinsic photosensitivity. Science 2002;295:1065–70.

[35] Provencio I, Rollag MD, Castrucci AM. Photoreceptive net in the mammalian retina. Nature 2002;415:493.

[36] Berson DM, Dunn FA, Takao M. Phototransduction by retinal ganglion cells that set the circadian clock. Science 2002;295:1070–3.

[37] Provencio I, Rodriguez IR, Jiang G, et al. A novel human opsin in the inner retina. J Neurosci 2000;20:600–5.

[38] Ruby NF, Brennan TJ, Xie X, et al. Role of melanopsin in circadian responses to light. Science 2002;298:2211–3.

[39] Panda S, Sato TK, Castrucci AM, et al. Melanopsin (Opn4) requirement for normal light-induced circadian phase shifting. Science 2002;298:2213–6.

[40] Sancar A. Cryptochrome: the second photoactive pigment in the eye and its role in circadian photoreception. Annu Rev Biochem 2000;69:31–67.

[41] Gander PH, Nguyen D, Rosekind MR, et al. Age, circadian rhythms, and sleep loss in flight crews. Aviat Space Environ Med 1993;64:189–95.

[42] Yamazaki S, Numano R, Abe M, et al. Resetting central and peripheral circadian oscillators in transgenic rats. Science 2000;288:682–5.

[43] Crowley SJ, Lee C, Tseng CY, et al. Complete or partial circadian re-entrainment improves performance, alertness, and mood during night-shift work. Sleep 2004;27:1077–87.

[44] Boulos Z, Campbell SS, Lewy AJ, et al. Light treatment for sleep disorders: consensus report. VII. Jet lag. J Biol Rhythms 1995;10:167–76.

[45] Czeisler CA, Duffy JF, Shanahan TL, et al. Stability, precision, and near-24-hour period of the human circadian pacemaker. Science 1999;284:2177–81.

[46] Waterhouse J, Reilly T, Atkinson G. Jet-lag. Lancet 1997;350:1611–6.

[47] Takahashi T, Sasaki M, Itoh H, et al. Re-entrainment of circadian rhythm of plasma melatonin on an 8-h eastward flight. Psychiatry Clin Neurosci 1999;53:257–60.

[48] Gundel A, Wegmann HM. Transition between advance and delay responses to eastbound transmeridian flights. Chronobiol Int 1989;6:147–56.

[49] Takahashi T, Sasaki M, Itoh H, et al. Re-entrainment of the circadian rhythms of plasma melatonin in an 11-h eastward bound flight. Psychiatry Clin Neurosci 2001;55:275–6.

[50] Daan S, Lewy AJ. Scheduled exposure to daylight: a potential strategy to reduce "jet lag" following transmeridian flight. Psychopharmacol Bull 1984;20:566–8.

[51] Boivin DB, Duffy JF, Kronauer RE, et al. Dose-response relationships for resetting of human circadian clock by light. Nature 1996;379:540−2.

[52] Boivin DB, James FO. Phase-dependent effect of room light exposure in a 5-h advance of the sleep-wake cycle: implications for jet lag. J Biol Rhythms 2002;17:266−76.

[53] Van Cauter E, Moreno-Reyes R, Akseki E, et al. Rapid phase advance of the 24-h melatonin profile in response to afternoon dark exposure. Am J Physiol 1998;275:E48−54.

[54] Crowley SJ, Lee C, Tseng CY, et al. Combinations of bright light, scheduled dark, sunglasses, and melatonin to facilitate circadian entrainment to night shift work. J Biol Rhythms 2003;18: 513−23.

[55] Campbell SS, Dijk DJ, Boulos Z, et al. Light treatment for sleep disorders: consensus report. III. Alerting and activating effects. J Biol Rhythms 1995;10:129−32.

[56] Wehr TA, Aeschbach D, Duncan Jr WC. Evidence for a biological dawn and dusk in the human circadian timing system. J Physiol 2001;535:937−51.

[57] Cajochen C, Krauchi K, Danilenko KV, et al. Evening administration of melatonin and bright light: interactions on the EEG during sleep and wakefulness. J Sleep Res 1998;7:145−57.

[58] Cajochen C, Zeitzer JM, Czeisler CA, et al. Dose-response relationship for light intensity and ocular and electroencephalographic correlates of human alertness. Behav Brain Res 2000; 115:75−83.

[59] Yokoi M, Aoki K, Shimomura Y, et al. Effect of bright light on EEG activities and subjective sleepiness to mental task during nocturnal sleep deprivation. J Physiol Anthropol Appl Human Sci 2003;22:257−63.

[60] Campbell SS, Dawson D. Enhancement of nighttime alertness and performance with bright ambient light. Physiol Behav 1990;48:317−20.

[61] Costa G, Ghirlanda G, Minors DS, et al. Effect of bright light on tolerance to night work. Scand J Work Environ Health 1993;19:414−20.

[62] Daurat A, Foret J, Benoit O, et al. Bright light during nighttime: effects on the circadian regulation of alertness and performance. Biol Signals Recept 2000;9:309−18.

[63] Foret J, Daurat A, Tirilly G. Effect of bright light at night on core temperature, subjective alertness and performance as a function of exposure time. Scand J Work Environ Health 1998; 24(Suppl 3):S115−20.

[64] Babkoff H, French J, Whitmore J, et al. Single-dose bright light and/or caffeine effect on nocturnal performance. Aviat Space Environ Med 2002;73:341−50.

[65] Wright Jr KP, Badia P, Myers BL, et al. Combination of bright light and caffeine as a countermeasure for impaired alertness and performance during extended sleep deprivation. J Sleep Res 1997;6:26−35.

[66] Horne JA, Donlon J, Arendt J. Green light attenuates melatonin output and sleepiness during sleep deprivation. Sleep 1991;14:233−40.

[67] Hayashi M, Masuda A, Hori T. The alerting effects of caffeine, bright light and face washing after a short daytime nap. Clin Neurophysiol 2003;114:2268−78.

[68] Landstrom U, Akerstedt T, Bystrom M, et al. Effect on truck drivers' alertness of a 30-min. exposure to bright light: a field study. Percept Mot Skills 2004;98:770−6.

[69] Perrin F, Peigneux P, Fuchs S, et al. Nonvisual responses to light exposure in the human brain during the circadian night. Curr Biol 2004;14:1842−6.

[70] Badia P, Myers B, Boecker M, et al. Bright light effects on body temperature, alertness, EEG and behavior. Physiol Behav 1991;50:583−8.

[71] Phipps-Nelson J, Redman JR, Dijk DJ, et al. Daytime exposure to bright light, as compared to dim light, decreases sleepiness and improves psychomotor vigilance performance. Sleep 2003; 26:695−700.

[72] Lafrance C, Dumont M, Lesperance P, et al. Daytime vigilance after morning bright light exposure in volunteers subjected to sleep restriction. Physiol Behav 1998;63:803−10.

[73] O'Brien PM, O'Connor PJ. Effect of bright light on cycling performance. Med Sci Sports Exerc 2000;32:439−47.

[74] Goldman BD. Mammalian photoperiodic system: formal properties and neuroendocrine mechanisms of photoperiodic time measurement. J Biol Rhythms 2001;16:283−301.

[75] Rosenthal NE, Sack DA, Gillin JC, et al. Seasonal affective disorder. A description of the syndrome and preliminary findings with light therapy. Arch Gen Psychiatry 1984;41:72–80.

[76] Cashmore AR, Jarillo JA, Wu YJ, et al. Cryptochromes: blue light receptors for plants and animals. Science 1999;284:760–5.

[77] Thresher RJ, Vitaterna MH, Miyamoto Y, et al. Role of mouse cryptochrome blue-light photoreceptor in circadian photoresponses. Science 1998;282:1490–4.

[78] Wehr T. Photoperiodism in humans and other primates: evidence and implications. J Biol Rhythms 2001;16:348–64.

[79] Marx H. Zur Klinik des Hypophysenzwischenhirnsystems: Hypophysäre Insuffizienz bei Lichtmangel. Klinische Wochenschrift 1946;24/25:18–21.

[80] Lewy AJ, Wehr TA, Goodwin FK, et al. Light suppresses melatonin secretion in humans. Science 1980;210:1267–9.

[81] Lewy AJ, Kern HA, Rosenthal NE, et al. Bright artificial light treatment of a manic-depressive patient with a seasonal mood cycle. Am J Psychiatry 1982;139:1496–8.

[82] Eastman C, Young MA, Fogg LF, et al. Bright light treatment of winter depression. Arch Gen Psychiatry 1998;55:883–9.

[83] Terman M, Terman JS, Ross DC. A controlled trial of timed bright light and negative air ionization for treatment of winter depression. Arch Gen Psychiatry 1998;55:875–82.

[84] Wehr TA, Duncan Jr WC, Sher L, et al. A circadian signal of change of season in patients with seasonal affective disorder. Arch Gen Psychiatry 2001;58:1108–14.

[85] Magnusson A, Stefansson JG. Prevalence of seasonal affective disorder in Iceland. Arch Gen Psychiatry 1993;50:941–6.

[86] Magnusson A, Axelsson J. The prevalence of seasonal affective disorder is low among descendants of Icelandic emigrants in Canada. Arch Gen Psychiatry 1993;50:947–51.

[87] Ozaki N, Ono Y, Ito A, et al. Prevalence of seasonal difficulties in mood and behavior among Japanese civil servants. Am J Psychiatry 1995;152:1225–7.

[88] Foster FG, Kupfer DJ, Coble P, et al. Rapid eye movement sleep density. An objective indicator in severe medical-depressive syndromes. Arch Gen Psychiatry 1976;33:1119–23.

[89] Wirz-Justice A, Tobler I, Kafka MS, et al. Sleep deprivation: effects on circadian rhythms of rat brain neurotransmitter receptors. Psychiatry Res 1981;5:67–76.

[90] Agumadu CO, Yousufi SM, Malik IS, et al. Seasonal variation in mood in African American college students in the Washington, D.C., metropolitan area. Am J Psychiatry 2004;161: 1084–9.

[91] Magnusson A. An overview of epidemiological studies on seasonal affective disorder. Acta Psychiatr Scand 2000;101:176–84.

[92] Madden PA, Heath AC, Rosenthal NE, et al. Seasonal changes in mood and behavior. The role of genetic factors. Arch Gen Psychiatry 1996;53:47–55.

[93] Lam RW, Beattie C, Mador JA, et al. The effects of light therapy on retinal electrophysiologic tests in winter depression. Bethesda, Maryland: SLTBR; 1993.

[94] Sher L, Matthews JR, Turner EH, et al. Early response to light therapy partially predicts long-term antidepressant effects in patients with seasonal affective disorder. J Psychiatry Neurosci 2001;26:336–8.

[95] Jang KL, Lam RW, Livesley WJ, et al. Gender differences in the heritability of seasonal mood change. Psychiatry Res 1997;70:145–54.

[96] Enoch MA, Goldman D, Barnett R, et al. Association between seasonal affective disorder and the 5-HT2A promoter polymorphism, -1438G/A. Mol Psychiatry 1999;4:89–92.

[97] Rosenthal NE, Mazzanti CM, Barnett RL, et al. Role of serotonin transporter promoter repeat length polymorphism (5- HTTLPR) in seasonality and seasonal affective disorder. Mol Psychiatry 1998;3:175–7.

[98] Wirz-Justice A, Richter R. Seasonality in biochemical determinations: a source of variance and a clue to the temporal incidence of affective illness. Psychiatry Res 1979;1:53–60.

[99] Swade C, Coppen A. Seasonal variations in biochemical factors related to depressive illness. J Affect Disord 1980;2:249–55.

[100] Lambert GW, Reid C, Kaye DM, et al. Effect of sunlight and season on serotonin turnover in the brain. Lancet 2002;360:1840–2.

[101] Carlsson A, Svennerholm L, Winblad B. Seasonal and circadian monoamine variations in human brains examined post mortem. Acta Psychiatr Scand Suppl 1980;280:75–85.

[102] Brewerton TD, Berrettini WH, Nurnberger Jr JI, et al. Analysis of seasonal fluctuations of CSF monoamine metabolites and neuropeptides in normal controls: findings with 5HIAA and HVA. Psychiatry Res 1988;23:257–65.

[103] Lam RW, Zis AP, Grewal A, et al. Effects of rapid tryptophan depletion in patients with seasonal affective disorder in remission after light therapy. Arch Gen Psychiatry 1996;53: 41–4.

[104] Neumeister A, Praschak-Rieder N, Besselmann B, et al. Effects of tryptophan depletion on drug-free patients with seasonal affective disorder during a stable response to bright light therapy. Arch Gen Psychiatry 1997;54:133–8.

[105] Neumeister A, Turner EH, Matthews JR, et al. Effects of tryptophan depletion vs catecholamine depletion in patients with seasonal affective disorder in remission with light therapy. Arch Gen Psychiatry 1998;55:524–30.

[106] Depue RA, Arbisi P, Spoont MR, et al. Seasonal and mood independence of low basal prolactin secretion in premenopausal women with seasonal affective disorder. Am J Psychiatry 1989;146: 989–95.

[107] Depue RA, Arbisi P, Krauss S, et al. Seasonal independence of low prolactin concentration and high spontaneous eye blink rates in unipolar and bipolar II seasonal affective disorder. Arch Gen Psychiatry 1990;47:356–64.

[108] Oren DA, Moul DE, Schwartz PJ, et al. A controlled trial of levodopa plus carbidopa in the treatment of winter seasonal affective disorder: a test of the dopamine hypothesis. J Clin Psychopharmacol 1994;14:196–200.

[109] Rudorfer MV, Skwerer RG, Rosenthal NE. Biogenic amines in seasonal affective disorder: effects of light therapy. Psychiatry Res 1993;46:19–28.

[110] Schwartz PJ, Murphy DL, Wehr TA, et al. Effects of meta-chlorophenylpiperazine infusions in patients with seasonal affective disorder and healthy control subjects. Diurnal responses and nocturnal regulatory mechanisms. Arch Gen Psychiatry 1997;54:375–85.

[111] Skwerer RG, Jacobsen FM, Duncan CC, et al. Neurobiology of seasonal affective disorder and phototherapy. J Biol Rhythms 1988;3:135–54.

[112] Anderson JL, Vasile RG, Mooney JJ, et al. Changes in norepinephrine output following light therapy for fall/winter seasonal depression. Biol Psychiatry 1992;32:700–4.

[113] Wehr TA, Moul DE, Barbato G, et al. Conservation of photoperiod-responsive mechanisms in humans. Am J Physiol 1993;265:R846–57.

[114] Wehr TA, Jacobsen FM, Sack DA, et al. Phototherapy of seasonal affective disorder. Time of day and suppression of melatonin are not critical for antidepressant effects. Arch Gen Psychiatry 1986;43:870–5.

[115] Lewy AJ, Bauer VK, Cutler NL, et al. Morning vs evening light treatment of patients with winter depression. Arch Gen Psychiatry 1998;55:890–6.

[116] Lewy AJ, Sack RL, Singer CM, et al. Winter depression and the phase-shift hypothesis for bright light's therapeutic effects: history, theory, and experimental evidence. J Biol Rhythms 1988;3:121–34.

[117] Lewy AJ, Sack RL. The phase-shift hypothesis of seasonal affective disorder. Am J Psychiatry 1988;145:1041–3.

[118] Lewy AJ, Bauer VK, Bish HA, et al. Antidepressant response correlates with phase advance in winter depression. Soc Light Treatment Biol Rhythms Abst 2000;12:22.

[119] Terman JS, Terman M, Lo ES, et al. Circadian time of morning light administration and therapeutic response in winter depression. Arch Gen Psychiatry 2001;58:69–75.

[120] Dahl K, Avery DH, Lewy AJ, et al. Dim light melatonin onset and circadian temperature during a constant routine in hypersomnic winter depression. Acta Psychiatr Scand 1993;88:60–6.

[121] Terman M, Terman JS, Quitkin FM, et al. Light therapy for seasonal affective disorder. A review of efficacy. Neuropsychopharmacology 1989;2:1–22.

[122] Vitaterna MH, Selby CP, Todo T, et al. Differential regulation of mammalian period genes and circadian rhythmicity by cryptochromes 1 and 2. Proc Natl Acad Sci USA 1999;96: 12114–9.

[123] Wirz-Justice A, Graw P, Krauchi K, et al. Light therapy in seasonal affective disorder is independent of time of day or circadian phase. Arch Gen Psychiatry 1993;50:929–37.

[124] Wirz-Justice A, Graw P, Pecker S. The seasonal pattern questionnaire (SPAQ): some comments. Bull Soc Light Treat Biol Rhythms 1993;5:257–87.

[125] Koorengevel KM, Beersma DG, Gordijn MC, et al. Body temperature and mood variations during forced desynchronization in winter depression: a preliminary report. Biol Psychiatry 2000;47:355–8.

[126] Koorengevel KM, Beersma DG, den Boer JA, et al. A forced desynchrony study of circadian pacemaker characteristics in seasonal affective disorder. J Biol Rhythms 2002;17:463–75.

[127] Depression Guideline Panel. Depression in primary care, volume 1. Detection and diagnosis. Clinical practice guideline, number 5. Rockville (MD): US Department of Health and Human Services, Agency for Health Care Policy and Research. AHCPR Publication No. 93-0550; April, 1993.

[128] Gabbard GO. Treatments of psychiatric disorders. Washington, DC: American Psychiatric Press; 1995.

[129] Postolache TT, Hardin TA, Myers FS, et al. Greater improvement in summer than with light treatment in winter in patients with seasonal affective disorder. Am J Psychiatry 1998;155: 1614–6.

[130] Rohan KJ, Lindsey KT, Roecklein KA, et al. Cognitive-behavioral therapy, light therapy, and their combination in treating seasonal affective disorder. J Affect Disord 2004;80:273–83.

[131] Kasper S, Rogers SL, Yancey A, et al. Phototherapy in individuals with and without subsyndromal seasonal affective disorder. Arch Gen Psychiatry 1989;46:837–44.

[132] Barbini B, Colombo C, Benedetti F, et al. The unipolar-bipolar dichotomy and the response to sleep deprivation. Psychiatry Res 1998;79:43–50.

[133] Levitt AJ, Lam RW, Levitan R. A comparison of open treatment of seasonal major and minor depression with light therapy. J Affect Disord 2002;71:243–8.

[134] Lam RW, Tam EM, Yatham LN, et al. Seasonal depression: the dual vulnerability hypothesis revisited. J Affect Disord 2001;63:123–32.

[135] Meesters Y, Jansen JH, Beersma DG, et al. An attempt to prevent winter depression by light exposure at the end of September. Biol Psychiatry 1994;35:284–6.

[136] Meesters Y, Jansen JH, Beersma DG, et al. Early light treatment can prevent an emerging winter depression from developing into a full-blown depression. J Affect Disord 1993;29:41–7.

[137] Kripke DF. Light treatment for nonseasonal depression: speed, efficacy, and combined treatment. J Affect Disord 1998;49:109–17.

[138] Tuunainen A, Kripke DF, Endo T. Light therapy for non-seasonal depression. Cochrane Database Syst Rev 2004:CD004050.

[139] Benedetti F, Colombo C, Pontiggia A, et al. Morning light treatment hastens the antidepressant effect of citalopram: a placebo-controlled trial. J Clin Psychiatry 2003;64:648–53.

[140] Drevets WC. Neuroimaging studies of mood disorders. Biol Psychiatry 2000;48:813–29.

[141] Cohen RM, Gross M, Nordahl TE, et al. Preliminary data on the metabolic brain pattern of patients with winter seasonal affective disorder. Arch Gen Psychiatry 1992;49:545–52.

[142] Matthew E, Vasile RG, Sachs G, et al. Regional cerebral blood flow changes after light therapy in seasonal affective disorder. Nucl Med Commun 1996;17:475–9.

[143] Postolache TT, Benson BE, Guzman A, et al. Acute effects of light treatment on cerebral blood flow in healthy subjects and patients with seasonal affective disorder. Presented at the Symposium on Healthy Lighting. Eindhoven, The Nederlands, Light & Health Research Foundation. 2002.

[144] Postolache TT, Benson BE, Guzman A, et al. Acute effects of light treatment on cerebral blood flow in healthy subjects. Chronobiol Int 2002;19:984–5.

[145] Davidson RJ. Affective style, psychopathology, and resilience: brain mechanisms and plasticity. Am Psychol 2000;55:1196–214.

[146] Rikli A. Arnold Rikli: A great-grandson's perspective. In: Holick M, editor. Biologic effects of light 2001. Boston: Kluwer Academic Publishers; 2002. p. XV–XX.

[147] Reme CE, Wirz-Justice A, Terman M. The visual input stage of the mammalian circadian pacemaking system: I. Is there a clock in the mammalian eye? J Biol Rhythms 1991;6:5–29.

[148] Wirz-Justice A, Graw P, Krauchi K, et al. 'Natural' light treatment of seasonal affective disorder. J Affect Disord 1996;37:109–20.

[149] Terman JS, Terman M, Schlager D, et al. Efficacy of brief, intense light exposure for treatment of winter depression. Psychopharmacol Bull 1990;26:3–11.

[150] Lee TM, Chan CC, Paterson JG, et al. Spectral properties of phototherapy for seasonal affective disorder: a meta-analysis. Acta Psychiatr Scand 1997;96:117–21.

[151] Terman M, Amira L, Terman JS, et al. Predictors of response and nonresponse to light treatment for winter depression. Am J Psychiatry 1996;153:1423–9.

[152] Levitt AJ, Joffe RT, Moul DE, et al. Side effects of light therapy in seasonal affective disorder. Am J Psychiatry 1993;150:650–2.

[153] Reme C, Reinboth J, Clausen M, et al. Light damage revisited: converging evidence, diverging views? Graefes Arch Clin Exp Ophthalmol 1996;234:2–11.

[154] Schwartz PJ, Brown C, Wehr TA, et al. Winter seasonal affective disorder: a follow-up study of the first 59 patients of the National Institute of Mental Health Seasonal Studies Program. Am J Psychiatry 1996;153:1028–36.

[155] Gallin PF, Terman M, Reme CE, et al. Ophthalmologic examination of patients with seasonal affective disorder, before and after bright light therapy. Am J Ophthalmol 1995; 119:202–10.

[156] Davis S, Mirick DK, Stevens RG. Night shift work, light at night, and risk of breast cancer. J Natl Cancer Inst 2001;93:1557–62.

[157] Pukkala E, Auvinen A, Wahlberg G. Incidence of cancer among Finnish airline cabin attendants, 1967–92. BMJ 1995;311:649–52.

[158] Tynes T, Hannevik M, Andersen A, et al. Incidence of breast cancer in Norwegian female radio and telegraph operators. Cancer Causes Control 1996;7:197–204.

[159] Rafnsson V, Tulinius H, Jonasson JG, et al. Risk of breast cancer in female flight attendants: a population-based study (Iceland). Cancer Causes Control 2001;12:95–101.

[160] Hansen J. Light at night, shiftwork, and breast cancer risk. J Natl Cancer Inst 2001;93:1513–5.

[161] Hahn RA. Profound bilateral blindness and the incidence of breast cancer. Epidemiology 1991; 2:208–10.

[162] Feychting M, Osterlund B, Ahlbom A. Reduced cancer incidence among the blind. Epidemiology 1998;9:490–4.

[163] Pukkala E, Verkasalo PK, Ojamo M, et al. Visual impairment and cancer: a population-based cohort study in Finland. Cancer Causes Control 1999;10:13–20.

[164] Verkasalo PK, Pukkala E, Stevens RG, et al. Inverse association between breast cancer incidence and degree of visual impairment in Finland. Br J Cancer 1999;80:1459–60.

[165] Kliukiene J, Tynes T, Andersen A. Risk of breast cancer among Norwegian women with visual impairment. Br J Cancer 2001;84:397–9.

[166] Poole C. The darkness at the end of the tunnel: summary and evaluation of an international symposium on light, endocrine systems and cancer. Neuro Endocrinol Lett 2002;23(Suppl 2): 71–8.

[167] Erren TC. Does light cause internal cancers? The problem and challenge of an ubiquitous exposure. Neuro Endocrinol Lett 2002;23(Suppl 2):61–70.

[168] Praschak-Rieder N, Neumeister A, Hesselmann B, et al. Suicidal tendencies as a complication of light therapy for seasonal affective disorder: a report of three cases. J Clin Psychiatry 1997; 58:389–92.

[169] Petridou E, Papadopoulos FC, Frangakis CE, et al. A role of sunshine in the triggering of suicide. Epidemiology 2002;13(1):106–9.

[170] Lam RW, Bowering TA, Tam EM, et al. Effects of rapid tryptophan depletion in patients with seasonal affective disorder in natural summer remission. Psychol Med 2000;30:79–87.

[171] Lam RW, Tam EM, Grewal A, et al. Effects of alpha-methyl-para-tyrosine-induced catechol-amine depletion in patients with seasonal affective disorder in summer remission. Neuro-psychopharmacology 2001;25(Suppl 5):S97–101.

[172] Neumeister A, Goessler R, Lucht M, et al. Bright light therapy stabilizes the antidepressant effect of partial sleep deprivation. Biol Psychiatry 1996;39:16–21.

[173] Neumeister A, Praschak-Rieder N, Hesselmann B, et al. Effects of tryptophan depletion in drug-free depressed patients who responded to total sleep deprivation. Arch Gen Psychiatry 1998;55:167–72.

[174] Leibenluft E, Turner EH, Feldman-Naim S, et al. Light therapy in patients with rapid cycling bipolar disorder: preliminary results. Psychopharmacol Bull 1995;31:705–10.

[175] Lewy AJ, Wehr TA, Goodwin FK, et al. Manic-depressive patients may be supersensitive to light. Lancet 1981;1:383–4.

[176] Lewy AJ, Nurnberger Jr JI, Wehr TA, et al. Supersensitivity to light: possible trait marker for manic-depressive illness. Am J Psychiatry 1985;142:725–7.

[177] Nurnberger Jr JI, Adkins S, Lahiri DK, et al. Melatonin suppression by light in euthymic bipolar and unipolar patients. Arch Gen Psychiatry 2000;57:572–9.

CLINICS
IN SPORTS
MEDICINE

ELSEVIER
SAUNDERS

Clin Sports Med 24 (2005) 415–456

Sports Chronobiology Consultation: From the Lab to the Arena

Teodor T. Postolache, MD[a,b,*], Tsung-Min Hung, PhD[c],
Richard N. Rosenthal, MD[d], Joseph J. Soriano[a],
Fernando Montes[e], John W. Stiller, MD[a,b,f,g]

[a]*Mood and Anxiety Program, Department of Psychiatry, University of Maryland School of Medicine,
685 West Baltimore Street, Baltimore, MD 21201, USA*
[b]*Institute for Sports Chronobiology, 2423 Pennsylvania Avenue, NW, Washington, DC 20037, USA*
[c]*Graduate Institute of Exercise & Sport Science, Taipei Physical Education College,
5 Tun-Hua North Road, Taipei, Taiwan, Republic of China*
[d]*Columbia University College of Physicians & Surgeons, St. Luke's Roosevelt Hospital Center,
Department of Psychiatry, 1090 Amsterdam Avenue, 16th Floor, New York, NY 10025, USA*
[e]*Texas Rangers Baseball Club, 1000 Ballpark Way, Arlington, TX 76011, USA*
[f]*Neurology Department, St. Elizabeth's Hospital, 2700 Martin Luther King Jr. Avenue,
Washington, DC 20032, USA*
[g]*Maryland State Athletic Commission, 500 North Calvert Street, Room 304,
Baltimore, MD 21202, USA*

Chronobiology is the science concerned with the investigation and objective quantification of biological rhythms, including the study of their manifestations, mechanisms, and consequences, and their experimental or clinical modification. Regular, robust, reproducible, and highly predictable biological fluctuations occur in all living things. In humans, these include fluctuations in physical and mental abilities. For elite and highly trained athletes, the slimmest

---

Because of the growing concern regarding use of stimulants in athletes of all ages to improve alertness, reduce fatigue, and maintain aggressiveness, several paragraphs in this article address this important doping issue.

Certain interventions for optimizing sleep/wake and aligning biological rhythms with competitive demands are safe and effective in improving qualities that are essential for competitive athletes (eg, alertness, attention, concentration, mood, reaction time, psychomotor learning). These interventions need to be evaluated and specifically tailored to the individual athlete, sport, and environmental conditions.

* Corresponding author. Department of Psychiatry, University of Maryland School of Medicine, 685 West Baltimore Street, Baltimore, MD 21201.
E-mail address: tpostolache@psych.umaryland.edu (T.T. Postolache).

0278-5919/05/$ – see front matter © 2005 Elsevier Inc. All rights reserved.
doi:10.1016/j.csm.2005.01.001
sportsmed.theclinics.com

of margins in performance, almost imperceptible to a casual observer, may be the difference between winning and failing even to qualify. Some pseudoscientific concepts of peaks and troughs, such as the now-debunked theory of biorhythms, have been postulated for sports. The biorhythms theory, introduced by Swoboda and Fliess at the turn of the twentieth century, proposed that infradian cycles of emotion, physical well-being, and intellectual functioning each had distinct and fixed periods, starting from birth and continuing throughout life. However, the principles of this theory were subsequently proved useless in predicting athletic performance [1–3]. Therefore, it is important not to confuse the well-recognized science of biological rhythms with the theory of biorhythms that has no accepted scientific basis.

Although there have been previous efforts to launch sports chronobiology as a scientific discipline [1], the overall impact on the world of sports was minimal.

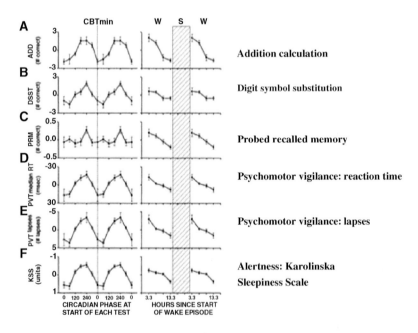

Fig. 1. Circadian variation in performance. Laboratory protocol consisting of 24 repetitions of a 20-hour rest/activity cycle, resulting in desynchrony between the sleep/wake cycle and the circadian rhythms of body temperature. Double plots of main effects of circadian phase relative to minimum of core body temperature (*left*) and duration of prior scheduled wakefulness (*right*) on neurobehavioral measures. Plotted points show deviation from mean values during forced desynchrony section of protocol and their respective SE. For all panels, values plotted lower in panel represent impairment on that neurobehavioral measure. Addition calculation test (ADD, *A*), Digit symbol substitution test (DSST, *B*), and Probed recalled memory test (PRM, *C*) scores are derived from total number of correct responses. PVT results represent median reaction time (*D*) and total number of lapses (*E*, reaction time > 500 milliseconds). KSS scores (*F*) represent responses a 1 through 9 Likert-type scale. (*From* Wyatt JK, Ritz-De Cecco A, Czeisler CA, et al. Circadian temperature and melatonin rhythms, sleep, and neurobehavioral function in humans living on a 20-h day. Am J Physiol 1999;277(4 Pt 2):R1152–63; with permission.)

Now, however, there are new conditions and opportunities that suggest it is time to revisit this field. First, sophisticated, reproducible laboratory investigations have defined a significant influence of various rhythms on human performance. For instance, certain abilities, including some of particular importance for athletic performance (ie, psychomotor vigilance and subjective alertness), deteriorate the longer one stays awake but tend to improve during the later part of the active circadian phase (Fig. 1) [4].

Second, there have been recent major advances in the understanding of biological rhythms at the molecular level. Of particular importance are the discovery of molecular processes of the "biological clock." Several studies have shown that preferences for morning versus evening performance are linked with the CLOCK gene. Morningness–eveningness in humans is linked with polymorphisms in the CLOCK gene [5] and Per genes [6], and recently a mouse animal model for morningness–eveningness has been developed [7]. Taken together, these seminal findings that link genes with circadian behavior provide a powerful theoretical framework for practical applications of chronobiology.

Third, technological advances have taken place in recording rest–activity rhythms with small ambulatory devices, repeating measurements of mental and physical abilities at different times, and measuring hormones in the saliva for circadian phase determination.

These advances, coupled with the desire of highly motivated athletes and coaches to predictably perform at their best at critical moments, suggest that the ground is now fertile to reexamine and expand on the science of biological rhythms in competitive sports.

The scope of this article is limited to practical applications of sports chronobiology. Articles found elsewhere in this issue provide a detailed understanding of the basis of sports chronobiology.

Goals of a sports chronobiology consultation

Minimizing adversity

The minimum goals of a sports chronobiology consultation are to avoid or reduce potential decrements in performance related to circadian (eg, early morning, early afternoon, or late evening dips in performance caused by jet lag), menstrual, or seasonal adversity, and to prevent or minimize the effects of less-than-optimal quantity or quality of sleep [8].

Maximizing performance

A key point of sports chronobiology is that peak performance, known as the "greatest moments," "flow," "individual zone of optimal functioning," and "being in the zone" [8–11], is more readily achieved during certain time intervals and duration of prior wakefulness. Specifically, the broader goals of a sports chronobiology consultation include aligning the endogenous circadian peak in athletic performance with the timing of the competitive event, and competing with a minimum or no sleep "debt."

Before the impact of biological rhythms on alertness is addressed, methods of measuring sleepiness/alertness, alertness enhancing drugs, and alterations in sleep/alertness associated with mood disorders are discussed.

Measurement of sleepiness and alertness

Subjective scales of sleep, sleepiness, and alertness

To assess sleepiness/alertness, a number of subjective questionnaires have been developed. The Epworth Sleepiness Scale (ESS) [12] asks for a self-report of sleepiness over time, varying from several weeks to a month, and normative data are available.

A number of scales have been used for assessing sleepiness (ie, the immediate urge to sleep), such as the Karolinska Sleepiness Scale (KSS) and Stanford Sleepiness Scale. The KSS [13] is a nine-point sleepiness scale ranging from 1 (very alert) to 9 (very sleepy, difficulty staying awake, or fighting sleep).

Objective tests of sleep, sleepiness, and alertness

Laboratory tests include the polysomnogram, multiple sleep latency test, and maintenance of wakefulness test, which are further discussed in the article by Dement elsewhere in this issue. Ambulatory tests include the psychomotor vigilance test (PVT) [14] and actigraphy.

The PVT is a portable, easy-to-use reaction time test with a high stimulus load (visual or auditory) that can yield rapid (ie, in 10 minutes) and reliable measurements of psychomotor vigilance [15,16]. The PVT, administered at brief intervals (usually 2 hours), has generally been used in the laboratory to precisely measure the changes in psychomotor vigilance performance resulting from sleep loss and circadian rhythmicity. For further discussion of these changes, see the article by Van Dongen and Dinges elsewhere in this issue. Because of its reliability, convenience, and portability, the PVT can be taken outside of the laboratory for practical use in the study of sports chronobiology.

Athletes and coaches may use the PVT to measure psychomotor vigilance during certain favorable and adverse conditions, and several important features of psychomotor vigilance were found in athletes as a result of its use. First, motivation is essential; the visual feedback of the achieved reaction time is very important, as it may be used to stimulate the athlete's competitive spirit. Second, the average reaction time varies between different sports. There is also a considerable variation in reaction time between individuals at baseline and as a consequence of sleep loss, as Van Dongen and Dinges describe elsewhere in this issue.

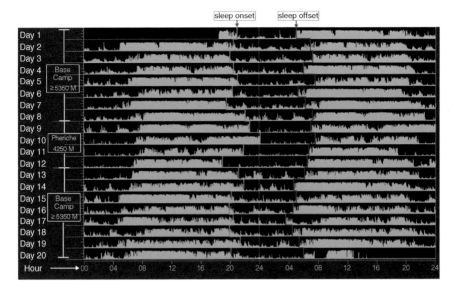

Fig. 2. Actigraphy documents moderate sleep disruption even in a well adjusted high altitude climber at the Base Camp of Mount Everest. Double plots of motor activity recorded using a Motionlogger Actigraph (Ambulatory Monitoring, Ardsley, New York). Hours are marked horizontally, days and altitudes vertically. Sleep onset and offset are marked with orange and red, respectively. Activity is in green and lack of activity in black. In this acclimatized climber, restless nights marked by awakenings were observed at the level of the Base Camp of Mount Everest (5350 m), becoming markedly quieter after descending to Pheriche (4250 m) for 3 days. Sleep became interrupted again after return to Base Camp.

Actigraphs are small devices (like tiny seismographs) that accurately record movement. Collected data is downloaded for display and analysis. Although the initial actigraphs that were first developed in 1970s were large, current actigraphs are no bigger than a watch and have sufficient memory to record continuously for up to several weeks. Computer programs are used to derive periods of activity/inactivity, levels of activity, certain circadian parameters such as acrophase (time of the daily peak), and sleep/wake parameters such as total sleep time, percent of time asleep, total wake time, and number of awakenings. Actigraphy can be useful in monitoring athletes and is reliable in monitoring sleep in extreme environments, as demonstrated in Appendix 1 and Figs. 2 and 3. For an in-depth discussion of actigraphy, see the article by Ancoli-Israel et al in the Further Readings section.

Alertness-enhancing drugs

Because some professional athletes use stimulants to improve performance, sports medicine practitioners should be constantly aware of this possibility.

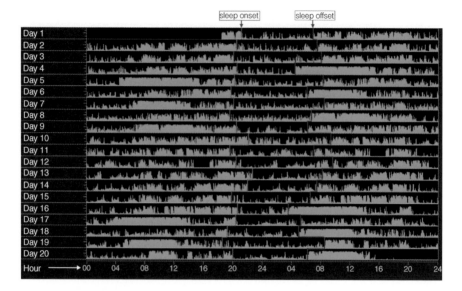

Fig. 3. Actigraphy documents moderate sleep disruption even in a well adjusted high altitude climber at the Base Camp of Mount Everest. Double plots of motor activity recorded using a Motionlogger Actigraph (Ambulatory Monitoring, Ardsley, New York). Hours are marked horizontally, days and altitudes vertically. Sleep onset and offset are marked with orange and red, respectively. Activity is in green and lack of activity in black. In this poorly acclimatized climber, restless nights with multiple awakenings and multiple daytime periods of inactivity were observed. This climber manifested periodic breathing and severe daytime fatigue, with need to rest and nap several times during daytime.

Use of stimulants can induce major fluctuations in alertness and mood, in addition to rarely inducing a frank psychosis and bizarre behavior. By World Anti-Doping Agency (WADA) standards, stimulant use to improve performance is considered doping [17].

Athletes may take stimulant drugs to improve performance, to mask fatigue, for recreation, or occasionally as self-medication for a mood disorder. For performance enhancement, potent stimulants such as amphetamines may improve vigilance and concentration, enhance speed, power, energy, and endurance, and aid in the control of appetite and weight [18,19]. The increased vigilance and energy are associated with a decreased need for sleep, frank insomnia, and perturbation of the circadian processes. The National Football League (NFL), the National Basketball Association (NBA), International Soccer Federation (FIFA), and the International Olympic Committee (IOC) each conduct random tests for steroids and amphetamines. However, the current regulations in Major League Baseball are more lax with steroids and nonexistent with stimulants. Although the use of ephedrine has been discouraged by Major League Baseball, there is no testing for amphetamines, which are the most prevalent drugs used for performance enhancement [20].

Emotional and behavioral motivations may also underlie stimulant use. In the short-term, stimulants may induce a sense of well-being and improve self-confidence, providing a competitive psychologic edge [18]. Unfortunately, the positive subjective effects of stimulants are generally rapidly reversed as the levels drop, and most dramatically after chronic administration. Stimulant dependence often occurs when doses are initially escalated in an attempt to reproduce the "high" or "rush," and then again to avoid crashing with the associated dysphoria. Although the acute effects of amphetamines often include a sense of well-being or euphoria with increased energy and initiative [21], higher or chronic doses can induce anxiety, irritability, tremor, and seizures, as shown in Box 1. In addition, a frank psychosis characterized by persecutory delusions, hypervigilance, ideas of reference, and multiple modalities of hallu-cinations may also occur [22]. Taking multiple doses of, or binging on, amphetamines typically results in a crash, along with depressed mood, fatigue, hypersomnia, and craving for the drug. Less potent stimulants, such as methylphenidate, phenylpropanolamine, and ephedrine, tend to induce milder intoxication and withdrawal symptoms. However, in higher doses, they are still capable of creating acute and potentially severe disturbances in cardiovascular functioning, including hypertension; myocardial infarction and arrhythmia; mood disturbances such as anxiety and irritability; and severe central nervous system (CNS) consequences such as stroke, cerebral hemorrhage, and confu-sional states [18].

Cocaine is a stimulant drug that is highly reinforcing and may result in a dependence syndrome. It is also associated with a host of medical sequelae, including the potential for significant cardiac and CNS toxicity. Because increased circulating catecholamines are associated with cocaine use and physiologic stress, the athlete may be particularly vulnerable to catecholamine-induced toxicity associated with cocaine use [18]. Although cocaine is not usually used as a performance-enhancing drug, athletes may use it to "amp up" in preparation for competition or to alleviate dysphoria after a loss.

Stimulant abuse often results in behavioral changes, such as those described in Box 2. When these types of changes are observed, the sports medicine practitioner should recommend abstinence, follow up in a professional manner, and encourage treatment. Box 3 outlines a basic approach to the evaluation and treatment of the athlete with substance-related problems. The importance of the clinician making an appropriate and timely referral for an athlete when a substance use or other mental disorder is uncovered cannot be overstated, because, among other things, it may be life saving. In our view, clinicians should never prescribe stimulants for performance enhancement, in any sports, at any level. Even in situations in which stimulants would address decrements in alert-ness (eg, secondary to severe sleep restriction), they would be unethical because stimulants may improve performance beyond just restoring it. In addition, clinicians should be mindful of the current ethical principles, rules, regulations, and legislation when treating a disorder with an approved but potentially per-formance enhancing substance in an athlete who currently is or is expected to

Box 1. Stimulant effects

Acute Stimulant use

  Euphoria
  Vigilance
  Anorexia
  Increased activity
  Insomnia
  Irritability
  Aggressiveness
  Increased speech
  Elevated blood pressure

Stimulant intoxication

  Grandiosity
  Hypervigilance
  Anorexia
  Psychomotor agitation
  Insomnia
  Anxiety
  Aggression
  Speech pressure
  Hypertension
  Tremor
  Hyperthermia
  Seizures
  Cardiotoxicity
  Stereotypies
  Psychosis
  Nausea and vomiting
  Confusion

Stimulant withdrawal

  Dysphoria
  Poor attention
  Hyperphagia
  Fatigue
  Hypersomnia
  Irritability, craving
  Social withdrawal
  Decreased speech

Box 2. Warning signs of stimulant dependence

New behavioral patterns

Irritability
Moodiness
Suspiciousness
Argumentative with coaches and teammates
Frequent absences from practices and meetings
Use of illness or social crisis as excuses
Periodically unreachable during the day
Difficult to contact

Changes in personal behavior

Unkempt appearance
Poor hygiene
Trembling
Bloodshot or bleary eyes
Poor memory
Poor concentration
Isolation from friends
Bizarre behavior

---

become subject to anti-doping testing, even if it is a bona fide treatment. For instance, the WADA prohibited list should be consulted before any pharmacologic treatment is prescribed in a national or international athlete subject to WADA regulation [17]. If a team physician is included in the treatment plan and follows the proper process for obtaining a therapeutic use exemption (TUE) [17], exceptions can be approved for certain medications in certain conditions.

Often there are other classes of medications that are not banned and can be used for specific medical conditions. For instance, an athlete from a national testing pool (maintained by a national antidoping organization) or an international testing pool (maintained by an international federation) may require pharmacologic treatment for attention deficit/hyperactivity disorder (ADHD). This athlete, although not permitted to receive amphetamines (which is a mainstream treatment of ADHD), may be treated with atomoxetine or bupropion, which are on the WADA monitoring program along with caffeine and pseudoephedrine. However, because of the dynamic nature of the banned list, and because certain agents are prohibited only in certain sports, it is essential for the clinician and athlete to be diligent in keeping up with these lists. If any doubt exists, they should directly contact the national antidoping federations for national-level athletes, the international antidoping federations or WADA for

Box 3. Substance treatment

How to treat the substance-dependent athlete

- Safety first: a complete medical evaluation
- Evaluation by a clinician/program knowledgeable in addiction
- If behavioral disturbance, work-up by a psychiatrist, preferably an addiction psychiatrist (www.aaap.org)
- Nonthreatening approach to engage the athlete in treatment
- Treatment requiring education, development of new behavioral skills, and attention to emotional, medical, and amateur/professional sequelae
- Judicious use of discipline/consequences to support compliance with treatment, with graded penalties for infractions
- Routine urine or other toxicologic testing to support compliance with abstinence
- Attention to confidentiality if a diagnosis is made to assist athlete in treatment engagement

How to treat the substance-abusing athlete

- Safety first: a complete medical evaluation
- Evaluation by a clinician/program knowledgeable in addiction
- A program including drug education, promotion of healthy pleasures, and secondary prevention of drug dependence
- Judicious use of discipline/consequences to support compliance with program, with graded penalties for infractions
- Routine urine or other toxicologic testing to support compliance with abstinence

How to treat the doping athlete

- Safety first: a complete medical and behavioral evaluation
- Referral to clinician/educator knowledgeable about substance use in sports
- A program including education about drugs and drug effects, the ethics of doping, doping awareness, and promotion of healthy pleasures
- Judicious use of discipline/consequences to support compliance with abstinence, with graded penalties for infractions
- Routine urine or other toxicologic testing to support compliance with abstinence

international-level athletes, and the national or international federation for the particular sport involved. In particular cases, such as with the treatment of asthma, athletes or their physicians could apply for a TUE. A TUE for international- or national-level athletes should be reported to WADA by the national antidoping organizations and international federations. WADA may review the information and reverse the decision, either revoking a granted TUE or granting a previously revoked TUE, if the international standards for TUE have been violated. However, the athlete and the national antidoping federations can appeal a decision by WADA. The criteria for granting a TUE are as follows:

- The medical condition, its diagnosis, and treatment are clearly documented.
- An application for a TUE is submitted by the athlete no less than 21 days before participation in an event.
- The athlete would experience a significant impairment to health if the prohibited substance were withheld in treating an acute or chronic medical condition.
- The use of the prohibited substance or method would produce no improvement in performance beyond that which may be expected by returning to a normal state of health following the treatment of a medical condition; increasing a "low normal" level of any hormone does not qualify.
- There is no reasonable therapeutic alternative to the prohibited substance or method.
- The necessity for the use of the prohibited substance is not a consequence of the prior nontherapeutic use of the substance.

If an athlete discloses his nontherapeutic use of stimulants to his clinician, an unequivocal recommendation to stop use must be immediately made; consideration for a medical taper of the stimulants *while the athlete is competing or training* should never be applied, as it would infringe on one of the principles of the World Anti-Doping Code (ie, that performance enhancers are to *never* be used by national or international athletes). Some believe that stopping a stimulant cold turkey would result in deterioration of performance and that prescribing smaller amounts of the stimulant would prevent deterioration of alertness and concentration, reduction of the pain threshold, and a significant increase in appetite and weight gain. However, prescribing the stimulant would in fact contravene the first principle mentioned above because there is no indication to treat withdrawal of stimulants with stimulants, as may be the case under certain circumstances such as with alcohol, benzodiazepines, or opiates. In his book, Mandel [23] describes how prescribing amphetamines to football players for the purpose of tapering, even with the best of intentions, resulted in disaster for the doctor, management, and players.

Pseudoephedrine and caffeine

Pseudoephedrine is a stimulant frequently used as a decongestant in the treatment of nasal congestion caused by infection or allergy. It also carries all the potential risks and adverse effects of stimulants, and has been used for performance enhancement. In 2004, it was taken off the list of prohibited medications by WADA, although it remains on the monitoring list. For further discussion about alternative treatments of allergy and upper airway inflammation in athletes, see the article on seasonal allergy by Komarow and Postolache elsewhere in this issue.

Caffeine is one of the most frequently used stimulants in the world. Caffeine is present in coffee, tea, cocoa, chocolate, sodas, sports drinks, and many nutritional supplements. Caffeine has been widely reported to increase alertness and levels of cognitive performance, and when taken before exercise has demonstrated ergogenic properties. Caffeine can be used to restore function affected by sleep debt or can be used to boost performance. Previously classified as a substance with a threshold between nutritional and doping category, caffeine has been downgraded from the WADA Prohibited List to the monitoring program. For an in-depth discussion about the performance implications of caffeine, see review by Rogers and Dinges elsewhere in this issue.

Sleep/wake considerations in athletes with mood disorders

Dysfunctional sleep is a cardinal symptom associated with depression. Although insomnia [24] is common in depression, increased sleepiness is not rare. Atypical depression is characterized by increased sleep, increased rather than decreased appetite, and weight gain rather than weight loss. Disturbances of circadian rhythms are also common in depression [24], and a variety of chronobiologic interventions have been used in the treatment of depression. Of particular importance is bright light treatment, which has become a first-line treatment for a winter-type seasonal depression. Further discussion of seasonal depression and bright light treatment is provided in the article by Postolache and Oren elsewhere in this issue.

Any losses could represent a trigger for depression in vulnerable individuals, and losses are inherent to athletic life. Losing in competition, which may affect an athlete's sense of self-worth/competence, and loss of physical function through injury can potentially trigger depression. An injury to the athlete may cause a chain of circumstances associated with a significant decrease in exercise, light exposure, and social interaction, all of which may contribute to triggering depression in a vulnerable individual. Successfully coping with injury often requires a positive, supportive atmosphere with help from family, teammates, coaches, and health care professionals.

More commonly, prolonged and excessive training with insufficient recovery time results in an overtraining syndrome (OTS) accompanied by performance decrements. OTS affects a large percentage of athletes at least once during their careers and is remarkably similar to clinical depression. OTS and clinical depression share the same clinical signs and symptoms associated with similar changes in neurotransmitters, endocrine, and immunological functions [25]. Armstrong and VanHeest [25] have proposed that athletes who have OTS should be treated with antidepressant medications and psychologic counseling, the common treatments for depression.

An in-depth discussion of the treatment of mood and anxiety disorders and their relationship to sleep is beyond the scope of this article. However, sports physicians, coaches, and trainers should be mindful that sleep disturbances and excessive daytime sleepiness might be symptoms of a larger problem, which, if properly diagnosed, may be treatable with appropriate psychotherapeutic and pharmacologic interventions. Therefore, as opposed to just attempting to correct the sleep complaints, a referral to either a sports psychologist or a psychiatrist for a confidential consultation should be considered. A psychiatrist is essential when medications may be used (eg, when depression is moderate to severe, persistent, or of a bipolar type). The psychiatrist should be knowledgeable of the effects of psychotropic medications on sports performance and thermoregulation and their enhanced toxicity in conditions of dehydration and heat stress, in addition to doping considerations.

It is our impression that undiagnosed, untreated, and undertreated mood and anxiety disorders are as common in athletes as they are in the general population, causing unnecessary psychologic suffering, adverse health consequences, and underachievement. If sleep impairment or daytime sleepiness is accompanied by symptoms such as persistent sadness, lack of pleasure from playing, an inability to enjoy activities that were previously pleasurable, reduced self-esteem, a pessimistic view of the future, or excessive guilt (eg, an exaggerated view of one's role in a team's loss), a specialty consultation is necessary. If an athlete talks about life not being worth living or makes reference to a suicidal intent or plan, that individual should not be left alone and should undergo an immediate evaluation.

Homeostatic and circadian impairments in alertness and sports performance

Impairment in alertness could be the consequence of a homeostatic and circadian hardship. The homeostatic hardship relates to the appetitive function of sleep (ie, sleep being like thirst, appetite, and so forth), in that its behavior increases with its absence and decreases with its abundance. The circadian hardship relates to less-favorable time windows for performance associated with an internal promotion of the propensity to sleep under the control of the "body clock," or the suprachiasmatic nucleus of the hypothalamus. Stiller and Postolache, Van Dongen and Dinges, and Dement provide in-depth discussions of the functional neuroanatomy of sleep and circadian rhythms; the interaction between homeostatic and circadian processes; and sleep extension, respectively, elsewhere in this issue.

Impairment of alertness as cause for increased appetite for sleep: homeostatic adversity

Sleep restriction

Often sleep is restricted at various times for academic purposes, such as with high school and college athletes recreationally and during training. For instance, many athletes who have early morning practice do not go to bed early enough to allow for an adequate sleep duration.

Insomnia

Screening for insomnia involves asking athletes about their ability to fall asleep within 15 minutes, tendency to wake up several times during the night, inability to get back to sleep, tendency to wake 1 or 2 hours earlier than desired, feelings of anxiety about being able to go to sleep (often anxiety which itself may reduce the ability to fall asleep), and habit of watching a clock while attempting to fall asleep. For a detailed discussion of the workup and management of insomnia, see the article by Leger et al elsewhere in this issue.

Athletes should be asked about sleep difficulties associated with evening or nighttime practices and competitions, and whether any self-corrective measures (including drinking alcohol after the game) are used. It is also important to inquire about pain, stiffness, and urinary frequency, all of which may affect the quality and duration of sleep.

Obstructive sleep apnea

To screen for possible obstructive sleep apnea, prior to indicating a confirmatory sleep study, the athlete should be asked about snoring, witnessed apnea, frequent awakenings, awakening from sleep with shortness of breath or with a feeling of being choked, and the degree of excessive daytime sleepiness. A detailed history and workup of sleep apnea is provided by Emsellem and Murtagh elsewhere in this issue.

Importance of monitoring sleep at high altitude

Hypoxia of high altitude impairs physical performance, mental performance, and sleep. Sleep impairment is often reported to be the most distressing challenge during high-altitude exposure [26].

Sleep disturbance is a frequent feature of an acute ascent at high altitude, with the most common symptoms being frequent awakening and waking up unrefreshed [27]. An increased number of awakenings, periodic breathing, and a shift from deeper to lighter sleep stages (ie, decreases in stages 3 and 4, increases in stage 1, and inconsistently reported changes in rapid eye movement [REM] sleep), are all associated with sleep at high altitude. This fragmentation of sleep is not accompanied by alterations of sleep duration and is not explained by either paradoxical sleepiness at high altitude or by either hypoxia or hypocapnia secondary to hyperventilation. Periodic breathing associated with high altitude occurs most commonly in stages 1 and 2 sleep and is promptly terminated by REM sleep.

Acetazolamide is used as a prophylactic treatment for many of the sequelae associated with high altitude exposure, including periodic breathing. Several mechanisms have been proposed for its action, but it is likely that the induction of a mild acidosis results in the lowering of the apneic threshold [27]. Acclimatization reduces but does not abolish the effects of hypoxia (it is a common misconception that acclimatization returns the body to its sea level physiologic state) (see Fig. 2). The sleep impairment associated with high altitude climbing exacerbates symptomatology already present as a result of brain hypoxia and includes such characteristics as fatigue, cognitive difficulties (eg, problems concentrating, planning, organizing), and personality changes (eg, impulsivity, irritability). The principle "climb high, sleep low" is largely accepted. However, as Appendix 1 demonstrates, the current strategies applied by most climbers of Mount Everest may not sufficiently emphasize the need to pay the sleep debt by an adequate descent before the summit attempt. Sleep debt cannot be paid at the Base Camp, because despite acclimatization, the sleep remains somewhat impaired in most climbers at that level (see Fig. 2). At the same time, chronic sleep debt cannot be nullified in one nap or even in one night, as Dement discusses in his article elsewhere in this issue. Because the hematologic benefits of acclimatization persist over several weeks, a feasible descent to a low altitude to pay sleep debt before returning for a summit attempt requires further study and may be a critical concept that could reduce mortality in high altitude climbers. Thus, the "climb high, sleep low" concept should perhaps be changed to "climb high, sleep *very* low" before a summit attempt.

Certain elite and highly trained athletes use a combination of living and sleeping in conditions of hypobaric hypoxia and training at low altitude as a supplement to endurance training. This training philosophy is the *live high, train low* (LHTL) model. Living at a relatively high altitude can stimulate an increase in red blood cell mass and hemoglobin, whereas training at a low altitude allows a greater level of intensity and avoids potential hypoxia-induced muscle damage. LHTL has been achieved naturally in a few geographic locations around the world, and by the use of artificial means, such as normobaric hypoxic apartments and hypoxic sleeping devices (tents). For instance, the running economy of elite runners after 20 days of simulated altitude training on the LHTL regimen (high: 2000 to 3100 meters) improved compared with control conditions [28]. Nevertheless, certain other studies failed to find an advantage for the LHTL regimen. For a further review of these studies, see the article by Wilber in the Further Readings section. Because the altitudes achieved with simulated altitude training may disrupt sleep, impaired sleep may impair performance, and sleep disruption was not quantified and adjusted for, sleep disruption may account for the inconsistent findings of high altitude training studies. The ethical considerations involving the use of these devices are a matter of ongoing debate: on one hand, an unfair advantage is given to the athlete using them, on the other hand, a real-life LHTL model is available in only a few places in the world and not affordable for most athletes. It is the our belief that sleep monitoring should be an integral part of an altitude exposure program and that the degree of altitude exposure needs to be titrated to a level that avoids the disruption of sleep. Specifically, it may be possible to minimize sleep debt by choosing an altitude (after an initial period of acclimatization) that does not cause perturbation of sleep, which could be conveniently monitored actigraphically.

Addressing the homeostatic adversity

Sleep as a marker of fitness to perform

Sleep is an important marker of well-being, so any issue concerning the quality of sleep may signal a correctable factor affecting the athlete's performance. For instance, many underlying physical and emotional problems associated with overtraining, including fatigue, anxiety, or depression, may initially present as sleep-related complaints. Less than average ratings of sleep quality should be followed up as soon as possible with an interview by an experienced practitioner. Important points to cover during the interview (or by more detailed questionnaires) include difficulty falling asleep, time of "lights out," number and times of awakenings, presence and degree of snoring, and inappropriate excessive sleepiness.

Sleep reserves and satiation

Sleeping less than one needs may result in metabolic and endocrine alterations, such as lower glucose tolerance, lower thyrotropin concentration, and elevated cortisol and sympathetic nervous system activity [29]. Even small amounts of less-than-optimal sleep may be accompanied by a worsening of reaction time, as described in the articles by Dement, and Van Dongen and Dinges, elsewhere in this issue. This is a particularly relevant observation in that reaction time is a ubiquitous element of sports performance. In addition, because sleep is important for memory consolidation, including in retaining psychomotor skills, sleep loss may be associated with a decreased ability to learn and improve skills essential for maximizing individual and team performance. Studies have demonstrated that there are people, referred to as *short sleepers*, who consistently require less than 6 hours of sleep, and *long sleepers*, who consistently need more than 9 hours of sleep, and that their respective physiologies may be different [30–33]. Furthermore, the vulnerability to sleep deprivation shows a distinct individual variation, as the article by Van Dongen and

Dinges discusses elsewhere in this issue. Currently, rest/activity and sleep/wake scheduling (if done at all) is generated for an entire team. However, it may be useful to use individualized schedules. At the very least, identification of and intervention for long sleepers who are getting less-than-optimal amounts of sleep will provide a chance for those individuals to significantly improve their performance and will reduce the risk for insufficient recovery.

Sleep inertia

Paradoxically, people's psychomotor and cognitive abilities are worse for a short period of time after they wake up than before going to sleep. Because it is usually easy to reinitiate sleep during this time, the phenomenon is called *sleep inertia* [34]. Reported decrements associated with sleep inertia involve simple reaction time; grip strength; steadiness and coordination; time estimates; and visual/perceptual, memory, and complex behavior–simulation tasks [34]. Sleep inertia is greater when the person awakens from deep sleep, such as non–rapid eye movement (NREM) stages 3 and 4 sleep. The impairments in functioning are also greater if prolonged wakefulness preceded the episode of sleep, the episode of sleep is interrupted during the first few hours of nocturnal sleep, or it is interrupted around the time of the body temperature minimum [34].

Naps

Although sleep supplementation and satiation may be difficult to implement given the general difficulty in changing lifestyles, particularly with elite athletes involved in team sports (because of the necessary synchrony with teammates, coaching personnel, and so forth), strategic napping is a simple and underused technique to enhance functioning. For instance, a short nap of 20 minutes may normalize the performance on a PVT that had diminished after a 4-hour nocturnal sleep curtailment, and markedly reduces sleepiness [35]. How does a 20-minute nap decrease several hours of sleep debt? This can be understood by viewing the graph of process S, which is the homeostatic, appetitive aspect of sleep (Fig. 4). The abrupt exponential decay of process S (which can be measured by delta power in the electroencephalogram tracing during sleep) contrasts to the slow saturating accumulation in process S that occurred during wakefulness. Thus, sleepiness caused by several hours of sleep deprivation is rapidly dissipated by a short nap.

Naps have been demonstrated to improve (30-minute nap) and restore (60-minute nap) deterioration from information overload as a consequence of excessive training on a cognitive task during 1 day [36]. Longer naps (eg, hours) appear to have more potent effects than short naps (eg, 15–30 minutes) [37]. In addition, longer naps more often include components of REM and delta-wave sleep, which are considered necessary for memory consolidation processes

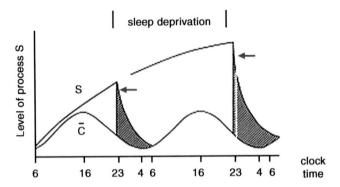

Fig. 4. Two process model of sleep. The original description of process C (circadian) and process S (sleep homeostat). Process S is reflected in delta activity during sleep, which decreases exponentially, and expresses appetite for sleep and sleepiness. Note that although the appetite for sleep tends to saturate in time, its decrement during the initial sleep is represented by an exponential decay and starts abruptly (*red arrow*). This is why the accumulated sleep debt of several hours can be paid with a short nap. (*From* Borbely AA. A two-process model of sleep regulation. Hum Neurobiol 1982;1(3): 195–204; with permission.)

(memory consolidation thus far has only been studied in longer naps). See the article by Walker and Stickgold elsewhere in this issue for further discussion of memory consolidation.

Longer naps are advisable when learning of skills, strategy, or tactic is desired. However, the price to pay for a longer nap is the burden of additional sleep inertia, during which time there is a suboptimal level of functioning. It is important to consider that the additional sleep inertia associated with long naps, when added to the sleep inertia after morning awakening, may add up to a considerable amount of time being spent at a suboptimal level of functioning. However, because showering, hygiene, grooming, and dressing are activities that may take longer than sleep inertia, which usually lasts less than 30 minutes, it is our opinion that the benefits of a longer nap often exceeds the risks. Nevertheless, longer naps that end less than 2 hours before any competition should be avoided, as minor elements of sleep inertia may persist in a small number of individuals for up to 2 hours after awakening.

If a longer nap is not logistically possible (considering the duration of the nap and sleep inertia associated with it), a short nap may be beneficial. For instance, a 15-minute nap may reduce sleepiness in conditions of prior sleep deficit [38]. Similarly, a recent study demonstrated that a 10-minute nap, but not naps lasting 30 or 90 minutes, resulted in immediately improved alertness and performance compared with controls who did not nap [39]. Furthermore, although improvements in alertness and vigor and decreased fatigue occurred with 10-minute and 30-minute naps, the 10-minute nap was not followed by sleep inertia whereas the 30-minute nap was associated with temporary decrements in cognitive function [40].

Sleep induction

Not everyone can nap, and most cannot nap on command, anywhere, at anytime. Furthermore, increasing the amount of sleep by going to bed earlier than usual is exceedingly difficulty because this earlier time (during the earlier evening hours) normally occurs during the *wake maintenance zone*, a sleep refractory period that is discussed later. Stiller and Postolache provide further exploration of this topic elsewhere in this issue. For many athletes who have insomnia, especially precompetition insomnia, falling asleep is not easy even at the regular sleep time. For these reasons, the current issue dedicates one article to nonpharmacologic methods of inducing sleep, authored by Cole, and another article to a discussion of the pharmacologic agents used for sleep induction in insomnia, authored by Leger et al. Furthermore, Kräuchi et al provides an in-depth understanding of the thermoregulatory considerations underlying some sleep-promoting interventions elsewhere in this issue. Some recommendations for sleep induction are summarized in Box 4, and Appendix 2 illustrates the significance of naps in sports performance.

Circadian adversity

A biological rhythm has been defined as an alternating sequence of events, which in a steady state repeat themselves in a constant order and interval. Rhythms with a period of approximately 24 hours are called circadian. If a phenomenon shows a variation between different times of the day, but does not manifest a repeated rhythm, it is said to have diurnal variations. Many view sine waves as a prototype rhythm with maximums (peak), minimums (troughs), acrophase (timing of the peak), and mesor (midline of the rhythm). However, this description seems to better describe a *cycle*. The sine-wave rhythm view is an appropriate representation of the core body temperature cycle, with minimums at 4 AM to 5 AM and maximums just after 6 PM in most individuals. However, more often than not, *rhythms* are not cycles, as in sine-wave fluctuations, but regular alternation between distinct states (eg, internal night and internal day) [41]. In this view, rhythms can only be accurately described for each individual subject, as opposed to averaging the rhythm across subjects, which would result in blurred borders between states. Articles by Stiller and Postolache, Van Dongen and Dinges, Kräuchi et al, Monk, and Reilly et al found elsewhere in this issue all provide detailed discussions of circadian rhythms. This article focuses on the applicative aspects of circadian rhythms.

Sleep gates, wake maintenance zones, and performance

Over 24 hours there are predictable distinct periods of time when it is relatively easy to fall asleep, and these periods alternate with other distinct

Box 4. Recommendations for sleep induction, naps, and the avoidance of sleep inertia

- Keep the room dark or use eye shades.
- Keep the room quiet (if not possible, use ear plugs).
- Keep the air in the room cool and keep extremities warm (covered with a blanket).
- Use horizontal position, ideally with the legs slightly elevated.
- Take a hot bath shortly before nocturnal sleep (ie, not nap).
- Be sure that there is no discomfort associated with hunger, thirst, need to urinate, and so forth.
- Turn phones off.
- Have someone wake you up. The anxiety of not waking up on time may decrease the capability of falling asleep, and the need to hear an alarm clock may prohibit the use of earplugs or the reduction of noise.
- Minimize and shorten sleep inertia after a long sleep episode with a hot shower, caffeinated drinks in moderation, bright light, and light exercise.
- Soft relaxing music and/or a monotonous recitation (eg, a mantra) may help induce a state of deep relaxation and sleep.
- Do not use sleep-inducing medications for napping, as their after-effects last longer than needed.
- Do not attempt to nap early in the evening. The gate for sleep is commonly closed 1 to 3 hours before the habitual bedtime (a "forbidden zone" for sleep) and late morning, unless there is considerable sleep debt. The best time to nap is during early afternoon.
- For athletes who have a competition that starts early morning and ends on the same day (eg, Taekwondo in the Olympics), bring a mat, a blanket, perhaps some mittens, pillows (including some for the legs), eyeshades, earplugs, and a player loaded with relaxing music. It is important to create a personal space.
- For athletes who travel a lot and have problems falling asleep in unfamiliar environments, especially with mattresses that do not fit their preferences, carrying a portable foam mattress to place on top of the hotel bed may prove beneficial.
- If napping for longer than 20 minutes, make sure there is at least a 2-hour period between the end of the nap and the beginning of the competition.

periods when it is relatively difficult to fall asleep. The two distinct periods when it is easy to fall asleep can be viewed as *sleep gates*. The first of these periods is the *postprandial dip*, which usually occurs between 1300 and 1600 and occurs more frequently, but not exclusively, in morning individuals (Fig. 5). Monk provides a detailed discussion of the postprandial dip elsewhere in this issue. A 20-minute nap has positive effects on subjective sleepiness and cognitive performance deterioration associated with the postprandial dip [42]. Naps may be combined with caffeine, bright light, and temperature manipulations. For instance, caffeine (200 mg) and bright light (2000 lux for 1-minute duration) augmented and consolidated the effect of a nap on midafternoon sleepiness and the postprandial dip in cognitive performance [43].

The second period, which is the nocturnal period that starts in the late evening when the "biological night" sets in, is much longer and omnipresent (see Fig. 5). Certain interventions can decrease sleepiness during the biological night, including bright light, caffeine, and temperature manipulations, either individually or in various combinations. See the articles by Postolache and Oren, Rogers and Dinges, and Kräuchi et al elsewhere in this issue for further exploration of these measures. Using stimulants, including modafinil, to improve performance during these adverse circadian times is unethical because stimulants may enhance performance beyond normal.

Performance level is at its minimum during these windows or sleep gates, even if it is not obvious to the individual. If a performance occurs during a sleep gate (as in a typical afternoon NFL football game, an occasional late-night baseball game, the finals in figure skating, or a major championship in pro-

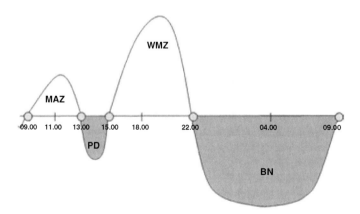

Fig. 5. Sleep gates and alertness peaks. Sleep gates are in gray below the baseline, and peaks of alertness in white above the baseline. In general, sleep gates are associated with poorer performance, and peaks of alertness with better performance. A superior player during a sleep gate may perform worse compared with an inferior player during a peak of alertness. MAZ, morning alertness zone (late morning); WMZ, wake maintenance zone (late afternoon/early evening); PD, postprandial dip (noon, early afternoon); BN, biological night (starts 2 hours before regular sleep onset time).

fessional boxing), the athletes will be unknowingly competing against circadian adversity. To avoid competing during this circadian adversity, athletes could shift their internal circadian rhythm with the intent of desynchronizing the internal sleep gate from the external competitive demand (time of the game). This may be accomplished in a manner similar to the treatment of jet lag using nonpharmacologic techniques, such as appropriately timed bright light exposure and avoidance.

Appendix 3 provides an example of how various nonpharmacologic methods to induce sleep affected one elite athlete's performance in competition.

Refractory periods for falling asleep

The refractory periods for sleep occur in the late morning and late afternoon/ evening. The evening refractory period is in fact paradoxical (ie, people are often more alert just before they usually go to bed than when they wake up), in that it usually occurs 3 hours before the habitual time for bed (under constant conditions) and is associated with the stimulating effect of the circadian system that compensates for the accumulated time awake and associated sleep pressure, as described by Stiller and Postolache elsewhere in this issue. The late evening refractory period for falling asleep is also called the *wake maintenance zone* (see Fig. 5), when psychomotor, cognitive, and physical functions are performed at or near their peak.

Evidence that the wake maintenance zone is optimal for sports performance

World records are usually broken by athletes competing in the later afternoon to early evening hours, as seen in runners, weight throwers, and 100- and 200-meter swimmers (see references [1,44]). These investigators also reviewed the methodological challenges related to laboratory studies of circadian effects on sports performance, and observed some consistent findings in diurnal variation. For instance, speed of reaction time and muscle strength peaked consistently in the early evening. However, accuracy without speed (as is necessary for golf or darts), fine motor control, and cognitive performances such as mental arithmetic and short-term memory (eg, recall of complex coaching instructions) tended to be better in the morning rather than the afternoon. Two peaks (late morning and early evening) have been described in isometric strength of the knee extensors and grip strength, with a drop in muscular strength during 1300 and 1400, coinciding with the *circadian dip*, a period when reaction time is also reduced in a sizeable proportion of athletes. In addition, late afternoon/early evening peaks in short-term power output were reported, with longer work times at 2200 than at 0630 and long jumps showing a late-afternoon peak (3.4% of the 24-hour average). These observations may be important for meeting certain performance standards to qualify for major events, or when attempting to set records or personal bests. Additionally, an evening peak in swimming performance with a rhythm of 11% to 14% of the 24-hour average, in excess of the effect of 3 hours of sleep deprivation for three successive nights, has been reported [1].

Morningness–eveningness

Some people tend to naturally wake up very early ("larks") and others to stay up very late ("owls"). Although environmental factors pay an important

---

Name: _____   Date: _____   Score: _____

Athlete's Morningness-Eveningness Scale (AMES)

Directions: This Scale is designed to help you identify your chronotype, that is, your tendency toward a morning ("lark"), mid-range or evening ("owl") performance pattern. To complete this Scale, first print out the document. Then, read each question and consider all of the responses carefully. Then, complete each of the six items on this Scale as accurately as you can; circle only one response per item.

1. At what time in the evening do you usually start feeling tired and in need of sleep?

    (7) A. 8:00 PM–9:30 PM
    (6) B. 9:31 PM–10:45 PM
    (5) C. 10:46 PM–12:30 AM
    (4) D. 12:31 AM–1:45 AM
    (3) E. 1:46 AM–3:00 AM

2. Suppose that you were able to choose your own competition hours. For some athletes, it might be useful to think about the 3-hour block when there would be a greater chance of feeling "in the zone," or performing "at peak." Which one of the following 3-hour blocks would be your most preferred time?

    (8) A. 6:00 AM–9:00 a.m.
    (7) B. 9:00 AM–Noon
    (6) C. Noon–3:00 PM
    (5) D. 3:00 PM–6:00 PM
    (4) E. 6:00 PM–9:00 PM.
    (3) F. 9:00 PM–Midnight

3. One sometimes hears about "feeling best in the morning" or "feeling best in the evening" types of people. Which type do you consider yourself?

    (8) A. Definitely a "morning" type
    (6) B. More a "morning" than an "evening" type
    (3) C. More an "evening" than a "morning" type
    (1) D. Definitely an "evening" type

4. Suppose that you were able to choose your own training (practice) hours, and organize all other daily routines to protect those hours. Which one of the following 3-hour blocks would be your most preferred time?

    (8) A. 6:00 AM–9:00 AM
    (7) B. 9:00 AM–Noon
    (6) C. Noon–3:00 PM
    (5) D. 3:00 PM–6:00 PM
    (4) E. 6:00 PM–9:00 PM
    (3) F. 9:00 PM–Midnight

Calculate your sleep score by adding the values in parentheses beside your circled answers. **Total Score:**	10 to 12	=	Extreme Evening Type
	13 to 17	=	Moderate Evening Type
	18 to 23	=	Mid range
	24 to 28	=	Moderate Morning Type
	29 to 31	=	Extreme Morning Type

Fig. 6. The Athlete's Morningness–Eveningness Scale questionnaire. (*Adapted from* Horne JA, Ostberg O. A self-assessment questionnaire to determine morningness-eveningness in human circadian rhythms. Int J Chronobiol 1976;4(2):97–110.)

role, endogenous circadian rhythms have been shown to determine the *chronotype*, or the "morningness–eveningness" preference. Since the original formulation of a morningness-eveningness questionnaire by Horne and Ostberg [45], other questionnaires have been proposed, such as one by Torsvall and Akerstedt [46], and the one by Smith et al [47] that we recommend for non-athletes. For athletes, we recommend the Athlete's Morningness–Eveningness Scale (AMES) (Fig. 6). Nevertheless, each sport has specific demands, and the athletes may have passed many thresholds of selection before competing at an elite level. It is possible that athletes who were stellar at the high school and college level do not perform as well at the professional level because the different temporal demands are difficult given their particular chronotype, as opposed to any lack of abilities or training. Morningness–eveningness questionnaires need to be adapted with the particular sport in mind, as not all questionnaires are suitable for all sports. For instance, current morningness–eveningness questionnaires do not apply for Major League Baseball, with its exceptionally heavy schedule and evening demands.

Circadian markers

Certain physiologic markers are essential when designing interventions for shifting circadian rhythms. One of the most important circadian markers is the timing of the central temperature minimum (T_{min}). For this purpose, T_{min} should be measured in constant conditions during extended wakefulness using a rectal probe in a constant position at rest with regular intake of water and food. This should be monitored continuously to eliminate "masking" by the sleep/wake cycle, positional physiologic changes (eg, orthostatic noradrenergic activation), and food/water metabolism. This procedure is called *constant routine*, and it is essentially impractical except during well-designed circadian research study protocols.

Hormonal markers

Biological day–night alterations are characterized by predictable rhythmic changes of certain hormones. Two of the most important are melatonin and cortisol. Cortisol levels start and continue to increase during the biological night, and decrease during the biological day. Melatonin is a hormone secreted during darkness. Its secretion begins approximately 2 hours before the usual bedtime and is limited to the biological night. Because melatonin is suppressed by bright light, it should be collected for measurement in dim light. Because there is a relatively abrupt and predictable onset of melatonin secretion preceding the onset of sleep, the dim light melatonin onset is a conveniently measured circadian marker. However, because blood measurements are often inconvenient, dim light saliva melatonin onset (DLMO) is recommended as a highly replicated surrogate measure. The procedures for the collection of saliva for circadian phase assessments using dim light melatonin onset are as follows:

- Subject must remain awake in dim light (<10 lux) during assessment (eg, in a dark hotel room, a TV video is allowed if seen on a small screen from at least 4 meters).
- A 2 mL saliva sample should be obtained every 30 minutes.
- To prevent sample contamination, use of toothpaste or mouthwash during phase assessment is prohibited. Caffeine, chocolate, bananas, and use of lipstick must be avoided for 5 hours before testing.
- Small snacks and fluids are allowed except for 10 minutes before samples taken.
- Saliva sample should be centrifuged, frozen, and sent to a laboratory for analysis.

Jet lag

Transcontinental travel is potentially disruptive for sports performance. Chronobiology interventions are critical for shortening and minimizing these disturbances. Even crossing few time zones may result in changes in the performance levels. For example, Recht et al [48] showed that 1.24 more home runs were hit in a Major League Baseball game by the home team when playing against a visiting team that had traveled eastward.

Although it usually represents a liability, transmeridian travel may offer a circadian advantage by avoiding an alignment between a sleep gate and duration of the game or competition. In football, Smith et al [49] showed that the Monday Night Football games give West Coast teams an advantage in terms of playing during the wake maintenance zone (ie, peak of performance) compared with East Coast teams. The West Coast teams score more points during Monday Night Football, enhancing their home advantage when playing at home and eliminating the home field advantage when the game is played on the East Coast [49]. This is consistent with the finding of Jehue et al [50] that there was a similar advantage for West Coast teams over East and Central teams for night games, at home and away, but a disadvantage for the West Coast teams for day games played on the East Coast.

In basketball, when a team traveled west to east rather than east to west, the visiting team scored four more points ($P = .07$), almost nullifying the home-court advantage [51]. This effect, similar to findings for Monday Night Football games, may be caused by West Coast visitors playing night games at an earlier time according to their internal clock.

Reilly et al provide a detailed discussion of jet lag, and Postolache and Oren of bright light treatment, elsewhere in this issue. Furthermore, for in-depth discussion of the relationship of bright light administration to jet lag, see the article by Parry in the Further Readings section. Appendix 4 describes a program of management of jet lag and napping for Chinese Taipei Olympic archery team.

Light for 8 to 12 hours before T_{min} delays circadian rhythms, whereas light for 8 to 12 hours after T_{min} advances circadian rhythms (Fig. 7). The principles of bright light application are based on the phase response to light [52], and several laboratory simulation protocols and field studies [53]. Phase advances are desirable with eastward travel whereas phase delays are desirable with westward travel. A given T_{min} on the first day at the new destination (T_{min2}) can be calculated as:

$$\text{Eastward travel } T_{min2} = T_{min} \text{ (of origin)} + \text{number of time zones crossed}$$

$$\text{Westward travel } T_{min2} = T_{min} \text{ (of origin)} - \text{number of time zones crossed}$$

Based on the formulas above, one can design paradigms of light exposure and avoidance for jet lag. To apply these principles, because of the importance

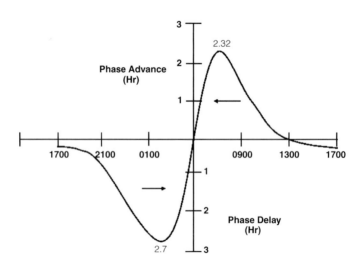

Fig. 7. PRC to bright light. PRC to the bright light phase advances (positive values) and delays (negative values) are plotted against the timing of the center of the light exposure relative to the core body temperature. Tics on the *y* axis are hours. The maximum phase delay (2.7 hours) exceeds the maximum phase advance (2.3 hours). (*Adapted from* Khalsa SB, Jewett ME, Cajochen C, et al. A phase response curve to single bright light pulses in human subjects. J Physiol 2003;549(Pt 3): 945–52.)

of the inflection point from when light phase-delays to when it phase-advances, it is crucial to ascertain T_{min}, but continuous monitoring of central temperature in constant conditions is practically and logistically infeasible in elite athletes. Nocturnal plasma melatonin and cortisol profiles are invasive measurements, involving a catheter and frequent blood sampling by way of a long catheter (to not disrupt sleep), and is too disruptive for athletes. Because T_{min} refers to temperature minimum measured in constant conditions in the absence of sleep, it is difficult to determine in real-life situations, especially in elite athletes. Therefore, surrogate measures must be used to estimate T_{min}, including the assumption that T_{min} falls between 4 AM and 5 AM in most individuals, 2 AM and 4 AM in morning types (larks), and 5 AM to 7 AM in evening types who were sleeping late in the morning for the last week. A more precise estimation of T_{min} (if sleep onset and offset have been generally regular for the last week) is to use a sleep-related measure, such as sleep duration midpoint, and add 1 to 2 hours. Furthermore, an even more precise estimation that allows some individualization involves measuring DLMO and adding 7 hours to the DLMO).

Preflight adjustment to travel is highly recommended especially to hasten adaptation [53], along with several days of shifting at the location of origin, although this is rarely feasible.

Room light and jet lag

Lower intensities of light, similar to those present in routine illumination conditions, have been shown to suppress melatonin and shift circadian rhythms [54]. For instance, room light in a jet-lag simulation has been shown to alter circadian rhythms [55]. Thus, exposure to room light in the hotel or at practice, if extended over several hours, should be considered active from a circadian standpoint and, depending on whether it occurs during a "favorable" or "unfavorable" interval, may either help or hurt the adjustment to the new time zone. During the favorable interval on the PRC, brighter light should be used in the room, and during the undesired portions on the PRC, lights should be dimmed. Because short-wavelength light is a more potent circadian shifter, sunglasses with overall high transmission but selectively low transmission in the blue-green range could be used indoors for reading or watching television during a potentially adverse time on the PRC (see Fig. 7), although no specific research is currently available to support this recommendation. Tables 1 and 2 provide general strategies for using light exposure and avoidance to alleviate jet lag.

Melatonin and jet lag

Although bright light exposure and avoidance is the most potent thera-peutic agent for shifting circadian rhythms, athletes and coaches, perhaps out

Table 1
General strategies for light exposure and avoidance for jet lag: eastward travel[a]

Interval	Description	Start range	End range
First day of arrival			
Desirable bright light avoidance	12 hr time interval	T_{min} + number time zones crossed − 12	T_{min} + number time zones crossed
Critical light avoidance	8 hr time interval	T_{min} + number time zones crossed − 9	T_{min} + number time zones crossed − 1
Desirable bright light exposure	At least 1 hr light exposure within 12 hr interval (earlier exposure in range more beneficial)	T_{min} + number time zones crossed	T_{min} + number time zones crossed + 12
Critical light exposure	At least 1 hr light exposure within 8 hr interval (earlier exposure in range more beneficial)	T_{min} + number time zones crossed + 1	T_{min} + number time zones crossed + 9

The following days: shift the time of bright light and dark exposure 2 hours earlier each day and stop the regimen of light avoidance when T_{min} coincides with the desired wake-up time, continuing bright light exposure as early as possible after awakening.

[a] The goal is to phase advance and to avoid phase delay.

of convenience or habit, often prefer to only take melatonin. Melatonin is synthesized from serotonin in the pineal gland, secreted during the internal nighttime, and suppressed by bright light to the eyes. In a sense, melatonin serves as a chemical "dark pulse," indicating to the rest of the body that the time is right for behaviors associated with nighttime (ie, sleep in diurnal species).

Table 2
General strategies for light exposure and avoidance for jet lag: westward travel[a]

Interval	Description	Start range	End range
First day of arrival			
Desirable bright light avoidance	12 hr time interval	T_{min} − number time zones crossed	T_{min} − number time zones crossed + 12
Critical light avoidance	8 hr time interval	T_{min} − number time zones crossed + 1	T_{min} − number time zones crossed + 9
Desirable bright light exposure	At least 1 hr light exposure within 12 hr interval (earlier exposure in range more beneficial)	T_{min} − number time zones crossed − 12	T_{min} − number time zones crossed
Critical light exposure	At least 1 hr light exposure within 8 hr interval (earlier exposure in range more beneficial)	T_{min} − number time zones crossed − 9	T_{min} − number time zones crossed − 1

The following days: shift the time of bright light and dark exposure 2 hours later every day, until the T_{min} falls within 2 to 3 hours before wake-up time, then stop the regimen.

[a] The goal is to phase delay and to avoid phase advance.

Melatonin shifts circadian rhythms according to a PRC that approximates a mirror image of the light PRC (Fig. 8) [56]. Specifically, when melatonin is administered during the internal late afternoon/early evening, it results in a phase advance of circadian rhythms, and if administered during the early morning, a phase delay occurs (see Fig. 8). When bright light and melatonin are strategically administered at phase-appropriate times, the combination may act additively. For instance, morning light in combination with evening melatonin will cause a phase advance, and evening light with morning melatonin a phase delay (see Figs. 7 and 8). For a review of these effects, see the article by Waterhouse et al in the Further Readings section.

Melatonin is marketed and sold as a food supplement in the United States; it is not approved for the treatment of any disorder by the US Food and Drug Administration. Smaller doses (0.5–1 mg) are sufficient for phase shifting, but larger doses (3–10 mg) are often used as a nonspecific soporific for sleep induction. For the optimal treatment of jet lag, the timing of melatonin administration is critical, and following a schedule such as the one presented in the review by Waterhouse et al [57] can be useful.

Pharmacologic doses of melatonin are associated with hypnotic and hypothermic responses, and may cause short-term reductions in mental and physical performance (eg, psychomotor vigilance) [58]. The decline in physical performance may be short-lived, but decrements in certain tasks requiring vigilance may persist for 3 to 5 hours or more after administration. However, the impairment in vigilance does not occur if the individual gets adequate sleep after

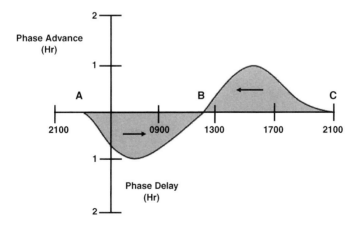

Fig. 8. PRC to melatonin. PRC to melatonin phase advances (positive values) and delays (negative values) are plotted against the timing of the center of the light exposure relative to the core body temperature. It can be observed that the PRC to melatonin is relatively less ample than the one to light (not more than 1 hour maximum), and that overall the effects are approximately mirror imaging the PRC to light (ie, late afternoon melatonin phase advances while light phase delays, and morning melatonin phase delays while light phase advances).

the administration, as discussed by Atkinson and Drust elsewhere in this issue. There is also experimental evidence supporting the claim that melatonin does not affect physical performance the day after taking even higher doses (5 mg) [59]. Although melatonin has been used successfully to alleviate symptoms of jet lag associated with sleep, there is no convincing data that melatonin improves athletic performance when used for jet lag, and the small amount of supportive evidence available is controversial. The most common mistakes made in melatonin use are:

- Wrong timing of melatonin administration. Indiscriminately taking melatonin as a sleep inducer can cause circadian shifts in an unwanted direction in certain circumstances;
- The administered dose being too high. For phase shifting, dosages of 0.5 to 1 mg are sufficient;
- Not checking the purity of the melatonin preparation. Although melatonin is not on the WADA Prohibited List, the preparation of melatonin may contain impurities that could result in a positive doping test.

The routine administration of melatonin to prevent or treat jet lag in athletes is not recommended, particularly if a correctly timed regime of light exposure and avoidance can be used. However, when the logistical circumstances do not provide enough time for adjustment at the destination and a preflight adjustment is not practical, for example with a particularly busy schedule (eg, tennis, golf), many athletes prefer to use melatonin. Under these circumstances, a small dose designed to induce circadian shifting should be administered carefully and according to appropriate timing. Large soporific doses should be avoided and the purity of the preparation needs to be assured to avoid the inadvertent contamination by banned substances.

Situations in which it may be detrimental to make a circadian phase adjustment to the destination time

One situation where circadian shifts to the new time zone should be avoided is when a short trip away from home is followed by an important competition or home game scheduled a short time after the return and there is not enough time to comfortably readjust. In this case, all efforts must be made during the short trip to avoid light exposure to the eyes (eg, using window shades, having minimal lights in the room, wearing dark sunglasses that ideally block or reflect short wavelength light, avoiding outdoor exposure) and to maintain as much as feasible the sleep/wake activity and meal schedule in sync with the home, rather than destination, schedule.

Another situation where a circadian shift to the new time zone should be avoided is when the competition occurs during the competitor's sleep gate, and the avoidance of shifting results in a better alignment between the time of the competition and the endogenous time of peak performance. For instance, when traveling from Western Europe for a match in the United States at 1300 (falling during the postprandial dip for a local player), the West European player may have a circadian advantage because, if they have not adjusted to the new time zone, they will play just as if it is 1900, which generally falls during the wake maintenance zone and is the peak time for alertness and psychomotor performance. To some degree, this advantage may counteract the effect of playing away and the travel fatigue.

Similarly, traveling from the West to the East Coast for a late-night competition (eg, figure skating) may offer an advantage to the West Coast athlete who, if not adjusted, will play during the wake maintenance zone, whereas the East Coast athlete, at least in the second part of the game, may be competing after the onset of internal night (ie, after the internal melatonin secretion has started) and may therefore experience impaired psychomotor vigilance [58].

Delayed sleep phase syndrome

Delayed sleep phase syndrome (DSPS) is a clinical syndrome commonly encountered by young high school and college athletes, and observed less frequently in adults. These athletes often cannot fall asleep until late at night, but still have to wake up early in the morning for practice and academic activities. Attempting to go to bed earlier does not work in most of these cases because the wake maintenance zone has shifted (delayed to a time when they would ideally be sleeping), and therefore it becomes difficult, if not impossible, to fall asleep naturally during this period. The DSPS may result in significant sleep debt and pronounced chronic underperformance in athletic and academic domains. Schedules of appropriately timed light exposure and avoidance, sleep hygiene, and a variety of other interventions may be necessary to bring the situation under control. A further discussion of this topic is provided in the article by Carskadon elsewhere in this issue.

Infradian rhythms

Infradian rhythms have a period longer than 24 hours (eg, menstrual, seasonal). For the implications of menstrual rhythms on athletic performance, see the article by Constantini et al on menstrual rhythms elsewhere in this issue. For a further discussion of the relevance of seasonal rhythms for athletes, see the article on seasonality of exercise by Atkinson and Drust, the article on bright light treatment by Postolache and Oren, and the article on the effect of seasonal allergies on athletic performance by Komarow and Postolache elsewhere in this issue. An inquiry about menstrual and seasonal variation in performance should be included in any sports chronobiology consultation.

Summary

In addition to preventing performance deterioration and contributing to better health, implementing chronobiologic methods to preserve alertness may help certain athletes avoid or discontinue unethical and illegal use of stimulants.

The science of chronobiology relies on precise measurements in highly controlled environments. Additional studies looking at relevant outcome measures using these standards of design for performance in sports are necessary. However, the practice of chronobiology (as with any medical practice), although striving for the utmost in the use of precise scientifically based approaches, must compromise in dealing with issues of logistics, feasibility, and compliance. It is essential to provide individualized assessments and recommendations that are specific to the particular athlete and sport.

Appendix 5 provides a list of Web-based resources that provide information on chronobiology and circadian rhythms and Appendix 6 offers information on actigraphy.

Acknowledgments

We acknowledge those individuals who directly or indirectly contributed to data we present in this article. We would like to thank Ev- K2- CNR (Italy), Harold Been, MD, Arnold Winston, MD, Agostino Da Polenza, Gian-Pietro Verza, William Gruen, and Mal Duff for their help in the high altitude sleep study.

Many thanks go to Dr. Der Chia Lin, the Director of the National Training Center and the Chief of Chinese Taipei Mission at the Athens 2004 Olympic games for his far-sighted understanding of the importance of chronobiology for elite performance, and his invitation to apply chronobiologic principles to the training of athletes who then won historic Olympic medals for their country. We are indebted to Tatiana Tarasova, coach of many Olympic and World champions, who invited us to work with her team and helped us in taking chronobiologic principles outside the laboratory into the arena of a sport where quantification of performance is very subjective and individual differences huge, thus decreasing our anxiety about quantification of outcome measurement. After figure skating, the quantification of outcome in almost every other sport became easier to accept.

We would like to thank Drs. Xiaolong Jiao and Steven Wolf, who, with their increased attention to the organizational and logistical aspects of our day-to-day responsibilities, allowed us to dedicate more time to this article.

Appendix 1. Descending 1100 m from the Base Camp of Mount Everest improves sleep in an acclimatized climber

Subjects exposed to higher altitudes awaken more frequently and complain of waking up unrefreshed. Sleep deprivation induces cognitive dysfunction and fatigue, which are factors that are already present at high altitude as a result of hypobaric hypoxia, increasing the potential for fatal miscalculation. In addition to restoring necessary physical strength before an extremely demanding task, sleep may be critical to survival on Mount Everest.

Actigraphy was previously employed to document sleep disturbances and recently used to document high-altitude sleep disturbances [2]. We used actigraphs to assess if sleep in mountain climbers who were already acclimatized to high altitude was disturbed at the level of the Everest Base Camp (5350 m), which is at an altitude where the amount of inspired percent of O_2 is only about half that of sea level. We were also interested to see if an optional descent below the level of Base Camp to a reasonable altitude for the intermediate rest period before attempting the summit would have a favorable impact on sleep.

Six climbers of an international expedition wore a basic waterproof Motionlogger Actigraph (Ambulatory Monitoring, Ardsley, New York). Actigraph data was collected for approximately 20 days. At the end of the acclimatization, climbers had the option to rest at the level of Base Camp or to descend for rest to Pheriche (4250 m). Only one climber from the six descended, the other five remained at the level of Base Camp. The instruments worked flawlessly. Downloading and reinitialization were performed once in the field without incident and with a minimal loss of data.

Although the climbers had completed the entire process of acclimatization, their sleep was disturbed at the level of Base Camp. For the climber who descended to Pheriche, a major improvement in sleep occurred only for the days he slept there. A later ascent to Base Camp resulted in increased nocturnal activity (see Fig. 2), arguing against the possibility that cumulative acclimatization, rather than descent to a lower altitude, was the cause of sleep improvement at Pheriche.

In one climber, we observed severe disruption of sleep, indicated by recurrent awakenings (see Fig. 3). The activity during the day was marked by high levels of fatigue and sleepiness and low vigor, factors markedly affecting physical and mental functioning. The climber, although renouncing plans to summit, did not want to descend or leave the team, and even refused a temporary descent to lower altitudes for the possibility of paying a portion of the accumulated sleep debt. He explained that he was too exhausted to go down and return in time for the team's scheduled summit attempt. His cognition appeared sluggish and his psychomotor performance on a finger-tapping test markedly deteriorated.

Impressions
1. Sleep appears to be very disturbed at the level of Everest Base Camp even in acclimatized climbers. Accumulated sleep debt may contribute to fatalities as a result of reduced concentration, motivation, and volition.

2. Individual differences exist, with some climbers displaying major debilitating sleep impairments.

3. Although it is counterintuitive to descend before attempting the Everest Summit, and the effectiveness of descending has been questioned, our report confirms an improvement in sleep with a viable 1100-m descent from the Base Camp for 3 days, used by only a minority of climbers on an empirical basis.

4. Actigraphy performed reliably in a hostile environment.
   (T.T. Postolache, R.N. Rosenthal)

Appendix 2. Naps in Major League Baseball pitchers

Several elite level players participated in a program of optimum training for pitchers. Starting in late spring of 2004, after a chronobiology consultation (TTP) with the Director of Strength and Conditioning of a Major League Baseball team, sleep hygiene and napping strategies were added to other previously used interventions, such as nutrition and mental preparation. Consideration was also given for travel across more than one time zone.

The daily training log includes self-reports from the player in the areas of: (1) sleep (on the top of the list), (2) physical status, (3) mental status, (4) family time, (5) personal time, (6) eating/nutritional habits, (7) injury, and (8) workout/ daily performance. These areas were rated overall with scores of 1 through 5, with 1 designating "poor," 2 designating "below average," 3 designating "average," 4 designating "good," and 5 designating "great."

The players' daily routines were also charted. Training adjustments where made on a daily basis according to the following factors: (1) daily omega-wave test data, (2) participation in the baseball game, (3) game outcome/extra innings, (4) travel, (5) feedback/observation from the strength and conditioning coach, and (6) special needs.

Naps took place in the strength and conditioning exam room. A 1-hour nap opportunity was used between approximately 2 PM and 3 PM. The naps were only used on the day of a night game, and never before a day game. As recommended by the chronobiology consultant (TTP), the nap took place after lunch, the room was dark, the extremities of the player were covered with a blanket, the air was cool, and the noise was kept to a minimum. With these techniques, all players reported success in falling asleep. They were awakened at or before 3:15 PM.

The players participating in the program reported improvements in strength, vigor, and level of energy. Key areas identified as contributing to positive outcomes were napping techniques, better sound nutritional habits, and sleep/ recovery strategies for travel, and early-morning arrivals to new cities. Further study of these areas is of the utmost importance. In the world of Major League Baseball, with its high expectations, million-dollar payrolls, and the pressure to win at all costs (unfortunately leading to the reliance on performance-enhancing substances for some players), the need to have quality performance training backed by sound medical science is critical for athletes' abilities, longevity, health, and sports ethics. There is a great deal more that needs to be done to help define the "Optimal Training Philosophy" for today's professional baseball player and break the myth that adding science to baseball is like adding oil to water. (F. Montes)

Appendix 3. Elite figure skater with challenging competition hours

An elite female figure skater preparing for the World Championships meets a challenging competitive schedule: qualifiers in the early morning, a short program in the early afternoon, and the finals late in the evening. The events are separated by 24 to 48 hours. She scored as an evening person on a morningness–eveningness questionnaire and reported feeling extremely drowsy with an inability to concentrate in the early afternoon.

A repeated PVT showed significant sleep inertia with a mean reaction time (MRT) 5 minutes after awakening of 326.1 milliseconds with a large SD of 194 milliseconds and five lapses (reaction time above 500 milliseconds). The reaction time and ratings of sleepiness improved in the late morning, as evidenced by a lower MRT of 249 milliseconds and a narrower SD at 37.1 milliseconds. This pattern, suggesting impairment in vigilance related to sleep inertia and circadian dip, was confirmed by measurements during two other days of testing. The challenge in the skater's case was that the early-morning performance in the opening of the championship might possibly prompt an unwanted phase advance caused by morning light exposure. This could result in her competing in the finals after the onset of biological night (past the time of her circadian peak). Additionally, the short program, possibly occurring during her postprandial dip, could have also jeopardized her standing.

The chronobiology consultation emphasized the need to wake up at least 2 hours before the beginning of the competition and for nonpharmacologic methods to induce sleep during the previous evening to secure adequate sleep duration (see Box 4). Caffeinated drinks and snacks and bright light exposure were used to improve alertness for the early-morning competition. Immediately after the qualifiers, dark sunglasses were used in the morning and early afternoon, with bright light exposure in the late afternoon and evening. This was expected to phase delay rhythms, with a delay of the onset of biological night that could have been previously advanced by the early exposure to morning light during the qualifiers. Incidentally, delaying the rhythms is easier than advancing them, and two evenings of exposure to light and avoidance of light in the morning might have resulted in 3 to 4 hours of phase delay. This phase delay was intended to push the postprandial dip later, resulting in the short program taking place during the internal morning alertness zone (MAZ on Fig. 5) instead of during the postprandial dip, and pushing back the start of the biological night (BN on Fig. 5) several hours later so she would be performing in the finals with a circadian advantage. We also advised against napping before the afternoon short program given her documented problems with sleep inertia. Additional short exposure to bright light and a nap of 90 minutes ending 2 hours before the evening final performance were also recommended. During the competition, the skater was compliant with the recommendations, reported a high level of confidence, stamina, and alertness and an increased ability to concentrate, and exceeded her specific competitive goals. (T.T. Postolache)

Appendix 4. Jet lag management and napping in medal-contending Olympic archers

Chinese Taipei archers won a silver medal in the men's team event, a bronze in the women's team event, fourth and sixth places in the women's single events, and seventh place in the men's single event in the Athens 2004 Olympic games. Although these results may not appear impressive for certain countries that obtained far more medals in the games, they were significant achievements for Chinese Taipei. These accomplishments were particularly impressive considering the inexperience of the team and its modest level of performance in the past. The best that Chinese Taipei had ever done in previous Olympics was seventh place in the men's team and women's singles competitions more than 10 years ago. Furthermore, the men's team did not even qualify for Sydney 2000. Coincidentally, this was the first Olympics for the coaches and the athletes. Cooperation between sport scientists and coaches started approximately 1.5 years before the Olympics. The fields of sport science that were integrated with the training regimen included biomechanics, exercise physiology, and sport psychology. A sport psychologist for the team worked closely with the athletes and the coaches and strongly attributes the practical application of sport science as a major contributing factor for their success.

The team had experienced major detrimental and disruptive effects of jet lag before and after returning from trips to Greece and Germany several months before the Olympics (a 5-hour difference exists between Taiwan and Greece). Jet lag had a significantly negative effect on concentration and alertness, which delayed practice for several days.

A sports chronobiology consultant (TTP) was invited to Taiwan to introduce sport chronobiology to the entire Chinese Taipei team by using a three-step approach during a 2-day educational program. The first seminar was for the sports psychologists and graduate sports psychology students working individually with each athlete. The second seminar was for the coaches and trainers, and the third for the athletes. The educational message was tailored for each group's level of training. To avoid dampening the athletes' confidence, the message to the athletes was focused not on circadian adversity but on the motivating goal of competing at the peak of athletic ability.

Jet lag was only one aspect of the seminar. Other issues discussed at the seminar included the importance of proper sleep hygiene for optimal performance, nonpharmacologic methods for sleep induction, morningness–eveningness concepts, and reducing exposure (especially eye exposure) to seasonal allergens expected to be present in Athens during the Olympics. The seminar concluded with pragmatic techniques for maintaining performance, such as timed naps, jet lag management, and the use of sunglasses to protect the eyes and to assist in chronobiologic interventions (none of the archers used sunglasses before the seminar). Certain interventions, such as assessing the influence of menstrual rhythms on performance, were not applied because of time constraints. After the seminar, the chronobiology recommendations were applied by a sports psychologist who regularly discussed the results of the tests and interventions with the chronobiology consultant through e-mail and telephone conferences.

In addition to the educational approach, an individualized approach to the diagnosis and treatment phases of intervention was adopted and several baseline investigations were conducted. Initially, athletes were asked to complete morningness–eveningness questionnaires. Subsequently, DLMO was established for each archer to obtain a baseline circadian marker. Sleep quality was monitored by actigraphy and individual reaction times were used to measure psychologic vigilance at four different times of the day.

One chronobiologic technique the archers used was to start the adaptation processes 1 night before their trip to Athens. Several archers agreed to "jumpstart" the process by staying 2 hours later in the evening and through exposure to standard artificial light during the delaying portion of the PRC, as demonstrated on the actigraphic tracing in Fig. 9. Sunglasses were also used to avoid light early in the morning, when light would otherwise phase advance circadian rhythms and aggravate jet lag. Each archer received specific recommendations on bright light exposure and use of shades or sunglasses, which were derived from the specific flight schedule and the individual's melatonin onset time.

Because the athletes and coaches requested that melatonin be integrated into the regimen, the timing of its administration was decided according to the PRC for melatonin and the specific DLMO. The chronobiology consultant recommended the use of very small doses (0.5 mg) for phase-shifting purposes (in addition to the timed light exposure and avoidance). The coaches and the athletes considered the advice extremely beneficial. Generally, the coaches' impression was that intervention mitigated circadian adaptation by approximately 2 days compared with the previous trip. The hastened adaptation also helped these athletes resume regular training at an earlier time before the Olympics started and may be one of the factors contributing to the excellent performance.

In addition to the jet lag intervention, napping was another initiative used to help the archers. As a result of the competition schedule, napping was not applied during the preliminary round and single events. However, because the group competition was scheduled in the morning and the afternoon, napping was applied 3 hours before the afternoon competition. Results for the men's

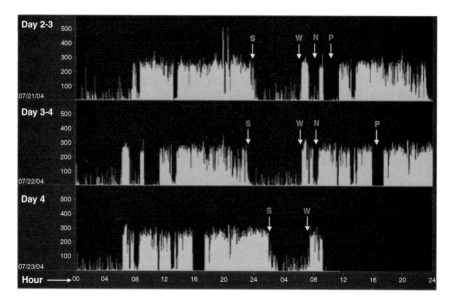

Fig. 9. Actigraphy in an elite archer from Chinese Taipei (team medalist) preparing for departure for Athens Olympics. Raw actigraphic tracing using a Motionlogger Actigraph (Ambulatory Monitoring, Ardsley, New York). Three days of double-plotted actigraphic tracings are visible (ie, two 24-hour periods per raw; with the nocturnal rest period intercalated by two diurnal activity periods). On day 4 of the tracing, (the lowest raw), an extension of wakefulness by approximately 2 hours compared with days 2 to 3 and 3 to 4 can be seen. Although this tracing could be attributed in other cases to sleep onset insomnia, often caused by anxiety/excitement before travel to a highly important competition, in this case it represented compliance with the jet lag program that required a more rapid delay of circadian rhythms. The phase delaying started with staying up later that night, with exposure to room light while playing video games with her coach. This jump-start of the jet lag program was followed with timed sunglass application, natural light exposure and avoidance, small dose melatonin administration, and schedules of sleep–wake. The sleep deprivation created by going to bed later allows the athlete to sleep longer and wake up later, thus diminishing the counter-therapeutic phase-advancing effect of morning exposure to light. S, sleep onset; W, wake-up time; N, an early morning postbreakfast rest/nap opportunity, part of an individually tailored approach; P, practice when the actigraphs were turned off (no activity).

team were encouraging: after napping, they outperformed their rivals in the semifinals. Although the women's team lost in the semifinals, they considered napping to be effective in raising their mental sharpness. One female archer even extolled the virtues of napping by admitting she would not have been able to perform in the afternoon otherwise.

In summary, the education and chronobiology intervention resulted in a degree of positive effects on the archers. Although these effects do not necessarily have a causal link to performance, and multiple factors may have been responsible for the archers' remarkable results, they did plausibly contribute to optimizing the archers' physical and mental state during competition. (T.M. Hung)

Appendix 5. Web-based resources that provide information on chronobiology and circadian rhythms

Organization	Description	Web site
American Association of Medical Chronobiology and Chronotherapeutics (AAMCC)	Provides an organizational framework for scientists and health care professionals interested in the medical application of chronobiology and chronotherapeutics.	www.aamcc.org
Center for Biological Timing Home Page	The National Science Foundation Center for Biological Timing. Tutorials and original papers on biological timing.	www.cbt.virginia.edu
Circadian Sleep Disorders Association	Supports and provides information to those affected by circadian sleep disorders, such as Delayed Sleep Phase Syndrome. Includes links, FAQs, message board, and a mailing list.	www.circadiandisorders.org
Society for Light Treatment and Biological Rhythms	A not-for-profit international organization founded in 1988 that aims to foster research, professional development, and clinical applications in the fields of light therapy and biological rhythms.	www.sltbr.org
Institute of Sports Chronobiology	Organization committed to educating the professional and amateur athletics in sleep hygiene, superior rest–activity schedules, and alignment between peak internal resources and external competitive demands.	www.sportschrono.org
World Anti-Doping Agency (WADA)	Seeks to foster a doping free culture in sport. It combines the resources of sport and government to enhance, supplement, and coordinate existing efforts to educate athletes about the harms of doping, reinforce the ideal of fair play, and sanction those who cheat.	www.wada-ama.org
Society for Research on Biological Rhythms	Formed in 1987 to promote the advancement of basic and applied research in all aspects of biological rhythms; to disseminate the important results of that research among scientists, to the agencies that fund research, and to the general public; to enhance the education and training of students and researchers in the field; and to foster interdisciplinary communication.	www.srbr.org
National Center on Sleep Disorders	Coordinating government-supported sleep research, training, and education to improve the health of Americans.	http://www.nhlbi.nih.gov/about/ncsdr/index.htm
Sleep Network	Educational site devoted to improving sleep health worldwide.	www.sleepnet.com

(continued on next page)

Appendix 5 (*continued*)

Organization	Description	Web site
National Sleep Foundation	Independent nonprofit organization dedicated to improving public health and safety by achieving a better understanding of sleep and sleep disorders, and supporting sleep related research and advocacy.	www.sleepfoundation.org

Appendix 6. Actigraphy information

Organization	Description	Web site
Ambulatory Monitoring, Inc., Ardsely, New York	Mini-Motionlogger Actigraph. Also has portable PVT devices available.	www.ambulatory-monitoring.com
Mini Mitter, Bend, Oregon	Actiwatch	www.minimitter.com
MTI ActiGraph, Fort Walton Beach, Florida	ActiGraph System	www.mtiactigraph.com
American Academy of Sleep Medicine review paper published in the journal *Sleep*	"The role of actigraphy in the study of sleep and circadian rhythms"	www.aasmnet.org/PDF/260315.pdf

References

[1] Atkinson G, Reilly T. Circadian variation in sports performance. Sports Med 1996;21:292–312.
[2] Quigley BM. "Biorhythms" and men's track and field world records. Med Sci Sports Exerc 1982;14:303–7.
[3] Quigley BM. "Biorhythms" and Australian track and field records. J Sports Med Phys Fitness 1981;21:81–9.
[4] Wyatt JK, Ritz-De Cecco A, Czeisler CA, et al. Circadian temperature and melatonin rhythms, sleep, and neurobehavioral function in humans living on a 20-h day. Am J Physiol 1999; 277:R1152–63.
[5] Katzenberg D, Young T, Finn L, et al. A CLOCK polymorphism associated with human diurnal preference. Sleep 1998;21:569–76.
[6] Katzenberg D, Young T, Lin L, et al. A human period gene (HPER1) polymorphism is not associated with diurnal preference in normal adults. Psychiatr Genet 1999;9:107–9.
[7] Sei H, Oishi K, Morita Y, Ishida N. Mouse model for morningness/eveningness. Neuroreport 2001;12:1461–4.
[8] Ravizza K. Peak experiences in sport. Journal of Humanistic Psychology 1977;17:35–40.
[9] Csikszentmihalyi M. Flow: the psychology of optimal experience. New York: Harper & Row; 1990.
[10] Jackson S, Csikszentmihalyi M. Flow in sports. Champaign, IL: Human Kinetics; 1999.
[11] Hanin YL. Individual zones of optimal functioning (IZOF) model: emotion-per-performance relationship in sport. In: Hanin YL, editor. Emotion in sport. Champaign, IL: Human Kinetics; 2000. p. 65–89.
[12] Johns MW. A new method for measuring daytime sleepiness: the Epworth Sleepiness Scale. Sleep 1991;14:540–5.

[13] Akerstedt T, Gillberg M. Subjective and objective sleepiness in the active individual. Int J Neurosci 1990;52:29–37.

[14] Dinges DF, Powell JW. Microcomputer analyses of performance on a portable, simple visual RT task during sustained operations. Behav Res Meth Instr Comp 1985;17:652–5.

[15] Doran SM, Van Dongen HP, Dinges DF. Sustained attention performance during sleep deprivation: evidence of state instability. Arch Ital Biol 2001;139:253–67.

[16] Dorrian J, Rogers NL, Dinges DF. Psychomotor vigilance performance: a neurocognitive assay sensitive to sleep loss. In: Kushida CA, editor. Sleep deprivation. New York: Marcel Dekker, Inc.; 2004.

[17] WADA. 2005 World Anti-Doping Code Prohibited List. Available at: www.wada-ama.org. Accessed October 2004.

[18] Jones AR, Pichot JT. Stimulant use in sports. Am J Addict 1998;7:243–55.

[19] Weiss B, Laties VG. Enhancement of human performance by caffeine and the amphetamines. Pharmacol Rev 1962;14:1–36.

[20] Freeman M, Olney B. New drug tests in baseball stir debate among players. Available at: http://query.nytimes.com/gst/abstract.html?res=F40F12F63B5E0C718EDDAD0894DB404482. Accessed April 22, 2003.

[21] CASA. Winning at any cost: doping in olympics sports. A report by the CASA National Commission on Sports and Substance Abuse; 2000. Available at http://www.casacolumbia.org/supportcasa/item.asp?cID=12&PID=119. Accessed March 7, 2005.

[22] Harris D, Batki SL. Stimulant psychosis: symptom profile and acute clinical course. Am J Addict 2000;9:28–37.

[23] Mandell AJ. The nightmare season. New York: Random House, Inc.; 1976.

[24] Riemann D, Berger M, Voderholzer U. Sleep and depression–results from psychobiological studies: an overview. Biol Psychol 2001;57:67–103.

[25] Armstrong LE, VanHeest JL. The unknown mechanism of the overtraining syndrome: clues from depression and psychoneuroimmunology. Sports Med 2002;32:185–209.

[26] West JB. American College of Physicians, American Physiological Society. The physiologic basis of high-altitude diseases. Ann Intern Med 2004;141:789–800.

[27] Weil JV. Sleep at high altitude. In: Kryger MH, Roth T, Dement WC, editors. Principles and practice of sleep medicine. 3rd edition. Philadelphia: W.B. Saunders Co.; 2000. p. 242–53.

[28] Saunders PU, Telford RD, Pyne DB, et al. Improved running economy in elite runners after 20 days of simulated moderate-altitude exposure. J Appl Physiol 2004;96:931–7.

[29] Spiegel K, Leproult R, Van Cauter E. Impact of sleep debt on metabolic and endocrine function. Lancet 1999;354:1435–9.

[30] Aeschbach D, Postolache TT, Sher L, et al. Evidence from the waking electroencephalogram that short sleepers live under higher homeostatic sleep pressure than long sleepers. Neuroscience 2001;102:493–502.

[31] Aeschbach D, Matthews JR, Postolache TT, et al. Two circadian rhythms in the human electroencephalogram during wakefulness. Am J Physiol 1999;277:R1771–9.

[32] Aeschbach D, Cajochen C, Landolt H, et al. Homeostatic sleep regulation in habitual short sleepers and long sleepers. Am J Physiol 1996;270:R41–53.

[33] Aeschbach D, Sher L, Postolache TT, et al. A longer biological night in long sleepers than in short sleepers. J Clin Endocrinol Metab 2003;88:26–30.

[34] Dinges DF, Orne MT, Orne EC. Assessing performance upon abrupt awakening from naps during quasi-continuous operations. Behav Res Methods Instrum Comput 1985;17:37–45.

[35] Gillberg M, Kecklund G, Axelsson J, et al. The effects of a short daytime nap after restricted night sleep. Sleep 1996;19:570–5.

[36] Mednick SC, Nakayama K, Cantero JL, et al. The restorative effect of naps on perceptual deterioration. Nat Neurosci 2002;5:677–81.

[37] Helmus T, Rosenthal L, Bishop C, et al. The alerting effects of short and long naps in narcoleptic, sleep deprived, and alert individuals. Sleep 1997;20:251–7.

[38] Takahashi M, Arito H. Maintenance of alertness and performance by a brief nap after lunch under prior sleep deficit. Sleep 2000;23:813–9.

[39] Tietzel AJ, Lack LC. The recuperative value of brief and ultra-brief naps on alertness and cognitive performance. J Sleep Res 2002;11:213–8.

[40] Tietzel AJ, Lack LC. The short-term benefits of brief and long naps following nocturnal sleep restriction. Sleep 2001;24:293–300.

[41] Wehr TA, Aeschbach D, Duncan Jr WC. Evidence for a biological dawn and dusk in the human circadian timing system. J Physiol 2001;535:937–51.

[42] Hayashi M, Watanabe M, Hori T. The effects of a 20 min nap in the mid-afternoon on mood, performance and EEG activity. Clin Neurophysiol 1999;110:272–9.

[43] Hayashi M, Masuda A, Hori T. The alerting effects of caffeine, bright light and face washing after a short daytime nap. Clin Neurophysiol 2003;114:2268–78.

[44] Reilly T, Atkinson G, Waterhouse JM. Biological rhythms and exercise. Oxford: Oxford University Press; 1997.

[45] Horne JA, Ostberg O. A self-assessment questionnaire to determine morningness-eveningness in human circadian rhythms. Int J Chronobiol 1976;4:97–110.

[46] Torsvall L, Akerstedt T. A diurnal type scale. Construction, consistency and validation in shift work. Scand J Work Environ Health 1980;6:283–90.

[47] Smith CS, Reilly C, Midkiff K. Evaluation of three circadian rhythm questionnaires with suggestions for an improved measure of morningness. J Appl Psychol 1989;74:728–38.

[48] Recht LD, Lew RA, Schwartz WJ. Baseball teams beaten by jet lag. Nature 1995;377:583.

[49] Smith RS, Guilleminault C, Efron B. Circadian rhythms and enhanced athletic performance in the National Football League. Sleep 1997;20:362–5.

[50] Jehue R, Street D, Huizenga R. Effect of time zone and game time changes on team performance: National Football League. Med Sci Sports Exerc 1993;25:127–31.

[51] Steenland K, Deddens JA. Effect of travel and rest on performance of professional basketball players. Sleep 1997;20:366–9.

[52] Khalsa SB, Jewett ME, Cajochen C, et al. A phase response curve to single bright light pulses in human subjects. J Physiol 2003;549:945–52.

[53] Burgess HJ, Crowley SJ, Gazda CJ, et al. Preflight adjustment to eastward travel: 3 days of advancing sleep with and without morning bright light. J Biol Rhythms 2003;18:318–28.

[54] Boivin DB, Duffy JF, Kronauer RE, et al. Dose-response relationships for resetting of human circadian clock by light. Nature 1996;379:540–2.

[55] Boivin DB, James FO. Phase-dependent effect of room light exposure in a 5-h advance of the sleep-wake cycle: implications for jet lag. J Biol Rhythms 2002;17:266–76.

[56] Lewy AJ, Ahmed S, Jackson JM, et al. Melatonin shifts human circadian rhythms according to a phase-response curve. Chronobiol Int 1992;9:380–92.

[57] Waterhouse J, Reilly T, Atkinson G. Jet-lag. Lancet 1997;350:1611–6.

[58] Reid K, Van den Heuvel C, Dawson D. Day-time melatonin administration: effects on core temperature and sleep onset latency. J Sleep Res 1996;5:150–4.

[59] Atkinson G, Buckley P, Edwards B, et al. Are there hangover-effects on physical performance when melatonin is ingested by athletes before nocturnal sleep? Int J Sports Med 2001;22:232–4.

Further readings

Ancoli-Israel S, Cole R, Alessi C, et al. The role of actigraphy in the study of sleep and circadian rhythms. Sleep 2003;26:342–92.

Parry BL. Jet lag: minimizing its effects with critically timed bright light and melatonin administration. J Mol Microbiol Biotechnol 2002;4:463–6.

Wilber RL. Current trends in altitude training. Sports Med 2001;31:249–65.

ELSEVIER
SAUNDERS

Clin Sports Med 24 (2005) 457–462

CLINICS
IN SPORTS
MEDICINE

Index

Note: Page numbers of article titles are in **boldface** type.

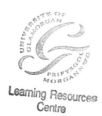

Order your subscription today. Simply complete and detach this card and drop it in the mail to receive the best clinical information in your field.

❑ **Adolescent Medicine Clinics**
❑ Individual $95
❑ Institutions $133
❑ *In-training $48

❑ **Anesthesiology**
❑ Individual $175
❑ Institutions $270
❑ *In-training $88

❑ **Cardiology**
❑ Individual $170
❑ Institutions $266
❑ *In-training $85

❑ **Chest Medicine**
❑ Individual $185
❑ Institutions $285

❑ **Child and Adolescent Psychiatry**
❑ Individual $175
❑ Institutions $265
❑ *In-training $88

❑ **Critical Care**
❑ Individual $165
❑ Institutions $266
❑ *In-training $83

❑ **Dental**
❑ Individual $150
❑ Institutions $242

❑ **Emergency Medicine**
❑ Individual $170
❑ Institutions $263
❑ *In-training $85
❑ Send CME info

❑ **Facial Plastic Surgery**
❑ Individual $199
❑ Institutions $300

❑ **Foot and Ankle**
Individual $160
Institutions $232

❑ **Gastroenterology**
❑ Individual $190
❑ Institutions $276

❑ **Gastrointestinal Endoscopy**
❑ Individual $190
❑ Institutions $276

❑ **Hand**
❑ Individual $205
❑ Institutions $319

❑ **Heart Failure (NEW in 2005!)**
❑ Individual $99
❑ Institutions $149
❑ *In-training $49

❑ **Hematology/ Oncology**
❑ Individual $210
❑ Institutions $315

❑ **Immunology & Allergy**
❑ Individual $165
❑ Institutions $266

❑ **Infectious Disease**
❑ Individual $165
❑ Institutions $272

❑ **Clinics in Liver Disease**
❑ Individual $165
❑ Institutions $234

❑ **Medical**
❑ Individual $140
❑ Institutions $244
❑ *In-training $70
❑ Send CME info

❑ **MRI**
❑ Individual $190
❑ Institutions $290
❑ *In-training $95
❑ Send CME info

❑ **Neuroimaging**
❑ Individual $190
❑ Institutions $290
❑ *In-training $95
❑ Send CME inf0

❑ **Neurologic**
❑ Individual $175
❑ Institutions $275

❑ **Obstetrics & Gynecology**
❑ Individual $175
❑ Institutions $288

❑ **Occupational and Environmental Medicine**
❑ Individual $120
❑ Institutions $166
❑ *In-training $60

❑ **Ophthalmology**
❑ Individual $190
❑ Institutions $325

❑ **Oral & Maxillofacial Surgery**
❑ Individual $180
❑ Institutions $280
❑ *In-training $90

❑ **Orthopedic**
❑ Individual $180
❑ Institutions $295
❑ *In-training $90

❑ **Otolaryngologic**
❑ Individual $199
❑ Institutions $350

❑ **Pediatric**
❑ Individual $135
❑ Institutions $246
❑ *In-training $68
❑ Send CME info

❑ **Perinatology**
❑ Individual $155
❑ Institutions $237
❑ *In-training $78
❑ Send CME inf0

❑ **Plastic Surgery**
❑ Individual $245
❑ Institutions $370

❑ **Podiatric Medicine & Surgery**
❑ Individual $170
❑ Institutions $266

❑ **Primary Care**
❑ Individual $135
❑ Institutions $223

❑ **Psychiatric**
❑ Individual $170
❑ Institutions $288

❑ **Radiologic**
❑ Individual $220
❑ Institutions $331
❑ *In-training $110
❑ Send CME info

❑ **Sports Medicine**
❑ Individual $180
❑ Institutions $277

❑ **Surgical**
❑ Individual $190
❑ Institutions $299
❑ *In-training $95

❑ **Thoracic Surgery (formerly Chest Surgery)**
❑ Individual $175
❑ Institutions $255
❑ *In-training $88

❑ **Urologic**
❑ Individual $195
❑ Institutions $307
❑ *In-training $98
❑ Send CME info

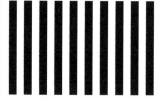

BUSINESS REPLY MAIL

FIRST-CLASS MAIL   PERMIT NO 7135   ORLANDO FL

POSTAGE WILL BE PAID BY ADDRESSEE

PERIODICALS ORDER FULFILLMENT DEPT
ELSEVIER
6277 SEA HARBOR DR
ORLANDO FL 32821-9816

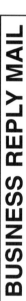

Your *Clinics* subscription just got better!

You can now access the FULL TEXT of this publication online at no additional cost! Activate your online subscription today and receive...

- Full text of all issues from 2002 to the present
- Photographs, tables, illustrations, and references
- Comprehensive search capabilities
- Links to MEDLINE and Elsevier journals

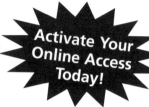
Activate Your Online Access Today!

Plus, you can also sign up for E-alerts of upcoming issues or articles that interest you, and take advantage of exclusive access to bonus features!

To activate your individual online subscription:

1. Visit our website at **www.TheClinics.com**.

2. Click on "Register" at the top of the page, and follow the instructions.

3. To activate your account, you will need your subscriber account number, which you can find on your mailing label (note: the number of digits in your subscriber account number varies from six to ten digits). See the sample below where the subscriber account number has been circled.

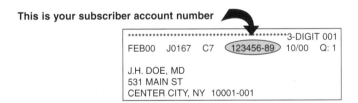

This is your subscriber account number

```
**************************************3-DIGIT 001
FEB00   J0167   C7   123456-89   10/00   Q: 1

J.H. DOE, MD
531 MAIN ST
CENTER CITY, NY  10001-001
```

4. That's it! Your online access to the most trusted source for clinical reviews is now available.

theclinics.com

ELSEVIER